Sacred Sexuality
Ancient
Egyptian Tantric Yoga

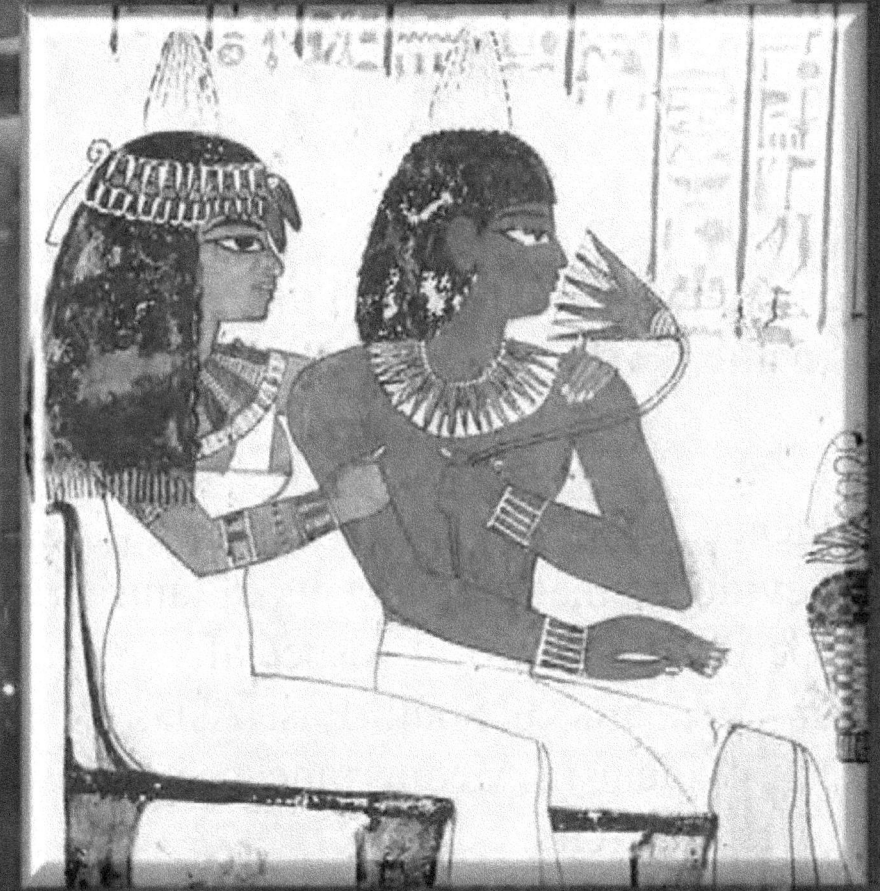

The Neterian Guide To
Love, Sexuality, Marriage, Relationships
and the Secrets of Sexual Energy Cultivation, Sublimation,
and Spiritual Enlightenment

Dr. Muata Ashby

Mystical Philosophy of Universal Consciousness

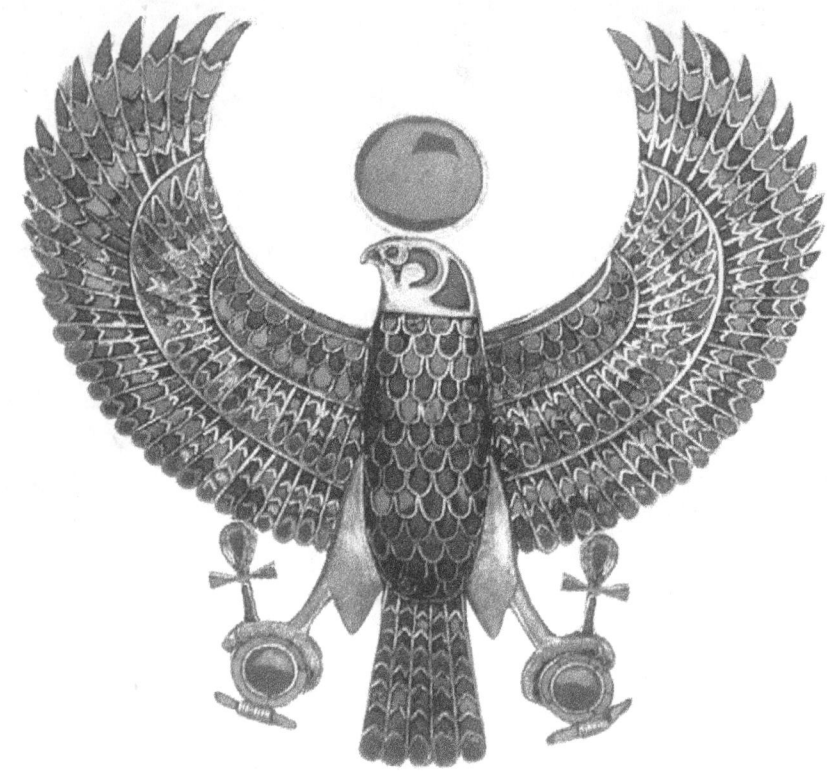

"Like is He unto that which he hath made, and which became his name."

Egyptian Book of Coming Forth By Day 17:20

Tantric influence, however, is not limited to India alone, and there is evidence that the precepts of tantrism traveled to various parts of the world, especially Nepal, Tibet, China, Japan and parts of South-East Asia; its influence has also been evident in Mediterranean cultures such as those of Egypt and Crete.

-Ajit Mookerjee (Indian Scholar-Author –from the book *The Tantric Way*)

Expanded Fourth Edition

EGYPTIAN TANTRIC YOGA

Sema Institute of Yoga / C.M. Books
P.O.Box 570459
Miami, Florida, 33257
(305) 378-6253 Fax: (305) 378-6253

First U.S. edition 1996

© 1998 Second Edition By Reginald Muata Ashby
© 1999 Third Edition
© 2003 Fourth Edition

All rights reserved. No part of this book may be used or reproduced in any manner whatsoever without written permission (address above) except in the case of brief quotations embodied in critical articles and reviews. All inquiries may be addressed to the address above.

The author is available for group lectures and individual counseling. For further information contact the publisher.

Ashby, Muata
Egyptian Tantra Yoga ISBN: 1-884564-03-8

Library of Congress Cataloging in Publication Data

1 Yoga 2 Egyptian Philosophy, 3 Tantrism, 4 Esoterism, 5 Meditation, 6 Self Help.

Check out the latest books, audio and video presentations on Egyptian Yoga and seminars, classes and courses now on the World Wide Web!
INTERNET ADDRESS: http://www.Egyptianyoga.com

E-MAIL ADDRESS: Semayoga@aol.com

Mystical Philosophy of Universal Consciousness

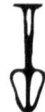

Temple of Shetaut Neter - Sema Institute

Sema (☥) is an ancient Egyptian word and symbol meaning *union*. The Sema Institute is dedicated to the propagation of the universal teachings of spiritual evolution which relate to the union of humanity and the union of all things within the universe. It is a non-denominational organization which recognizes the unifying principles in all spiritual and religious systems of evolution throughout the world. Our primary goals are to provide the wisdom of ancient spiritual teachings in books, courses and other forms of communication. Secondly, to provide expert instruction and training in the various yogic disciplines including Ancient Egyptian Philosophy, Christian Gnosticism, Indian Philosophy and modern science. Thirdly, to promote world peace and Universal Love.

A primary focus of our tradition is to identify and acknowledge the yogic principles within all religions and to relate them to each other in order to promote their deeper understanding as well as to show the essential unity of purpose and the unity of all living beings and nature within the whole of existence.

The Institute is open to all who believe in the principles of peace, non-violence and spiritual emancipation regardless of sex, race, or creed.

EGYPTIAN TANTRIC YOGA

About the author:

Muata Ashby D.D., P.C.

Sebai Dr. Muata Abhaya Ashby is a Priest of Shetaut Neter –African Kamitan Religion, Author, lecturer, poet, philosopher, musician, publisher, counselor and spiritual preceptor and founder of the Sema Institute-Temple of Aset, Muata Ashby was born in Brooklyn, New York City, and grew up in the Caribbean. His family is from Puerto Rico and Barbados. Displaying an interest in ancient civilizations and the Humanities, Sebai Maa began studies in the area of religion and philosophy and achieved doctorates in these areas while at the same time he began to collect his research into what would later become several books on the subject of the origins of Yoga Philosophy and practice in ancient Africa (Ancient Egypt) and also the origins of Christian Mysticism in Ancient Egypt.

Sebai Maa (Muata Abhaya Ashby) holds a Doctor of Philosophy Degree in Religion, and a Doctor of Divinity Degree in Holistic Health. He is a certified member of the American Alternative Medical Association as an Alternative Medical Practitioner. He is also a Pastoral Counselor and Teacher of Yoga Philosophy and Discipline. Dr. Ashby received his Doctor of Divinity Degree from and is an adjunct faculty member of Florida International University and the American Institute of Holistic Theology. Dr. Ashby is a certified as a PREP Relationship Counselor. Dr. Ashby has been an independent researcher and practitioner of Egyptian Yoga, Indian Yoga, Chinese Yoga, Buddhism and mystical psychology as well as Christian Mysticism. Dr. Ashby has engaged in Post Graduate research in advanced Jnana, Bhakti and Kundalini Yogas at the Yoga Research Foundation. He has extensively studied mystical religious traditions from around the world and is an accomplished lecturer, musician, artist, poet, screenwriter, playwright and author of over 25 books on Kemetic yoga and spiritual philosophy. He is an Ordained Minister and Spiritual Counselor and also the founder the Sema Institute, a non-profit organization dedicated to spreading the wisdom of Yoga and the Ancient Egyptian mystical traditions. Further, he is the spiritual leader and head priest of the Per Aset or Temple of Aset, based in Miami, Florida. Thus, as a scholar, Dr. Muata Ashby is a teacher, lecturer and researcher. However, as a spiritual leader, his title is *Sebai,* which means Spiritual Preceptor.

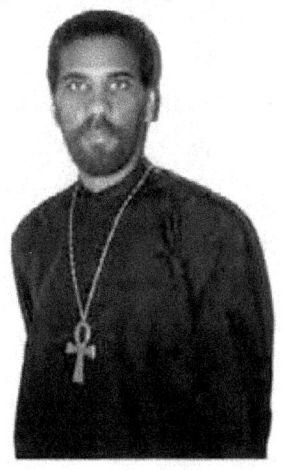

Dr. Muata Ashby

Sema Institute of Yoga/Cruzian Mystic Books P. O. Box 570459 Miami, Florida, 33257
(305) 378-6253 Fax: (305) 378-6253

Mystical Philosophy of Universal Consciousness
TABLE OF CONTENTS

TEMPLE OF SHETAUT NETER - SEMA INSTITUTE 3
AUTHOR'S FOREWORD 8
   What is Yoga Philosophy and Spiritual Practice 11
   How to study the wisdom teachings: 13

PART 1: INTRODUCTION TO SHETAUT NETER RELIGION AND SEMA TAWI PHILOSOPHY AND DISCIPLINES 15
   THE FUNDAMENTAL PRINCIPLES OF ANCIENT EGYPTIAN RELIGION 16
      Summary of Ancient Egyptian Religion 17
      "The practice of the Shedy disciplines leads to knowing oneself and the Divine. This is called being True of Speech" 17
      Neterian Great Truths 18
      Summary of The Great Truths and the Shedy Paths to their Realization 20
      The Spiritual Culture and the Purpose of Life: Shetaut Neter 21
   SHETAUT NETER 21
   WHO IS NETER IN KAMITAN RELIGION? 22
      Sacred Scriptures of Shetaut Neter 23
   NETER AND THE NETERU 24
   THE NETERU 24
      The Neteru and Their Temples 25
      The Neteru and Their Interrelationships 26
      Listening to the Teachings 27
      The Anunian Tradition 28
      The Theban Tradition 30
      The Goddess Tradition 31
      The Aton Tradition 33
      Akhnaton, Nefertiti and Daughters 33
   THE GENERAL PRINCIPLES OF SHETAUT NETER 34
      The Forces of Entropy 35
      The Great Awakening of Neterian Religion 36

PART 2: INTRODUCTION TO EGYPTIAN YOGA 37
   The Term "Egyptian Yoga" and The Philosophy Behind It 41
   The Yogic Postures in Ancient Egypt 53

PART 3: THE PHILOSOPHY OF TANTRA IN WORLD SPIRITUALITY 58
   SEXUAL ENERGY AND THE EVOLUTION OF HUMAN CONSCIOUSNESS 58
      Tantrism in Ancient Egypt and India 59
   INTRODUCTION TO TANTRIC PHILOSOPHY 64
      Sexual Energy and Yoga 64
      KUNDALINI YOGA 66
      LAYA YOGA 67
   THE TANTRIC ORIGINS OF CHRISTIAN GNOSTICISM IN ANCIENT EGYPT AND AFRICA 67
      The Gnostic Jesus and Mary: The New Phase of the Min and Hathor Tantrism 69

PART 4: THE TANTRA OF ANCIENT EGYPT 71

EGYPTIAN TANTRIC YOGA

A COMPENDIUM OF THE AUSARIAN RESURRECTION MYTH	73
Egyptian (Kemetic) Tantra Yoga In the Ancient Creation Myths	80
Egyptian (Kemetic) Tantra Yoga	83
The Tantric Symbolism of Creation in Neterian Spirituality	*84*
Sexuality in The Ausarian Iconography	*88*
Sexuality in The Ausarian Resurrection Myth	*89*
The Illusoriness of Sexuality	*100*
Discipline, Restraint and Control	*104*
The Tantra of the Soul and the Body	*106*
The Highest Tantra: Supreme Love	*106*
Tantric evolution through Kemetic Ritual	109
Ritual of the Journey of The Divine Boat	*109*
Ritual of the Dawn at Denderah Temple	*113*
Ritual of the Divine Embrace	*118*
Tantric Symbolism of Gods Hand	*119*
The Sublime Vision of Egyptian Tantra Yoga Part I	120

PART 5: ICONS AND SYMBOLS OF KEMETIC TANTRA MYSTICISM 121

The Tantric Menat Symbol of Ancient Egypt	*122*
Tantric Symbolism of The Mystical Ankh	*124*
Tantric Mysticism of the Hetep Offering Table	*127*
The Hetep Ritual Slab of Africa and the Lingam-Yoni of India	*128*
The Ithyphallic Symbol	*129*
The Lotus Symbol of Ancient Egypt	*130*
Tantric Symbolism of the Spinx	133
The Tantric Teachings of The Egyptian Book of Coming Forth By Day	*135*
The Role of Sexuality in Human Relationships and Society	*138*
Kemetic Tantra Yoga and the Serpent Power	142
The Teaching of the Caduceus	*145*
The Serpent Power and Tantra Yoga	*149*
The Mystical Implications of the Djed	*156*
The Mystical Sistrum	*159*
The Supreme Divinity: All-Encompassing and Eternal	161
The Sekhm Scepter	*162*

PART 6: THE SUBLIME VISION OF EGYPTIAN TANTRA YOGA 165

Marriage, Celibacy, Relationships, Conflicts and Spiritual Life	*166*
THE KEMETIC PRINCIPLES OF MARRIAGE	175
Marriage, Sexuality and Celibacy for Neterian Priests and Priestesses	*177*
Vegetarianism, Celibacy and Self-Control of the Neterian Clergy	*179*
CLOTHING AND SEXUALITY IN ANCIENT EGYPT	183

PART 7: THE ART OF KEMETIC SEX SUBLIMATION 190

SEX SUBLIMATION EXERCISES AND MEDITATIONS	191
One Last Word	209
INDEX	**210**

OTHER BOOKS FROM C M BOOKS 215
MUSIC BASED ON THE PRT M HRU AND OTHER KEMETIC TEXTS 222

EGYPTIAN TANTRIC YOGA

Author's Foreword

Who Were the Ancient Egyptians and What is Yoga Philosophy?

The Ancient Egyptian religion (*Shetaut Neter*), language and symbols provide the first "historical" record of Yoga Philosophy and Religious literature. Egyptian Yoga is what has been commonly referred to by Egyptologists as Egyptian "Religion" or "Mythology", but to think of it as just another set of stories or allegories about a long lost civilization is to completely miss the greatest secret of human existence. Yoga, in all of its forms and disciplines of spiritual development, was practiced in Egypt earlier than anywhere else in history. This unique perspective from the highest philosophical system which developed in Africa over seven thousand years ago provides a new way to look at life, religion, the discipline of psychology and the way to spiritual development leading to spiritual Enlightenment. Egyptian mythology, when understood as a system of Yoga (union of the individual soul with the Universal Soul or Supreme Consciousness), gives every individual insight into their own divine nature and also a deeper insight into all religions and Yoga systems.

Diodorus Siculus (Greek Historian) writes in the time of Augustus (first century B.C.):

"Now the Ethiopians, as historians relate, were the first of all men and the proofs of this statement, they say, are manifest. For that they did not come into their land as immigrants from abroad but were the natives of it and so justly bear the name of autochthones (sprung from the soil itself), is, they maintain, conceded by practically all men..."

"They also say that the Egyptians are colonists sent out by the Ethiopians, Osiris having been the leader of the colony. For, speaking generally, what is now Egypt, they maintain, was not land, but sea, when in the beginning the universe was being formed; afterwards, however, as the Nile during the times of its inundation carried down the mud from Ethiopia, land was gradually built up from the deposit...And the larger parts of the customs of the Egyptians are, they hold, Ethiopian, the colonists still preserving their ancient manners. For instance, the belief that their kings are Gods, the very special attention which they pay to their burials, and many other matters of a similar nature, are Ethiopian practices, while the shapes of their statues and the forms of their letters are Ethiopian; for of the two kinds of writing which the Egyptians have, that which is known as popular (demotic) is learned by everyone, while that which is called sacred (hieratic), is understood only by the priests of the Egyptians, who learnt it from their Fathers as one of the things which are not divulged, but among the Ethiopians, everyone uses these forms of letters. Furthermore, the orders of the priests, they maintain, have much the same position among both peoples; for all are clean who are engaged in the service of the gods, keeping themselves shaven, like the Ethiopian priests, and having the same dress and form of staff, which is shaped like a plough and is carried by their kings who wear high felt hats which end in a knob in the top and are circled by the serpents which they call asps; and this symbol appears to carry the thought that it will be the lot who shall dare to attack the king to encounter death-carrying stings. Many other

things are told by them concerning their own antiquity and the colony which they sent out that became the Egyptians, but about this there is no special need of our writing anything."

The ancient Egyptian texts state:

"Our people originated at the base of the mountain of the Moon, at the origin of the Nile river."

"KMT"
"Egypt", "Burnt", "Land of Blackness","Land of the Burnt People."

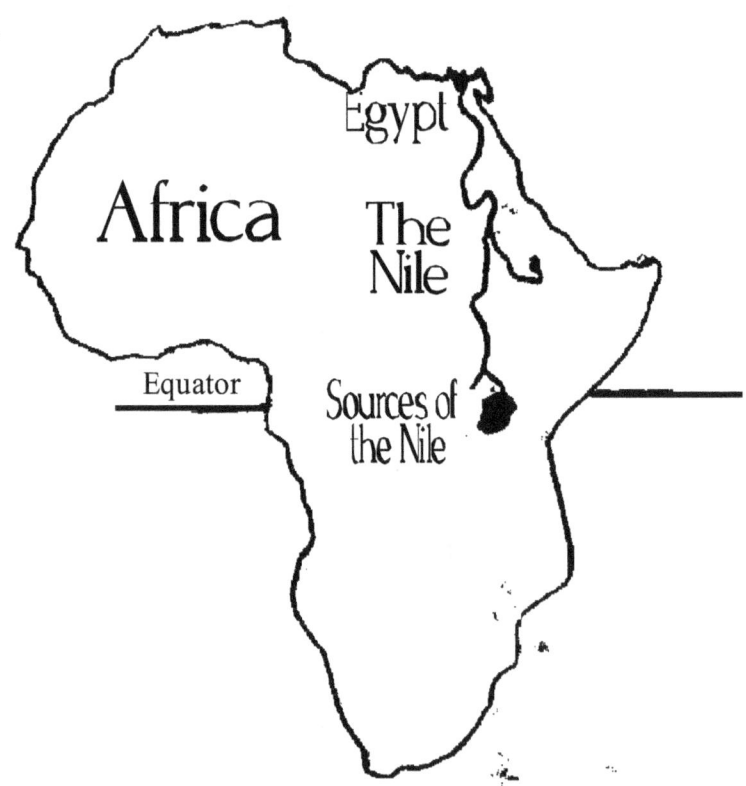

Historical evidence proves that Ethiopia-Nubia already had Kingdoms at least 300 years before the first Kingdom-Pharaoh of Egypt.

"Ancient Egypt was a colony of Nubia - Ethiopia. ...Osiris having been the leader of the colony..."

"And upon his return to Greece, they gathered around and asked, "tell us about this great land of the Blacks called Ethiopia." And Herodotus said, "There are two great Ethiopian nations, one in Sind (India) and the other in Egypt."

TANTRIC YOGA

Recorded by Egyptian high priest *Manetho* (300 B.C.)
also Recorded by *Diodorus* (Greek historian 100 B.C.)

...emselves however, cannot be dated, but indications are that they existed far ...uity. The Pyramid Texts (hieroglyphics inscribed on pyramid walls) and Coffin ...eroglyphics inscribed on coffins) speak authoritatively on the constitution of the human ...it, the vital Life Force along the human spinal cord (known in India as *"Kundalini"*), the immortality of the soul, reincarnation and the law of Cause and Effect (known in India as the Law of Karma).

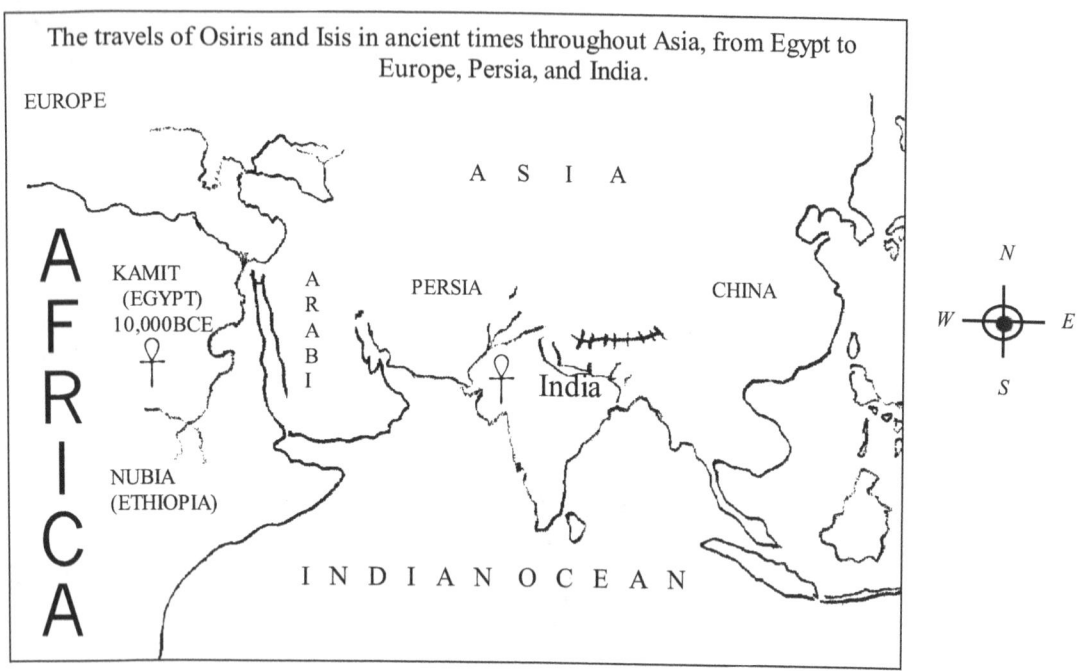

Mystical Philosophy of Universal Consciousness

What is Yoga Philosophy and Spiritual Practice

Since a complete treatise on the theory and practice of yoga would require several volumes, only a basic outline will be given here.

When we look out upon the world, we are often baffled by the multiplicity which constitutes the human experience. What do we really know about this experience? Many scientific disciplines have developed over the last two hundred years for the purpose of discovering the mysteries of nature, but this search has only engendered new questions about the nature of existence. Yoga is a discipline or way of life designed to promote the physical, mental and spiritual development of the human being. It leads a person to discover the answers to the most important questions of life such as Who am I?, Why am I here? and Where am I going?

The literal meaning of the word YOGA is to *"YOKE"* or to *"LINK"* back. The implication is: to link back to the original source, the original essence, that which transcends all mental and intellectual attempts at comprehension, but which is the essential nature of everything in CREATION. While in the strict or dogmatic sense, Yoga philosophy and practice is a separate discipline from religion, yoga and religion have been linked at many points throughout history. In a manner of speaking, Yoga as a discipline may be seen as a non-sectarian transpersonal science or practice to promote spiritual development and harmony of mind and body thorough mental and physical disciplines including meditation, psycho-physical exercises, and performing action with the correct attitude.

The disciplines of Yoga fall under five major categories. These are: *Yoga of Wisdom, Yoga of Devotional Love, Yoga of Meditation, Tantric Yoga* and *Yoga of Selfless Action*. Within these categories there are subsidiary forms which are part of the main disciplines. The important point to remember is that all aspects of yoga can and should be used in an integral fashion to effect an efficient and harmonized spiritual movement in the practitioner. Therefore, while there may be an area of special emphasis, other elements are bound to become part of the yoga program as needed. For example, while a yogin may place emphasis on the yoga of wisdom, they may also practice devotional yoga and meditation yoga along with the wisdom studies.

While it is true that yogic practices may be found in religion, strictly speaking, yoga is neither a religion or a philosophy. It should be thought of more as a way of life or discipline for promoting greater fullness and experience of life. Yoga was developed at the dawn of history by those who wanted more out of life. These special men and women wanted to discover the true origins of creation and of themselves. Therefore, they set out to explore the vast reaches of consciousness within themselves. They are sometimes referred to as "Seers", "Sages", etc. Awareness or consciousness can only be increased when the mind is in a state of peace and harmony. Thus, the disciplines of meditation (which are part of Yoga), and wisdom (the philosophical teachings for understanding reality as it is) are the primary means to controlling the mind and allowing the individual to mature psychologically and spiritually.

The teachings which were practiced in the ancient Egyptian temples were the same ones later intellectually defined into a literary form by the Indian Sages of Vedanta and Yoga. This was discussed in my book *Egyptian Yoga: The Philosophy of Enlightenment*. The Indian Mysteries of

EGYPTIAN TANTRIC YOGA

Yoga and Vedanta represent an unfolding and intellectual exposition of the Egyptian Mysteries. Also, the study of Gnostic Christianity or Christianity before Roman Catholicism will be useful to our study since Christianity originated in ancient Egypt and was also based on the ancient Egyptian Mysteries. Therefore, the study of the Egyptian Mysteries, early Christianity and Indian Vedanta-Yoga will provide the most comprehensive teaching on how to practice the disciplines of yoga leading to the attainment of Enlightenment.

The question is how to accomplish these seemingly impossible tasks? How to transform yourself and realize the deepest mysteries of existence? How to discover "who am I?" This is the mission of Yoga Philosophy and the purpose of yogic practices. Yoga does not seek to convert or impose religious beliefs on any one. Ancient Egypt was the source of civilization and the source of religion and Yoga. Therefore, all systems of mystical spirituality can coexist harmoniously within these teachings when they are correctly understood.

The goal of yoga is to promote integration of the mind-body-spirit complex in order to produce optimal health of the human being. This is accomplished through mental and physical exercises which promote the free flow of spiritual energy by reducing mental complexes caused by ignorance. There are two roads which human beings can follow, one of wisdom and the other of ignorance. The path of the masses is generally the path of ignorance which leads them into negative situations, thoughts and deeds. These in turn lead to ill health and sorrow in life. The other road is based on wisdom and it leads to health, true happiness and enlightenment.

Our mission is to extol the wisdom of yoga and mystical spirituality from the ancient Egyptian perspective and to show the practice of the teachings through our books, videos and audio productions. You may find a complete listing of other books by the author, in the back of this volume.

Mystical Philosophy of Universal Consciousness

How to study the wisdom teachings:

There is a specific technique which is prescribed by the scriptures themselves for studying the teachings, proverbs and aphorisms of mystical wisdom. The method is as follows:

The spiritual aspirant should read the desired text thoroughly, taking note of any particular teachings which resonates with him or her.

The aspirant should make a habit of collecting those teachings and reading them over frequently. The scriptures should be read and re-read because the subtle levels of the teachings will be increasingly understood the more the teachings are reviewed.

One useful exercise is to choose some of the most special teachings you would like to focus on and place them in large type or as posters in your living areas so as to be visible to remind you of the teaching.

The aspirant should discuss those teachings with others of like mind when possible because this will help to promote greater understanding and act as an active spiritual practice in which the teachings are kept at the forefront of the mind. In this way, the teachings can become an integral part of everyday life and not reserved for a particular time of day or of the week.

The study of the wisdom teachings should be a continuous process in which the teachings become the predominant factor of life rather than the useless and oftentimes negative and illusory thoughts of those who are ignorant of spiritual truths. This spiritual discipline should be observed until Enlightenment is attained.

May you discover supreme peace in this very lifetime!

MUATA ☉

(HETEP - Supreme Peace)

Mystical Philosophy of Universal Consciousness

Part 1: Introduction to Shetaut Neter Religion and Sema Tawi Philosophy and Disciplines

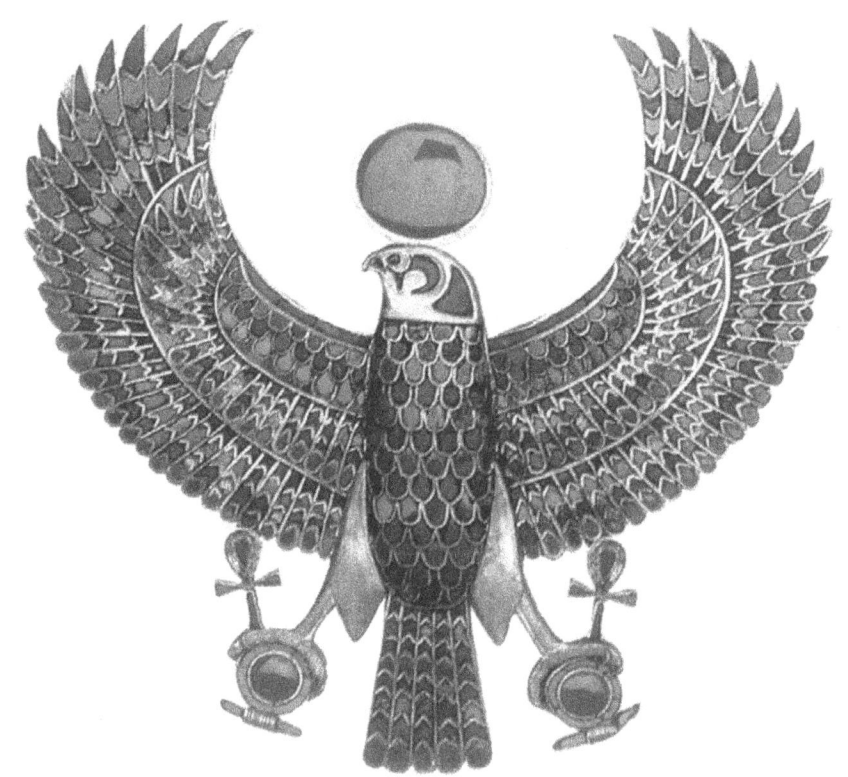

EGYPTIAN TANTRIC YOGA

The Fundamental Principles of Ancient Egyptian Religion

In order to fully understand the tantric philosophy and iconography that will be presented in this book it is necessary to have a working knowledge of what ancient Egyptian Religion consists in and the context in which it appears. Tantrism is a spiritual discipline within religion; in particular, the Ancient Egyptian Religion. There are other spiritual disciplines within Ancient Egyptian religion. The Spiritual disciplines are exercises, philosophical ways of thinking, meditations and rituals that allow a human being to discover the tantric reality of life and the underlying all-encompassing nature of Creation as well as the ever presence of the Divine (God/Goddess). All promote spiritual evolution and work together to elevate a spiritual practitioner. Egyptian Tantric Philosophy involves many aspects of Ancient Egyptian Religion and also spans across varied disciplines.

What is NETERIANISM?
(The Oldest Known Religion in History)

Shetaut Neter is the name given by the Ancient Egyptian-Africans to their religion. The term "Neterianism" is derived from the name "Shetaut Neter." Shetaut Neter means the "Hidden Divinity." It is the ancient philosophy and mythic spiritual culture that gave rise to the Ancient Egyptian civilization. Those who follow the spiritual path of Shetaut Neter are therefore referred to as "Neterians." The fundamental principles common to all denominations of Ancient Egyptian Religion may be summed up in four "Great Truths" that are common to all the traditions of Ancient Egyptian Religion.

Mystical Philosophy of Universal Consciousness

Summary of Ancient Egyptian Religion

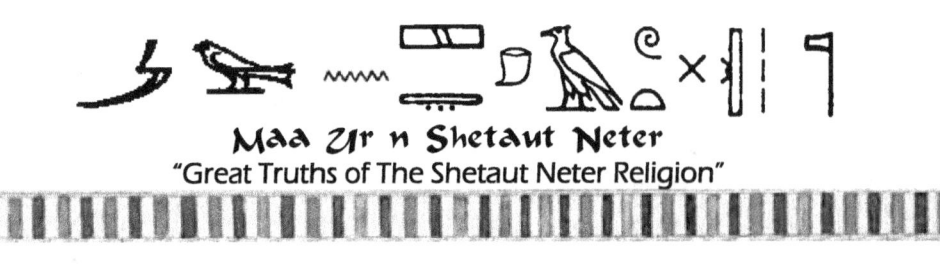

Maa Ur n Shetaut Neter

"Great Truths of The Shetaut Neter Religion"

I

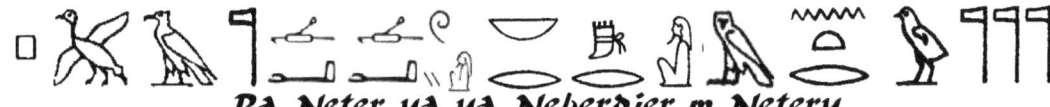

Pa Neter ua ua Neberdjer m Neteru

"The Neter, the Supreme Being, is One and alone and as Neberdjer, manifesting everywhere and in all things in the form of Gods and Goddesses."

II

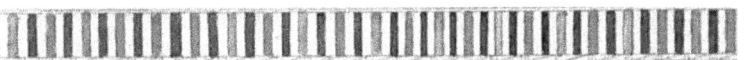

an-Maat swy Saui Set s-Khemn

"Lack of righteousness brings fetters to the personality and these fetters cause ignorance of the Divine."

III

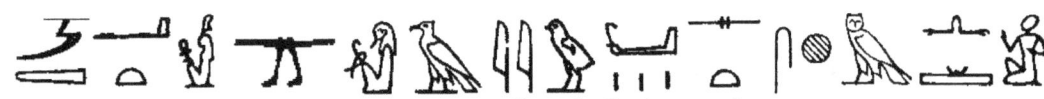

s-Uashu s-Nafu n saiu Set

"Devotion to the Divine leads to freedom from the fetters of Set."

IIII

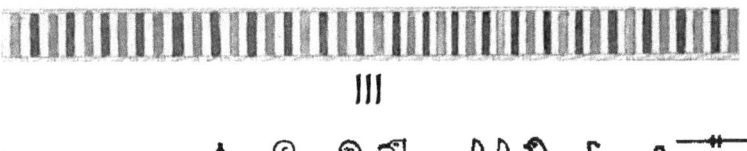

ari Shedy Rekh ab m Maakheru

"The practice of the Shedy disciplines leads to knowing oneself and the Divine. This is called being True of Speech"

EGYPTIAN TANTRIC YOGA

Neterian Great Truths

1. ***"Pa Neter ua ua Neberdjer m Neteru"*** -"The Neter, the Supreme Being, is One and alone and as Neberdjer, manifesting everywhere and in all things in the form of Gods and Goddesses."

Neberdjer means "all-encompassing divinity," the all-inclusive, all-embracing Spirit which pervades all and who is the ultimate essence of all. This first truth unifies all the expressions of Kamitan religion.

2. **"an-Maat swy Saui Set s-Khemn"** - "Lack of righteousness brings fetters to the personality and these fetters lead to ignorance of the Divine."

When a human being acts in ways that contradict the natural order of nature, negative qualities of the mind will develop within that person's personality. These are the afflictions of Set. Set is the neteru of egoism and selfishness. The afflictions of Set include: anger, hatred, greed, lust, jealousy, envy, gluttony, dishonesty, hypocrisy, etc. So to be free from the fetters of set one must be free from the afflictions of Set.

3. **"s-Uashu s-Nafu n saiu Set"** -"Devotion to the Divine leads to freedom from the fetters of Set."

To be liberated (Nafu - freedom - to breath) from the afflictions of Set, one must be devoted to the Divine. Being devoted to the Divine means living by Maat. Maat is a way of life that is purifying to the heart and beneficial for society as it promotes virtue and order. Living by Maat means practicing Shedy (spiritual practices and disciplines).

Uashu means devotion and the classic pose of adoring the Divine is called "Dua," standing or sitting with upraised hands facing outwards towards the image of the divinity.

4. **"ari Shedy Rekh ab m Maakheru"** - "The practice of the Shedy disciplines leads to knowing oneself and the Divine. This is called being True of Speech."

Doing Shedy means to study profoundly, to penetrate the mysteries (Shetaut) and discover the nature of the Divine. There have been several practices designed by the sages of Ancient Kamit to facilitate the process of self-knowledge. These are the religious (Shetaut) traditions and the Sema (Smai) Tawi (yogic) disciplines related to them that augment the spiritual practices.

All the traditions relate the teachings of the sages by means of myths related to particular gods or goddesses. It is understood that all of these neteru are related, like brothers and sisters, having all emanated from the same source, the same Supremely Divine parent, who is neither male nor female, but encompasses the totality of the two.

Mystical Philosophy of Universal Consciousness

The Great Truths of Neterianism are realized by means of Four Spiritual Disciplines in Three Steps

The four disciples are: Rekh Shedy (Wisdom), Ari Shedy (Righteous Action and Selfless Service), Uashu (Ushet) Shedy (Devotion) and Uaa Shedy (Meditation)

The Three Steps are: Listening, Ritual, and Meditation

SEDJM REKH SHEDY

LISTEN

- *Sedjm* **REKH** *Shedy* - **Listening** to the WISDOM of the Neterian Traditions

    - Shetaut Asar — Teachings of the Asarian Tradition
    - Shetaut Anu — Teachings of the Ra Tradition
    - Shetaut Menefer — Teachings of the Ptah Tradition
    - Shetaut Waset — Teachings of the Amun Tradition
    - Shetaut Netrit — Teachings of the Goddess Tradition
    - Shetaut Aton — Teachings of the Aton Tradition

ARI SHEDY

RITUAL

- *Ari Maat Shedy* – **Righteous Actions** – Purifies the GROSS impurities of the Heart

    - Maat Shedy — True Study of the Ways of hidden nature of Neter
    - Maat Aakhu — True Deeds that lead to glory
    - Maat Aru — True Ritual

UASHU (USHET) SHEDY

- *Ushet Shedy* – **Devotion to the Divine** – Purifies the EMOTIONAL impurities of the Heart

    - Shmai — Divine Music
    - Sema Paut — Meditation in motion
    - Neter Arit — Divine Offerings – Selfless-Service – virtue -

UAA SHEDY

MEDITATE

- *Uaa m Neter Shedy* - 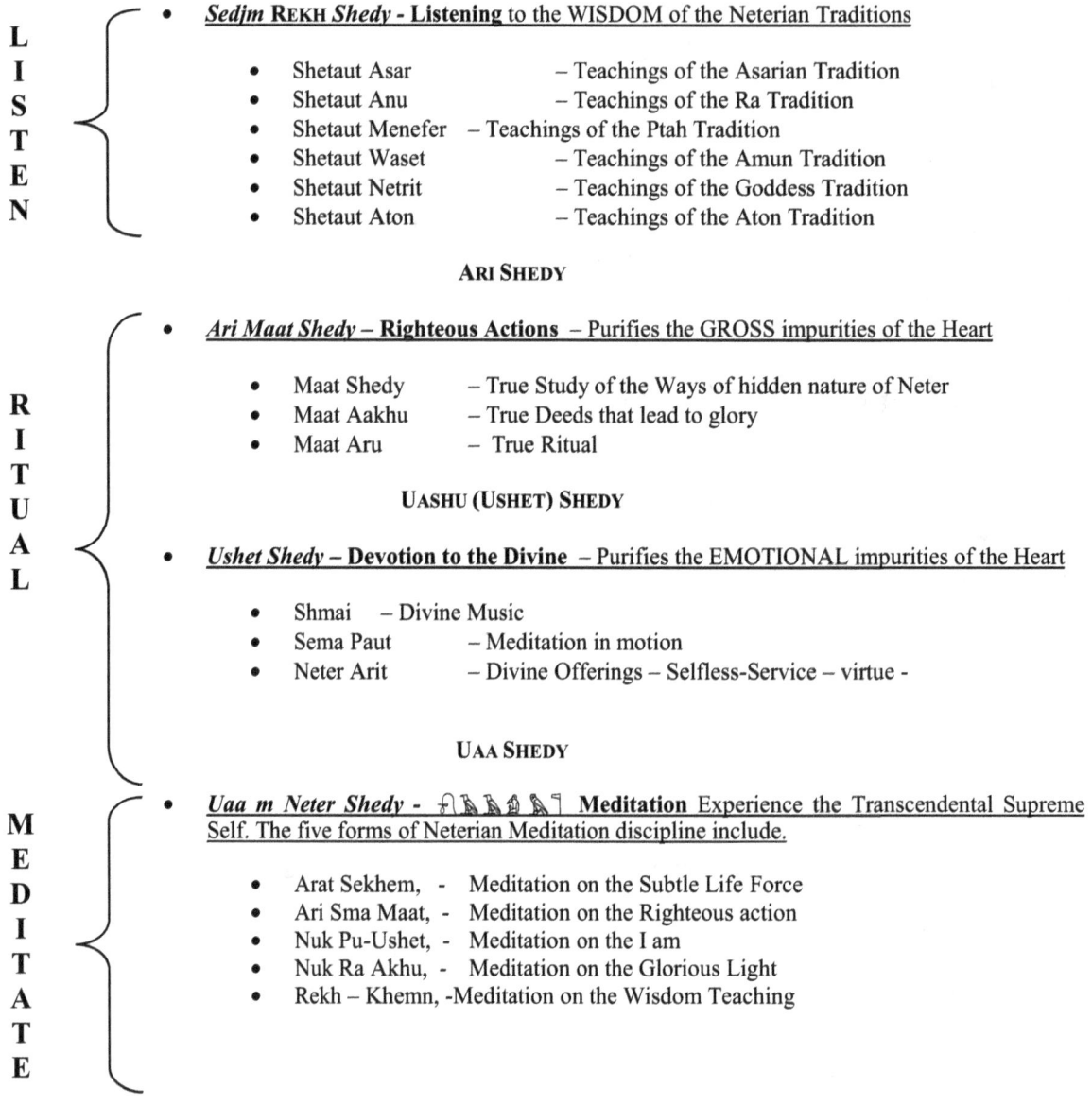 **Meditation** Experience the Transcendental Supreme Self. The five forms of Neterian Meditation discipline include.

    - Arat Sekhem, - Meditation on the Subtle Life Force
    - Ari Sma Maat, - Meditation on the Righteous action
    - Nuk Pu-Ushet, - Meditation on the I am
    - Nuk Ra Akhu, - Meditation on the Glorious Light
    - Rekh – Khemn, -Meditation on the Wisdom Teaching

EGYPTIAN TANTRIC YOGA

Summary of The Great Truths and the Shedy Paths to their Realization

Great Truths

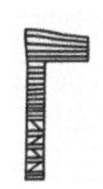

Shedy Disciplines

I
God is One and in all things manifesting through the Neteru

I
Listen to the Wisdom Teachings (Become Wise)
Learn the mysteries as taught by an authentic teacher which allows this profound statement to be understood.

I I
Unrighteousness brings fetters and these cause ignorance of truth
(#1)

I I
Acting (Living) by Truth
Apply the Philosophy of right action to become virtuous and purify the heart

I I I
Devotion to God allows the personality to free itself from the fetters

I I I
Devotion to the Divine
Worship, ritual and divine love allows the personality purified by truth to eradicate the subtle ignorance that binds it to mortal existence.

I I I I
The Shedy disciplines are the greatest form of worship of the Divine

I I I I
Meditation
Allows the whole person to go beyond the world of time and space and the gross and subtle ignorance of mortal human existence to discover that which transcends time and space.

Great Awakening
Occurs when all of the Great Truths have been realized by perfection of the Shedy disciplines to realize their true nature and actually experience oneness with the transcendental Supreme Being.

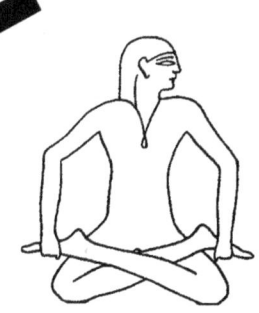

20

Mystical Philosophy of Universal Consciousness

The Spiritual Culture and the Purpose of Life: Shetaut Neter

> "Men and women are to become God-like through a life of virtue
> and the cultivation of the spirit through scientific knowledge,
> practice and bodily discipline."
>
> -Ancient Egyptian Proverb

The highest forms of Joy, Peace and Contentment are obtained when the meaning of life is discovered. When the human being is in harmony with life, then it is possible to reflect and meditate upon the human condition and realize the limitations of worldly pursuits. When there is peace and harmony in life, a human being can practice any of the varied disciplines designated as Shetaut Neter to promote {his/her} evolution towards the ultimate goal of life, which Spiritual Enlightenment. Spiritual Enlightenment is the awakening of a human being to the awareness of the Transcendental essence which binds the universe and which is eternal and immutable. In this discovery is also the sobering and ecstatic realization that the human being is one with that Transcendental essence. With this realization comes great joy, peace and power to experience the fullness of life and to realize the purpose of life during the time on earth. The lotus is a symbol of Shetaut Neter, meaning the turning towards the light of truth, peace and transcendental harmony.

Shetaut Neter

We have established that the Ancient Egyptians were African peoples who lived in the north-eastern quadrant of the continent of Africa. They were descendants of the Nubians, who had themselves originated from farther south into the heart of Africa at the Great Lakes region, the sources of the Nile River. They created a vast civilization and culture earlier than any other society in known history and organized a nation that was based on the concepts of balance and order as well as spiritual enlightenment. These ancient African people called their land Kamit, and soon after developing a well-ordered society, they began to realize that the world is full of wonders, but also that life is fleeting, and that there must be something more to human existence. They developed spiritual systems that were designed to allow human beings to understand the nature of this secret being who is the essence of all Creation. They called this spiritual system "Shtaut Ntr (Shetaut Neter)."

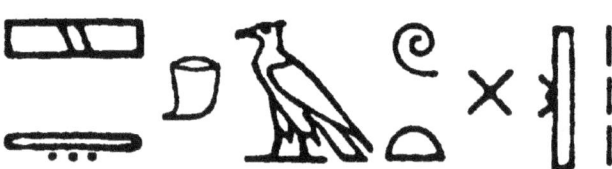

Shetaut means secret.

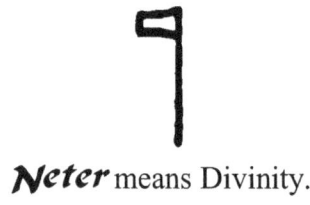

Neter means Divinity.

EGYPTIAN TANTRIC YOGA

Who is Neter in Kamitan Religion?

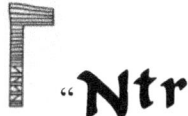

"**Ntr**

The symbol of Neter was described by an Ancient Kamitan priest as:
"That which is placed in the coffin"

The term Ntr, or Ntjr, comes from the Ancient Egyptian hieroglyphic language which did not record its vowels. However, the term survives in the Coptic language as *"Nutar."* The same Coptic meaning (divine force or sustaining power) applies in the present as it did in ancient times. It is a symbol composed of a wooden staff that was wrapped with strips of fabric, like a mummy. The strips alternate in color with yellow, green and blue. The mummy in Kamitan spirituality is understood to be the dead but resurrected Divinity. So the Nutar (Ntr) is actually every human being who does not really die, but goes to live on in a different form. Further, the resurrected spirit of every human being is that same Divinity. Phonetically, the term Nutar is related to other terms having the same meaning, such as the latin "Natura," the Spanish Naturalesa, the English "Nature" and "Nutriment", etc. In a real sense, as we will see, Natur means power manifesting as Neteru and the Neteru are the objects of creation, i.e. "nature."

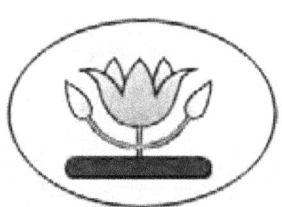

Mystical Philosophy of Universal Consciousness

Sacred Scriptures of Shetaut Neter

The following scriptures represent the foundational scriptures of Kamitan culture. They may be divided into three categories: *Mythic Scriptures*, *Mystical Philosophy* and *Ritual Scriptures*, and *Wisdom Scriptures* (Didactic Literature).

MYTHIC SCRIPTURES Literature	Mystical (Ritual) Philosophy Literature	Wisdom Texts Literature
SHETAUT ASAR-ASET-HERU The Myth of Asar, Aset and Heru (Asarian Resurrection Theology) - Predynastic **SHETAUT ATUM-RA** Anunian Theology Predynastic Shetaut Net/Aset/Hetheru Saitian Theology – Goddess Spirituality Predynastic **SHETAUT PTAH** Memphite Theology Predynastic Shetaut Amun Theban Theology Predynastic	**Coffin Texts** (C. 2040 B.C.E.-1786 B.C.E.) **Papyrus Texts** (C. 1580 B.C.E.- Roman Period)[1] Books of Coming Forth By Day Example of famous papyri: Papyrus of Any Papyrus of Hunefer Papyrus of Kenna Greenfield Papyrus, Etc.	**Wisdom Texts** (C. 3,000 B.C.E. – PTOLEMAIC PERIOD) Precepts of Ptahotep Instructions of Any Instructions of Amenemope Etc. **Maat Declarations** Literature (All Periods) **Blind Harpers Songs**

---

[1] After 1570 B.C.E they would evolve into a more unified text, the Egyptian Book of the Dead.

EGYPTIAN TANTRIC YOGA

Neter and the Neteru

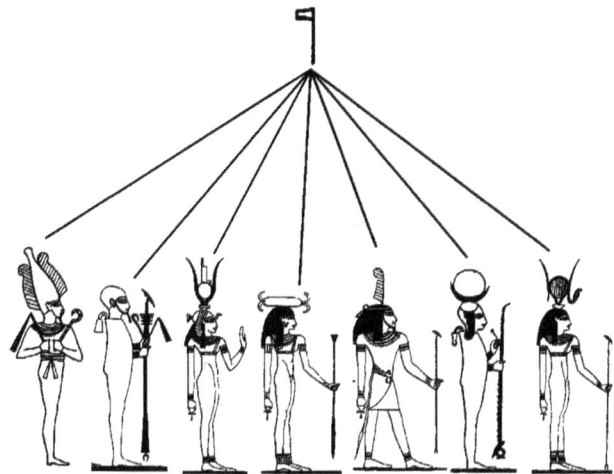

The Neteru (Gods and Goddesses) proceed from the Neter (Supreme Being)

As stated earlier, the concept of Neter and Neteru binds and ties all of the varied forms of Kamitan spirituality into one vision of the gods and goddesses all emerging from the same Supreme Being. Therefore, ultimately, Kamitan spirituality is not polytheistic, nor is it monotheistic, for it holds that the Supreme Being is more than a God or Goddess. The Supreme Being is an all-encompassing Absolute Divinity.

The Neteru

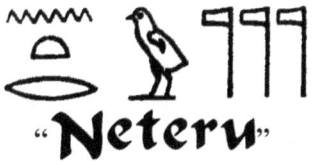

The term "Neteru" means "gods and goddesses." This means that from the ultimate and transcendental Supreme Being, "Neter," come the Neteru. There are countless Neteru. So from the one come the many. These Neteru are cosmic forces that pervade the universe. They are the means by which Neter sustains Creation and manifests through it. So Neterianism is a monotheistic polytheism. The one Supreme Being expresses as many gods and goddesses. At the end of time, after their work of sustaining Creation is finished, these gods and goddesses are again absorbed back into the Supreme Being.

All of the spiritual systems of Ancient Egypt (Kamit) have one essential aspect that is common to all; they all hold that there is a Supreme Being (Neter) who manifests in a multiplicity of ways through nature, the Neteru. Like sunrays, the Neteru emanate from the Divine; they are its manifestations. So by studying the Neteru we learn about and are led to discover their source, the Neter, and with this discovery we are enlightened. The Neteru may be depicted anthropomorphically or zoomorphically in accordance with the teaching about Neter that is being conveyed through them.

Mystical Philosophy of Universal Consciousness

The Neteru and Their Temples

Diagram 1: The Ancient Egyptian Temple Network

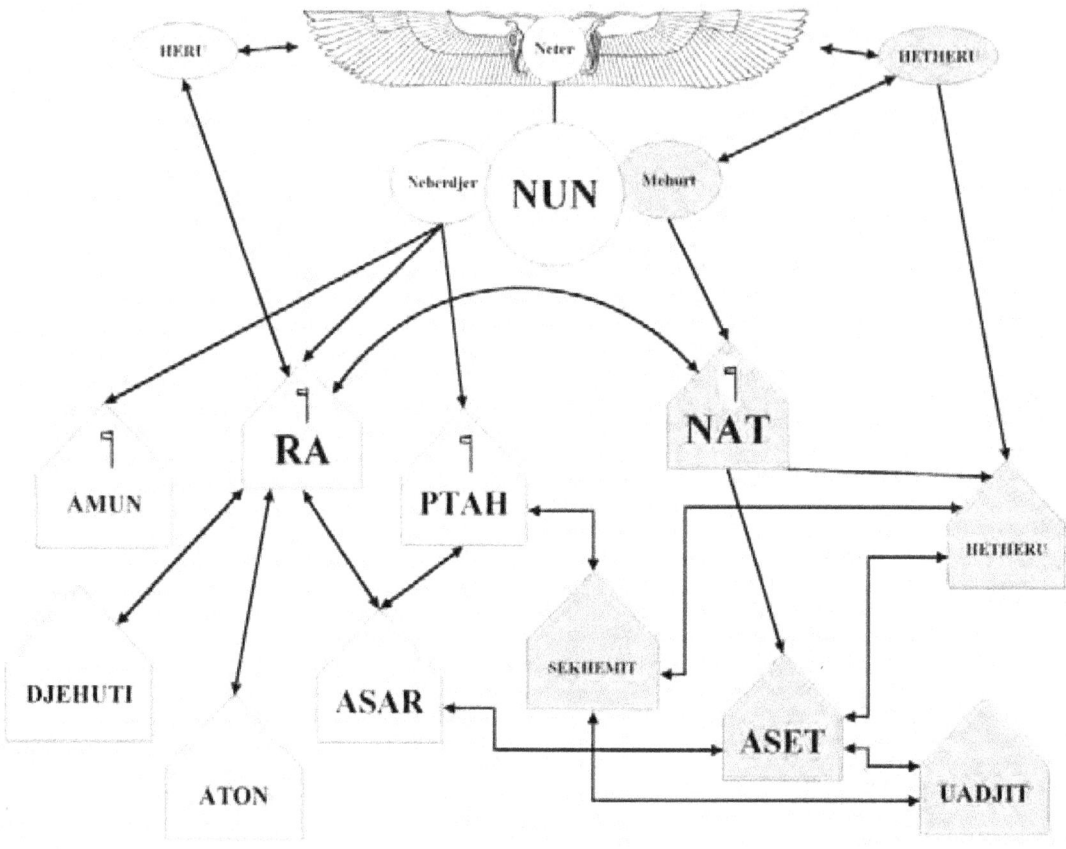

    The sages of Kamit instituted a system by which the teachings of spirituality were espoused through a Temple organization. The major divinities were assigned to a particular city. That divinity or group of divinities became the "patron" divinity or divinities of that city. Also, the Priests and Priestesses of that Temple were in charge of seeing to the welfare of the people in that district as well as maintaining the traditions and disciplines of the traditions based on the particular divinity being worshipped. So the original concept of "Neter" became elaborated through the "theologies" of the various traditions. A dynamic expression of the teachings emerged, which though maintaining the integrity of the teachings, expressed nuances of variation in perspective on the teachings to suit the needs of varying kinds of personalities of the people of different locales.

    In the diagram above, the primary or main divinities are denoted by the Neter symbol ( ). The house structure represents the Temple for that particular divinity. The interconnections with the other Temples are based on original scriptural statements espoused by the Temples that linked the divinities of their Temple with the other divinities. So this means that the divinities should be viewed not as separate entities operating independently, but rather as family members who are in the same "business" together, i.e. the enlightenment of society, albeit through variations in form of worship, name, form (expression of the Divinity), etc. Ultimately, all the divinities are referred to as Neteru and they are all said to be emanations from the ultimate and Supreme Being. Thus, the teaching from any of the Temples leads to an understanding of the others, and these all lead back to the source, the highest Divinity. Thus, the teaching within any of the Temple systems would lead to the attainment of spiritual enlightenment, the Great Awakening.

The Neteru and Their Interrelationships

Diagram : The Primary Kamitan Neteru and their Interrelationships

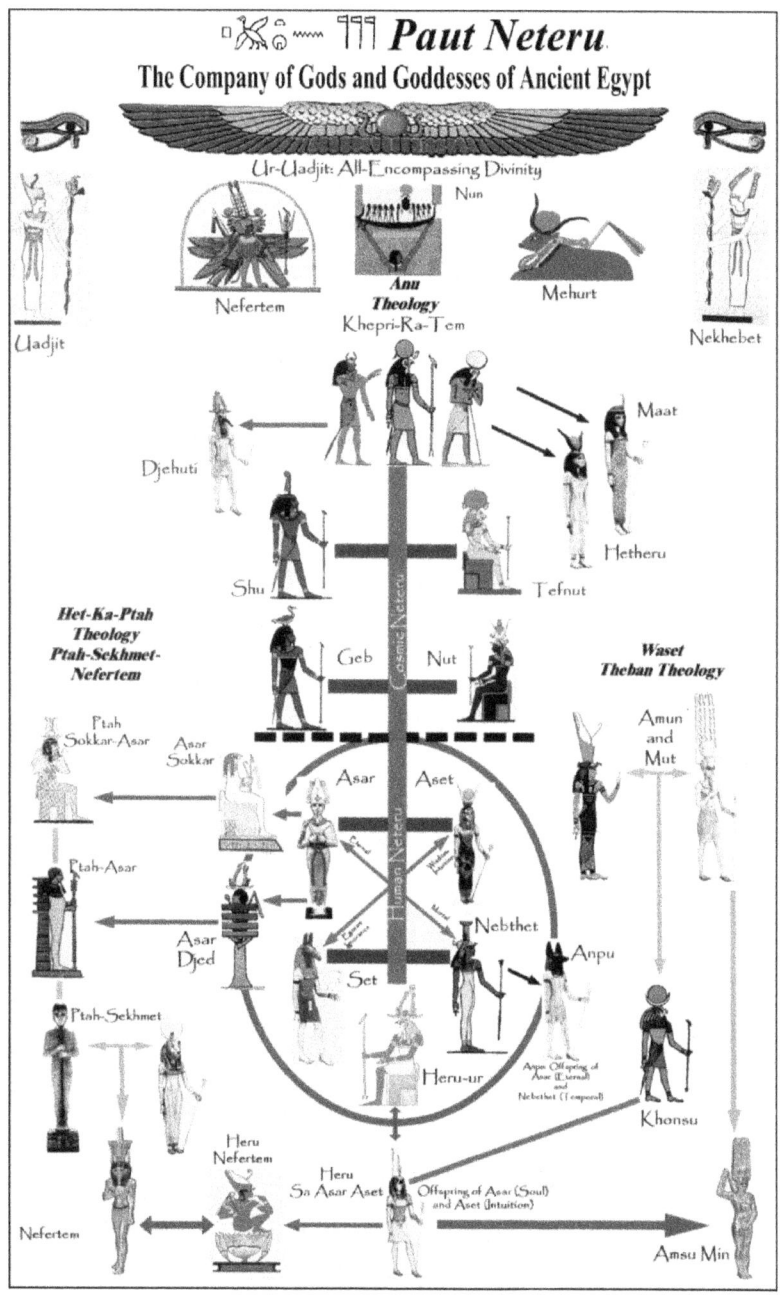

Mystical Philosophy of Universal Consciousness

The same Supreme Being, Neter, is the winged all-encompassing transcendental Divinity, the Spirit who, in the early history, is called "Heru." The physical universe in which the Heru lives is called "Hetheru" or the "house of Heru." This divinity (Heru) is also the Nun or primeval substratum from which all matter is composed. The various divinities and the material universe are composed from this primeval substratum. Neter is actually androgynous and Heru, the Spirit, is related as a male aspect of that androgyny. However, Heru in the androgynous aspect, gives rise to the solar principle and this is seen in both the male and female divinities.

The image above provides an idea of the relationships between the divinities of the three main Neterian spiritual systems (traditions): Anunian Theology, Wasetian (Theban) Theology and Het-Ka-Ptah (Memphite) Theology. The traditions are composed of companies or groups of gods and goddesses. Their actions, teachings and interactions with each other and with human beings provide insight into their nature as well as that of human existence and Creation itself. The lines indicate direct scriptural relationships and the labels also indicate that some divinities from one system are the same in others, with only a name change. Again, this is attested to by the scriptures themselves in direct statements, like those found in the *Prt m Hru* text Chapter 4 (17).[2]

Listening to the Teachings

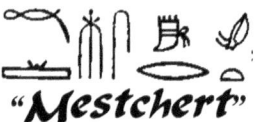
"*Mestchert*"

"Listening, to fill the ears, listen attentively-"

What should the ears be filled with?

The sages of Shetaut Neter enjoined that a Shemsu Neter (follower of Neter, an initiate or aspirant) should listen to the WISDOM of the Neterian Traditions. These are the myth related to the gods and goddesses containing the basic understanding of who they are, what they represent, how they relate human beings and to the Supreme Being. The myths allow us to be connected to the Divine.

An aspirant may choose any one of the 5 main Neterian Traditions.

- Shetaut Anu   – Teachings of the Ra Tradition
- Shetaut Menefer – Teachings of the Ptah Tradition
- Shetaut Waset   – Teachings of the Amun Tradition
- Shetaut Netrit   – Teachings of the Goddess Tradition
- Shetaut Asar   – Teachings of the Asarian Tradition
- Shetaut Aton   – Teachings of the Aton Tradition

---

[2] See the book *The Egyptian Book of the Dead* by Muata Ashby

EGYPTIAN TANTRIC YOGA

The Anunian Tradition

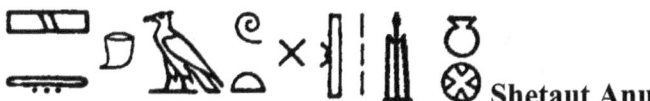 Shetaut Anu

The Mystery Teachings of the Anunian Tradition are related to the Divinity Ra and his company of Gods and Goddesses.[3] This Temple and its related Temples espouse the teachings of Creation, human origins and the path to spiritual enlightenment by means of the Supreme Being in the form of the god Ra. It tells of how Ra emerged from a primeval ocean and how human beings were created from his tears. The gods and goddesses, who are his children, go to form the elements of nature and the cosmic forces that maintain nature.

Below: The Heliopolitan Cosmogony.

The city of Anu (Amun-Ra)

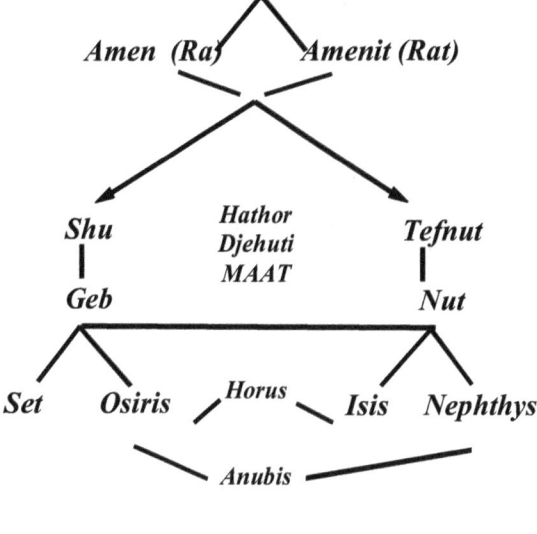

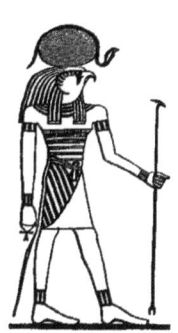

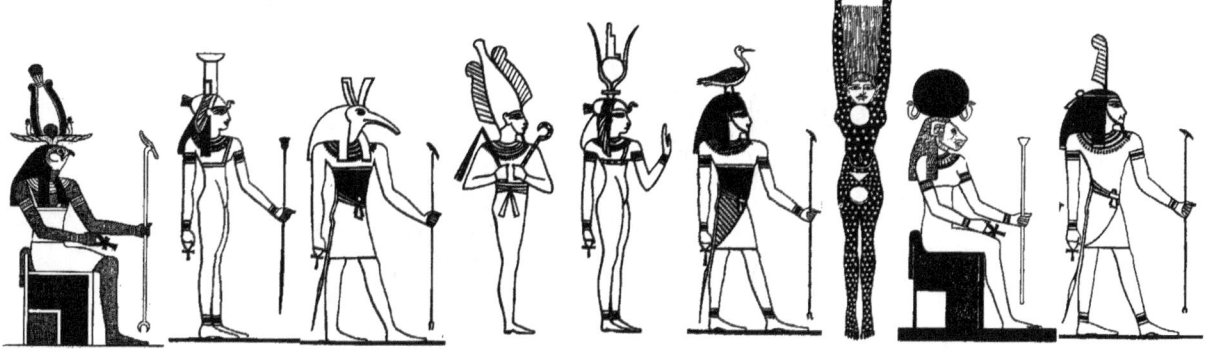

Top: Ra. From left to right, starting at the bottom level- The Gods and Goddesses of Anunian Theology: Shu, Tefnut, Nut, Geb, Aset, Asar, Set, Nebthet and Heru-Ur

---

[3] See the Book Anunian Theology by Muata Ashby

Mystical Philosophy of Universal Consciousness

The Memphite Tradition

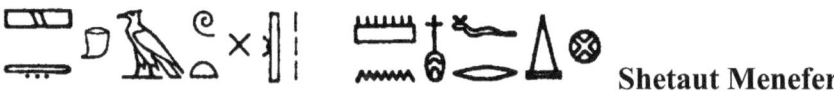 Shetaut Menefer

The Mystery Teachings of the Menefer (Memphite) Tradition are related to the Neterus known as Ptah, Sekhmit, Nefertem. The myths and philosophy of these divinities constitutes Memphite Theology.[4] This temple and its related temples espoused the teachings of Creation, human origins and the path to spiritual enlightenment by means of the Supreme Being in the form of the god Ptah and his family, who compose the Memphite Trinity. It tells of how Ptah emerged from a primeval ocean and how he created the universe by his will and the power of thought (mind). The gods and goddesses who are his thoughts, go to form the elements of nature and the cosmic forces that maintain nature. His spouse, Sekhmit has a powerful temple system of her own that is related to the Memphite teaching. The same is true for his son Nefertem.

Below: The Memphite Cosmogony.

The city of Hetkaptah (Ptah)

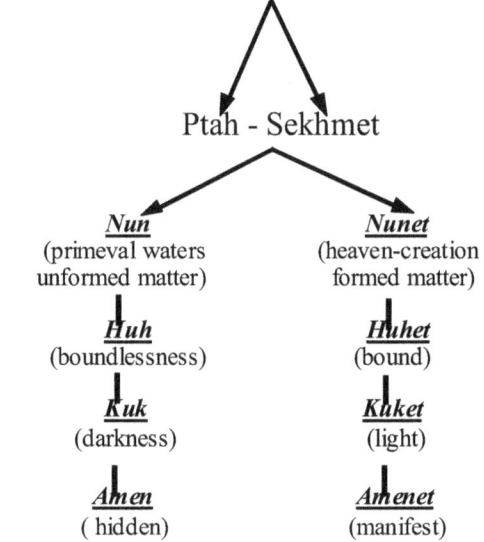

The Neters of Creation -
The Company of the Gods and Goddesses.
Neter Neteru
Nebertcher - Amun (unseen, hidden, ever present, Supreme Being, beyond duality and description)

Ptah - Sekhmet

Nun (primeval waters unformed matter)	*Nunet* (heaven-creation formed matter)
Huh (boundlessness)	*Huhet* (bound)
Kuk (darkness)	*Kuket* (light)
Amen (hidden)	*Amenet* (manifest)

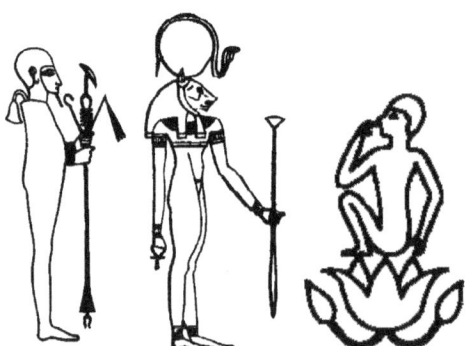

Ptah, Sekhmit and Nefertem

---
[4] See the Book Memphite Theology by Muata Ashby

EGYPTIAN TANTRIC YOGA

The Theban Tradition

Shetaut Amun

The Mystery Teachings of the Wasetian Tradition are related to the Neterus known as Amun, Mut Khonsu. This temple and its related temples espoused the teachings of Creation, human origins and the path to spiritual enlightenment by means of the Supreme Being in the form of the god Amun or Amun-Ra. It tells of how Amun and his family, the Trinity of Amun, Mut and Khonsu, manage the Universe along with his Company of Gods and Goddesses. This Temple became very important in the early part of the New Kingdom Era.

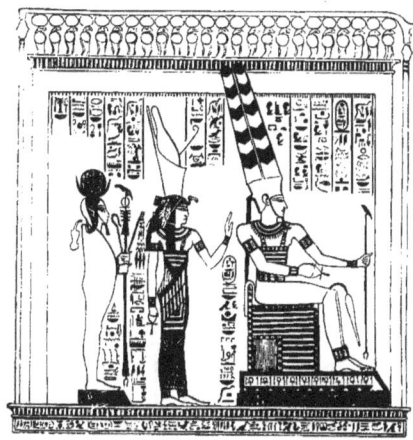

Below: The Trinity of Amun and the Company of Gods and Goddesses of Amun

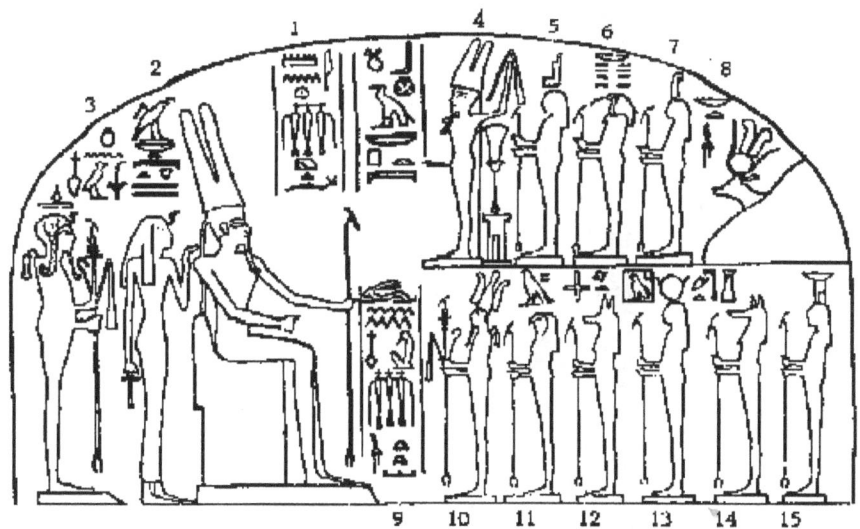

See the Book *Egyptian Yoga Vol. 2* for more on Amun, Mut and Khonsu by Muata Ashby

Mystical Philosophy of Universal Consciousness

The Goddess Tradition

Shetaut Netrit

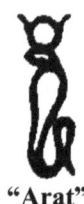

"Arat"

The hieroglyphic sign Arat means "Goddess." General, throughout ancient Kamit, the Mystery Teachings of the Goddess Tradition are related to the Divinity in the form of the Goddess. The Goddess was an integral part of all the Neterian traditions but special temples also developed around the worship of certain particular Goddesses who were also regarded as Supreme Beings in their own right. Thus as in other African religions, the goddess as well as the female gender were respected and elevated as the male divinities. The Goddess was also the author of Creation, giving birth to it as a great Cow. The following are the most important forms of the goddess.[5]

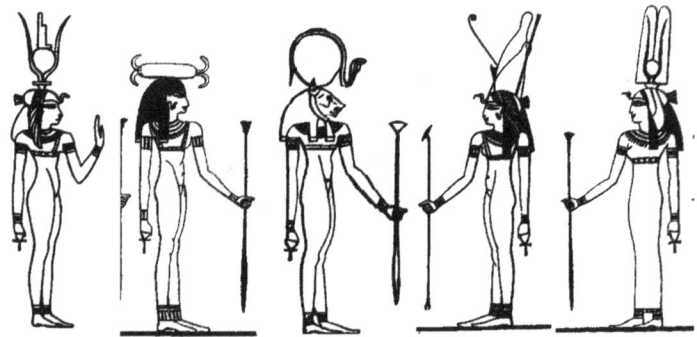

Aset, Net, Sekhmit, Mut, Hetheru

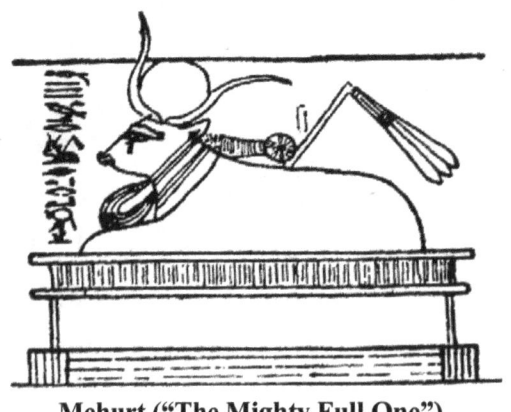

Mehurt ("The Mighty Full One")

---

[5] See the Books, *The Goddess Path, Mysteries of Isis, Glorious Light Meditation, Memphite Theology* and *Resurrecting Osiris* by Muata Ashby

EGYPTIAN TANTRIC YOGA
The Asarian Tradition

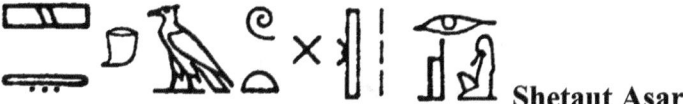 Shetaut Asar

This temple and its related temples espoused the teachings of Creation, human origins and the path to spiritual enlightenment by means of the Supreme Being in the form of the god Asar. It tells of how Asar and his family, the Trinity of Asar, Aset and Heru, manage the Universe and lead human beings to spiritual enlightenment and the resurrection of the soul. This Temple and its teaching were very important from the Pre-Dynastic era down to the Christian period. The Mystery Teachings of the Asarian Tradition are related to the Neterus known as: Asar, Aset, Heru (Osiris, Isis and Horus)

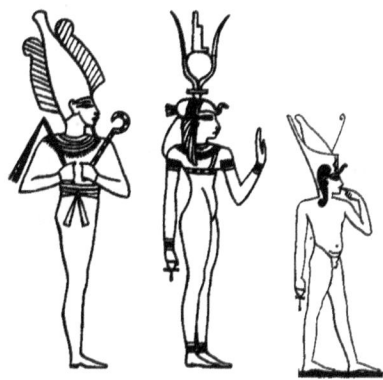

The tradition of Asar, Aset and Heru was practiced generally throughout the land of ancient Kamit. The centers of this tradition were the city of Abdu containing the Great Temple of Asar, the city of Pilak containing the Great Temple of Aset[6] and Edfu containing the Ggreat Temple of Heru.

---

[6] See the Book Resurrecting Osiris by Muata Ashby

Mystical Philosophy of Universal Consciousness

The Aton Tradition

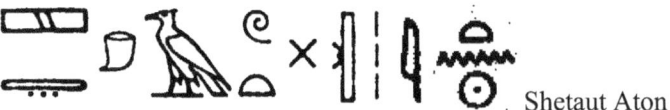 Shetaut Aton

This temple and its related temples espoused the teachings of Creation, human origins and the path to spiritual enlightenment by means of the Supreme Being in the form of the god Aton. It tells of how Aton with its dynamic life force created and sustains Creation. By recognizing Aton as the very substratum of all existence, human beings engage in devotional exercises and rituals and the study of the Hymns containing the wisdom teachings of Aton explaining that Aton manages the Universe and leads human beings to spiritual enlightenment and eternal life for the soul. This Temple and its teaching were very important in the middle New Kingdom Period. The Mystery Teachings of the Aton Tradition are related to the Neter Aton and its main exponent was the Sage King Akhnaton, who is depicted below with his family adoring the sundisk, symbol of the Aton.

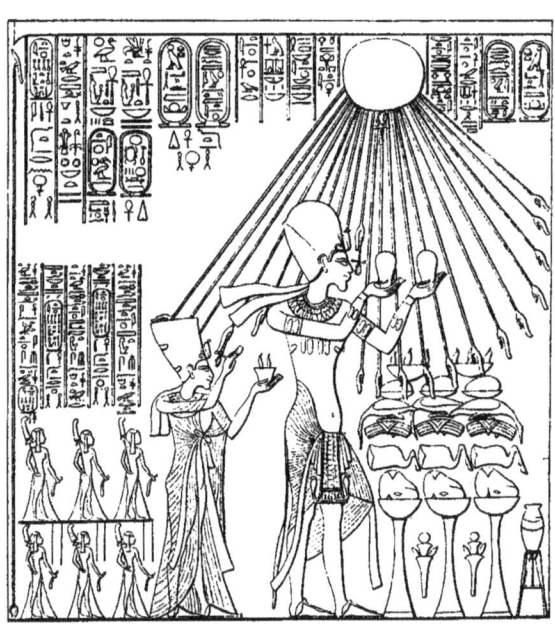

Akhnaton, Nefertiti and Daughters

For more on Atonism and the Aton Theology see the Essence of Atonism Lecture Series by Sebai Muata Ashby ©2001

EGYPTIAN TANTRIC YOGA

The General Principles of Shetaut Neter
(Teachings Presented in the Kamitan scriptures)

1. The Purpose of Life is to Attain the Great Awakening-Enlightenment-Know thyself.

2. SHETAUT NETER enjoins the Shedy (spiritual investigation) as the highest endeavor of life.

3. SHETAUT NETER enjoins that it is the responsibility of every human being to promote order and truth.

4. SHETAUT NETER enjoins the performance of Selfless Service to family, community and humanity.

5. SHETAUT NETER enjoins the Protection of nature.

6. SHETAUT NETER enjoins the Protection of the weak and oppressed.

7. SHETAUT NETER enjoins the Caring for hungry.

8. SHETAUT NETER enjoins the Caring for homeless.

9. SHETAUT NETER enjoins the equality for all people.

10. SHETAUT NETER enjoins the equality between men and women.

11. SHETAUT NETER enjoins the justice for all.

12. SHETAUT NETER enjoins the sharing of resources.

13. SHETAUT NETER enjoins the protection and proper raising of children.

14. SHETAUT NETER enjoins the movement towards balance and peace.

Mystical Philosophy of Universal Consciousness

The Forces of Entropy

In Neterian religion, there is no concept of "evil" as is conceptualized in Western Culture. Rather, it is understood that the forces of entropy are constantly working in nature to bring that which has been constructed by human hands to their original natural state. The serpent Apep (Apophis), who daily tries to stop Ra's boat of creation, is the symbol of entropy. This concept of entropy has been referred to as "chaos" by Western Egyptologists.

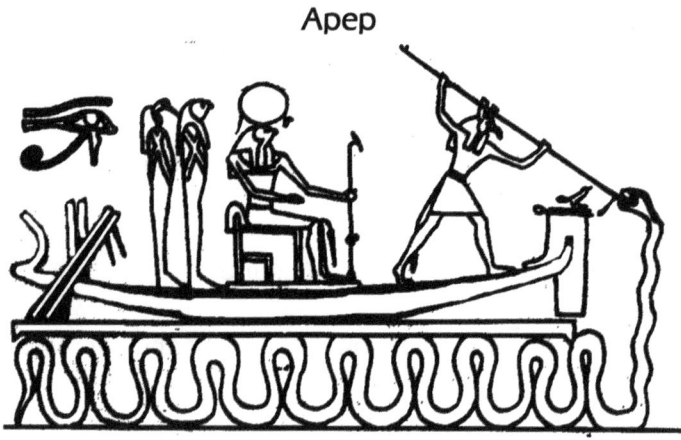

Above: Set protecting the boat of Ra from the forces of entropy (symbolized by the serpent Apep).

As expressed previously, in Neterian religion there is also no concept of a "devil" or "demon" as is conceived in the Judeo-Christian or Islamic traditions. Rather, it is understood that manifestations of detrimental situations and adversities arise as a result of unrighteous actions. These unrighteous actions are due to the "Setian" qualities in a human being. Set is the Neteru of egoism and the negative qualities which arise from egoism. Egoism is the idea of individuality based on identification with the body and mind only as being who one is. One has no deeper awareness of their deeper spiritual essence, and thus no understanding of their connectedness to all other objects (includes persons) in creation and the Divine Self. When the ego is under the control of the higher nature, it fights the forces of entropy (as above). However, when beset with ignorance, it leads to the degraded states of human existence. The vices (egoism, selfishness, extraverted ness, wonton sexuality (lust), jealousy, envy, greed, gluttony) are a result.

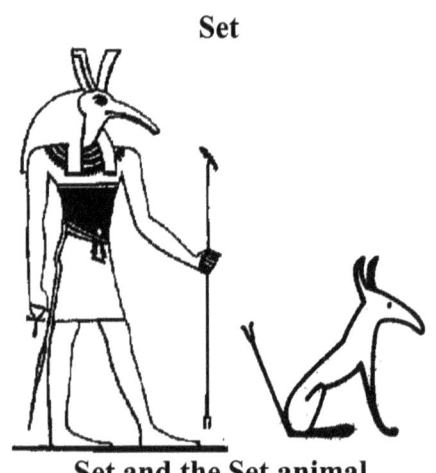

Set and the Set animal

EGYPTIAN TANTRIC YOGA

The Great Awakening of Neterian Religion

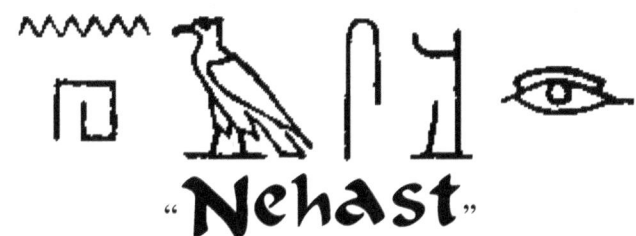

"Nehast"

Nehast means to "wake up," to Awaken to the higher existence. In the Prt m Hru Text it is said:

Nuk pa Neter aah Neter Ujah asha ren[7]

"I am that same God, the Supreme One, who has myriad of mysterious names."

The goal of all the Neterian disciplines is to discover the meaning of "Who am I?," to unravel the mysteries of life and to fathom the depths of eternity and infinity. This is the task of all human beings and it is to be accomplished in this very lifetime.

This can be done by learning the ways of the Neteru, emulating them and finally becoming like them, Akhus, (enlightened beings), walking the earth as giants and accomplishing great deeds such as the creation of the universe!

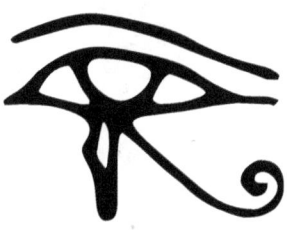

Udjat
The Eye of Heru is a quintessential symbol of awakening to Divine Consciousness, representing the concept of Nehast.

---

[7] (Prt M Hru 9:4)

Part 2: Introduction to Egyptian Yoga

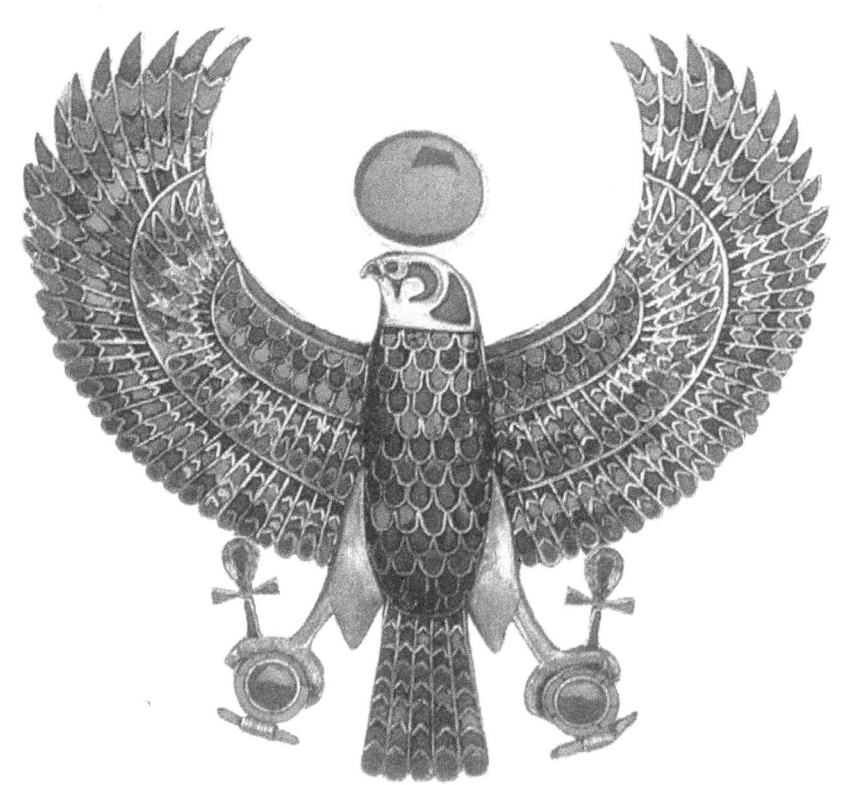

EGYPTIAN TANTRIC YOGA

Most students of yoga are familiar with the yogic traditions of India consider that the Indian texts such as the Bhagavad Gita, Mahabharata, Patanjali Yoga Sutras, etc. are the primary and original source of Yogic philosophy and teaching. However, upon examination, the teachings currently espoused in all of the major forms of Indian Yoga can be found in Ancient Egyptian scriptures, inscribed in papyrus and on temple walls as well as steles, statues, obelisks and other sources.

What is Yoga?

Yoga is the practice of mental, physical and spiritual disciplines which lead to self-control and self-discovery by purifying the mind, body and spirit, so as to discover the deeper spiritual essence which lies within every human being and object in the universe. In essence, the goal of Yoga practice is to unite or *yoke* one's individual consciousness with Universal or Cosmic consciousness. Therefore, Ancient Egyptian religious practice, especially in terms of the rituals and other practices of the Ancient Egyptian Temple system known as *Shetaut Neter* (the way of the hidden Supreme Being), also known in Ancient times as *Smai Tawi* "Egyptian Yoga," should as well be considered as universal streams of self-knowledge philosophy which influenced and inspired the great religions and philosophers to this day. In this sense, religion, in its purest form, is also a Yoga system, as it seeks to reunite the soul with its true and original source, God. In broad terms, any spiritual movement or discipline that brings one closer to self-knowledge is a "Yogic" movement. The main recognized forms of Yoga disciplines are:

- *Yoga of Wisdom,*
- *Yoga of Devotional Love,*
- *Yoga of Meditation,*
    - *Physical Postures Yoga*
- *Yoga of Selfless Action,*
- *Tantric Yoga*
    - *Serpent Power Yoga*

The diagram below shows the relationship between the Yoga disciplines and the path of mystical religion (religion practiced in its three complete steps: 1st receiving the myth {knowledge}, 2nd practicing the rituals of the myth {following the teachings of the myth} and 3rd entering into a mystical experience {becoming one with the central figure of the myth}).

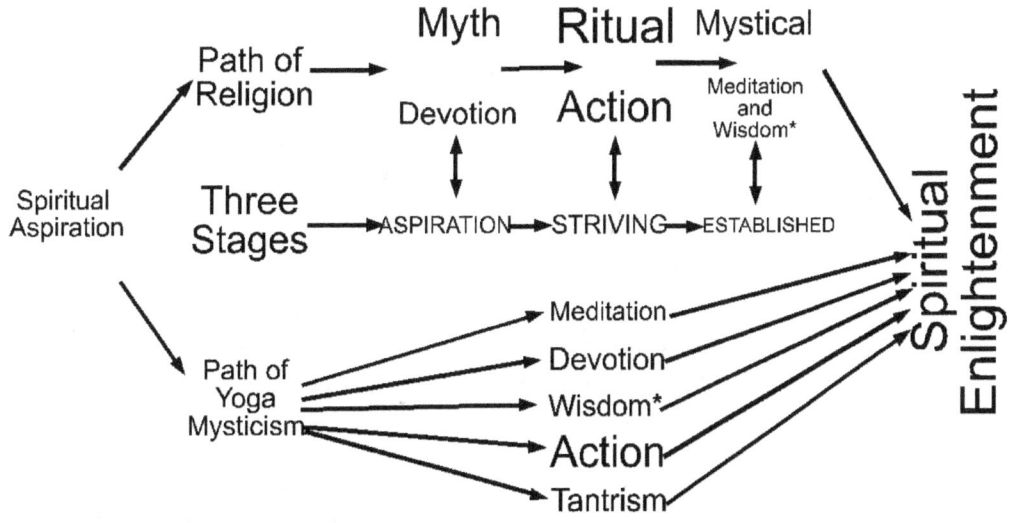

Mystical Philosophy of Universal Consciousness

The disciplines of Yoga fall under five major categories. These are: *Yoga of Wisdom, Yoga of Devotional Love, Yoga of Meditation, Tantric Yoga* and *Yoga of Selfless Action.* When these disciplines are practiced in a harmonized manner this practice is called "Integral Yoga." Within these categories there are subsidiary forms which are part of the main disciplines. The emphasis in the Kamitan Asarian (Osirian) Myth is on the Yoga of Wisdom, Yoga of Devotional Love and Yoga of Selfless Action. The important point to remember is that all aspects of Yoga can and should be used in an integral fashion to effect an efficient and harmonized spiritual movement in the practitioner. Therefore, while there may be an area of special emphasis, other elements are bound to become part of the Yoga program as needed. For example, while a Yogin (practitioner of Yoga, aspirant, initiate) may place emphasis on the Yoga of Wisdom, they may also practice Devotional Yoga and Meditation Yoga along with the wisdom studies. So the practice of any discipline that leads to oneness with Supreme Consciousness can be called Yoga. If you study, rationalize and reflect upon the teachings, you are practicing *Yoga of Wisdom*. If you meditate upon the teachings and your Higher Self, you are practicing *Yoga of Meditation.*

Thus, whether or not you refer to it as such, if you practice rituals which identify you with your spiritual nature, you are practicing *Yoga of Ritual Identification* (which is part of the Yoga of Wisdom {Kamitan-Rekh, Indian-Jnana} and the Yoga of Devotional Love {Kamitan-Ushet, Indian-Bhakti} of the Divine). If you develop your physical nature and psychic energy centers, you are practicing *Serpent Power* (Kamitan-*Uraeus* or Indian-*Kundalini*) *Yoga* (which is part of Tantric Yoga). If you practice living according to the teachings of ethical behavior and selflessness, you are practicing *Yoga of Action* (Kamitan-Maat, Indian-Karma) in daily life. If you practice turning your attention towards the Divine by developing love for the Divine, then it is called *Devotional Yoga* or *Yoga of Divine Love*. The practitioner of Yoga is called a Yogin (male practitioner) or Yogini (female practitioner), or the term "Yogi" may be used to refer to either a female or male practitioner in general terms. One who has attained the culmination of Yoga (union with the Divine) is also called a Yogi. In this manner, Yoga has been developed into many disciplines which may be used in an integral fashion to achieve the same goal: Enlightenment. Therefore, the aspirant is to learn about all of the paths of Yoga and choose those elements which best suit {his/her} personality or practice them all in an integral, balanced way.

Enlightenment is the term used to describe the highest level of spiritual awakening. It means attaining such a level of spiritual awareness that one discovers the underlying unity of the entire universe as well as the fact that the source of all creation is the same source from which the innermost Self within every human heart arises.

What is Egyptian Yoga?

The Term "Egyptian Yoga" and The Philosophy Behind It

As previously discussed, Yoga in all of its forms were practiced in Egypt apparently earlier than anywhere else in our history. This point of view is supported by the fact that there is documented scriptural and iconographical evidence of the disciplines of virtuous living, dietary purification, study of the wisdom teachings and their practice in daily life, psychophysical and psycho-spiritual exercises and meditation being practiced in Ancient Egypt, long before the evidence of its existence is detected in India (including the Indus Valley Civilization) or any other early civilization (Sumer, Greece, China, etc.).

The teachings of Yoga are at the heart of *Prt m Hru*. As explained earlier, the word "Yoga" is a Sanskrit term meaning to unite the individual with the Cosmic. The term has been used in

EGYPTIAN TANTRIC YOGA

certain parts of this book for ease of communication since the word "Yoga" has received wide popularity especially in western countries in recent years. The Ancient Egyptian equivalent term to the Sanskrit word yoga is: ***"Smai."*** *Smai* means union, and the following determinative terms give it a spiritual significance, at once equating it with the term "Yoga" as it is used in India. When used in conjunction with the Ancient Egyptian symbol which means land, ***"Ta,"*** the term "union of the two lands" arises.

In Chapter 4 and Chapter 17 of the *Prt m Hru,* a term "Smai Tawi" is used. It means "Union of the two lands of Egypt," ergo "Egyptian Yoga." The two lands refer to the two main districts of the country (North and South). In ancient times, Egypt was divided into two sections or land areas. These were known as Lower and Upper Egypt. In Ancient Egyptian mystical philosophy, the land of Upper Egypt relates to the divinity Heru (Heru), who represents the Higher Self, and the land of Lower Egypt relates to Set, the divinity of the lower self. So ***Smai Taui*** means "the union of the two lands" or the "Union of the lower self with the Higher Self. The lower self relates to that which is negative and uncontrolled in the human mind including worldliness, egoism, ignorance, etc. (Set), while the Higher Self relates to that which is above temptations and is good in the human heart as well as in touch with transcendental consciousness (Heru). Thus, we also have the Ancient Egyptian term ***Smai Heru-Set,*** or the union of Heru and Set. So Smai Taui or Smai Heru-Set are the Ancient Egyptian words which are to be translated as **"Egyptian Yoga."**

Above: the main symbol of Egyptian Yoga: *Sma*. The Ancient Egyptian language and symbols provide the first "historical" record of Yoga Philosophy and Religious literature. The hieroglyph Sma, "Sema," represented by the union of two lungs and the trachea, symbolizes that the union of the duality, that is, the Higher Self and lower self, leads to Non-duality, the One, singular consciousness.

The Ancient Egyptians called the disciplines of Yoga in Ancient Egypt by the term *"Smai Tawi."* So what does Smai Tawi mean?

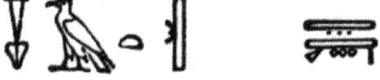

Smai Tawi
(From Chapter 4 of the *Prt m Hru*)

The Ancient Egyptian Symbols of Yoga

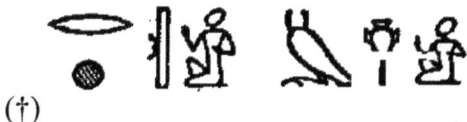

Mystical Philosophy of Universal Consciousness

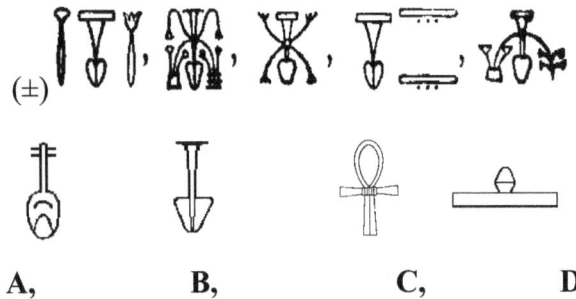

A,   B,   C,   D

The theme of the arrangement of the symbols above is based on the idea that in mythological and philosophic forms, Egyptian mythology and philosophy merge with world mythology, philosophy and religion. The hieroglyphic symbols at the very top (†) mean: *"Know Thyself," "Self knowledge is the basis of all true knowledge"* and (±) abbreviated forms of *Smai taui,* signifies "Egyptian Yoga." The next four below represent the four words in Egyptian Philosophy, which mean *"YOGA."* They are: (A) *"Nefer"* (B) *"Sema"* (C) *"Ankh"* and (D) *"Hetep."*

The Term "Egyptian Yoga" and The Philosophy Behind It

As previously discussed, Yoga in all of its forms were practiced in Egypt apparently earlier than anywhere else in our history. This point of view is supported by the fact that there is documented scriptural and iconographical evidence of the disciplines of virtuous living, dietary purification, study of the wisdom teachings and their practice in daily life, psychophysical and psycho-spiritual exercises and meditation being practiced in Ancient Egypt, long before the evidence of its existence is detected in India (including the Indus Valley Civilization) or any other early civilization (Sumer, Greece, China, etc.).

The teachings of Yoga are at the heart of *Prt m Hru*. As explained earlier, the word "Yoga" is a Sanskrit term meaning to unite the individual with the Cosmic. The term has been used in certain parts of this book for ease of communication since the word "Yoga" has received wide popularity especially in western countries in recent years. The Ancient Egyptian equivalent term to the Sanskrit word yoga is: *"Smai." Smai* means union, and the following determinative terms give it a spiritual significance, at once equating it with the term "Yoga" as it is used in India. When used in conjunction with the Ancient Egyptian symbol which means land, *"Ta,"* the term "union of the two lands" arises.

In Chapter 4 and Chapter 17 of the *Prt m Hru,* a term "Smai Tawi" is used. It means "Union of the two lands of Egypt," ergo "Egyptian Yoga." The two lands refer to the two main districts of the country (North and South). In ancient times, Egypt was divided into two sections or land areas. These were known as Lower and Upper Egypt. In Ancient Egyptian mystical philosophy, the land of Upper Egypt relates to the divinity Heru (Heru), who represents the Higher Self, and the land of Lower Egypt relates to Set, the divinity of the lower self. So *Smai Taui* means "the union of the two lands" or the "Union of the lower self with the Higher Self. The lower self relates to that which is negative and uncontrolled in the human mind including worldliness, egoism, ignorance, etc. (Set), while the Higher Self relates to that which is above temptations and is good in the human heart as well as in touch with transcendental consciousness (Heru). Thus, we also have the Ancient Egyptian term *Smai Heru-Set,* or the union of Heru and Set. So

41

EGYPTIAN TANTRIC YOGA

Smai Taui or Smai Heru-Set are the Ancient Egyptian words which are to be translated as **"Egyptian Yoga."**

Above: the main symbol of Egyptian Yoga: *Sma*. The Ancient Egyptian language and symbols provide the first "historical" record of Yoga Philosophy and Religious literature. The hieroglyph Sma, ↕ "Sema," represented by the union of two lungs and the trachea, symbolizes that the union of the duality, that is, the Higher Self and lower self, leads to Non-duality, the One, singular consciousness.

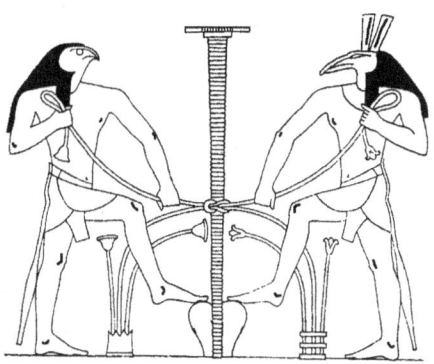

Above left: Smai Heru-Set, Heru and Set join forces to tie up the symbol of Union (Sema –see (B) above). The Sema symbol refers to the Union of Upper Egypt (Lotus) and Lower Egypt (Papyrus) under one ruler, but also at a more subtle level, it refers to the union of one's Higher Self and lower self (Heru and Set), as well as the control of one's breath (Life Force) through the union (control) of the lungs (breathing organs). The character of Heru and Set are an integral part of the Pert Em Heru.

The central and most popular character within Ancient Egyptian Religion of Asar is Heru, who is an incarnation of his father, Asar. Asar is killed by his brother Set who, out of greed and demoniac (Setian) tendency, craved to be the ruler of Egypt. With the help of Djehuti, the God of wisdom, Aset, the great mother and Hetheru, his consort, Heru prevailed in the battle against Set for the rulership of Kemit (Egypt). Heru's struggle symbolizes the struggle of every human being to regain rulership of the Higher Self and to subdue the lower self.

The most ancient writings in our historical period are from the Ancient Egyptians. These writings are referred to as hieroglyphics. The original name given to these writings by the Ancient Egyptians is *Metu Neter,* meaning "the writing of God" or *Neter Metu* or "Divine Speech." These writings were inscribed in temples, coffins and papyruses and contained the teachings in reference to the spiritual nature of the human being and the ways to promote spiritual emancipation, awakening or resurrection. The Ancient Egyptian proverbs presented in this text are translations from the original hieroglyphic scriptures. An example of hieroglyphic text was presented above in the form of the text of Smai Taui or "Egyptian Yoga."

Egyptian Philosophy may be summed up in the following proverbs, which clearly state that the soul is heavenly or divine and that the human being must awaken to the true reality, which is the Spirit, Self.

"Self knowledge is the basis of true knowledge."

Mystical Philosophy of Universal Consciousness

"Soul to heaven, body to earth."

"Man is to become God-like through a life of virtue and the cultivation of the spirit through scientific knowledge, practice and bodily discipline."

"Salvation is accomplished through the efforts of the individual. There is no mediator between man and {his/her} salvation."

"Salvation is the freeing of the soul from its bodily fetters, becoming a God through knowledge and wisdom, controlling the forces of the cosmos instead of being a slave to them, subduing the lower nature and through awakening the Higher Self, ending the cycle of rebirth and dwelling with the Neters who direct and control the Great Plan."

Egyptian Yoga is a revolutionary new way to understand and practice Ancient Egyptian Mysticism, the Ancient Egyptian mystical religion (*Shetaut Neter*). Egyptian Yoga is what has been commonly referred to by Egyptologists as Egyptian "Religion" or "Mythology," but to think of it as just another set of stories or allegories about a long lost civilization is to completely miss the greatest secret of human existence. What is Yoga? The literal meaning of the word YOGA is to *"YOKE"* or to *"LINK"* back. The implication is to link back individual consciousness to its original source, the original essence: Universal Consciousness. In a broad sense Yoga is any process which helps one to achieve liberation or freedom from the bondage to human pain and spiritual ignorance. So whenever you engage in any activity with the goal of promoting the discovery of your true Self, be it studying the wisdom teachings, exercise, fasting, meditation, breath control, rituals, chanting, prayer, etc., you are practicing yoga. If the goal is to help you to discover your essential nature as one with God or the Supreme Being or Consciousness, then it is Yoga. Yoga, in all of its forms as the disciplines of spiritual development, as practiced in Ancient Egypt earlier than anywhere else in history. The ancient scriptures describe how Asar, the first mythical king of Ancient Egypt, traveled throughout Asia and Europe establishing civilization and the practice of religion. This partially explains why the teachings of mystical spirituality known as Yoga and Vedanta in India are so similar to the teachings of Shetaut Neter (Ancient Egyptian religion - Egyptian Yoga. This unique perspective from the highest philosophical system which developed in Africa over seven thousand years ago provides a new way to look at life, religion, psychology and the way to spiritual development leading to spiritual Enlightenment. So Egyptian Yoga is not merely a philosophy but a discipline for promoting spiritual evolution in a human being, allowing him or her to discover the ultimate truth, supreme peace and utmost joy which lies within the human heart. These are the true worthwhile goals of life. Anything else is settling for less. It would be like a personality who owns vast riches thinking that he is poor and homeless. Every human being has the potential to discover the greatest treasure of all existence if they apply themselves to the study and practice of the teachings of Yoga with the proper guidance. Sema ( ) is the Ancient Egyptian word and symbol meaning *union or Yoga.* This is the vision of Egyptian Yoga.

The Study of Yoga

When we look out upon the world, we are often baffled by the multiplicity, which constitutes the human experience. What do we really know about this experience? Many scientific disciplines have developed over the last two hundred years for the purpose of discovering the mysteries of nature, but this search has only engendered new questions about the nature of existence. Yoga is a discipline or way of life designed to promote the physical, mental and spiritual development of the human being. It leads a person to discover the answers to the most important questions of life such as, Who am I? Why am I here? Where am I going?

As explained earlier, the literal meaning of the word *Yoga* is to *"Yoke"* or to *"Link"* back, the implication being to link the individual consciousness back to the original source, the original essence, that which transcends all mental and intellectual attempts at comprehension, but which is the essential nature of everything in Creation, termed "Universal Consciousness. While in the strict sense, Yoga may be seen as a separate discipline from religion, yoga and religion have been linked at many points throughout history and continue to be linked even today. In a manner of speaking, Yoga as a discipline may be seen as a non-sectarian transpersonal science or practice to promote spiritual development and harmony of mind and body thorough mental and physical disciplines including meditation, psycho-physical exercises, and performing action with the correct attitude.

The teachings which were practiced in the Ancient Egyptian temples were the same ones later intellectually defined into a literary form by the Indian Sages of Vedanta and Yoga. This was discussed in our book *Egyptian Yoga: The Philosophy of Enlightenment*. The Indian Mysteries of Yoga and Vedanta may therefore be understood as representing an unfolding exposition of the Egyptian Mysteries.

The question is how to accomplish these seemingly impossible tasks? How to transform yourself and realize the deepest mysteries of existence? How to discover "Who am I?" This is the mission of Yoga Philosophy and the purpose of yogic practices. Yoga does not seek to convert or impose religious beliefs on any one. Ancient Egypt was the source of civilization and the source of religion and Yoga. Therefore, all systems of mystical spirituality can coexist harmoniously within these teachings when they are correctly understood.

The goal of yoga is to promote integration of the mind-body-spirit complex in order to produce optimal health of the human being. This is accomplished through mental and physical exercises which promote the free flow of spiritual energy by reducing mental complexes caused by ignorance. There are two roads which human beings can follow, one of wisdom and the other of ignorance. The path of the masses is generally the path of ignorance which leads them into negative situations, thoughts and deeds. These in turn lead to ill health and sorrow in life. The other road is based on wisdom and it leads to health, true happiness and enlightenment.

The central and most popular character within ancient Egyptian Religion of Asar is Heru who is an incarnation of his father, Asar. Asar is killed by his brother Set who, out of greed and demoniac (Setian) tendency, craves to be the ruler of Egypt. With the help of Djehuti, the God of wisdom, Aset, the great mother and Hetheru, his consort, Heru prevails in the battle against Set for the rulership of Egypt. Heru' struggle symbolizes the struggle of every human being to regain rulership of the Higher Self and to subdue the lower self. With this understanding, the land of Egypt is equivalent to the Kingdom/Queendom concept of Christianity.

The most ancient writings in our historical period are from the ancient Egyptians. These writings are referred to as hieroglyphics. Also, the most ancient civilization known was the ancient Egyptian civilization. The proof of this lies in the ancient Sphinx which is over 12,000 years old. The original name given to these writings by the ancient Egyptians is *Metu Neter*, meaning "the writing of God" or *Neter Metu* or "Divine Speech." These writings were inscribed

Mystical Philosophy of Universal Consciousness

in temples, coffins and papyruses and contained the teachings in reference to the spiritual nature of the human being and the ways to promote spiritual emancipation, awakening or resurrection. The —Ancient Egyptian Proverbs presented in this text are translations from the original hieroglyphic scriptures. An example of hieroglyphic text is presented on the front cover.

Egyptian Philosophy may be summed up in the following proverbs which clearly state that the soul is heavenly or divine and that the human being must awaken to the true reality which is the spirit Self.

"Self knowledge is the basis of true knowledge."

"Soul to heaven, body to earth."

"Man is to become God-like through a life of virtue and the cultivation of the spirit through scientific knowledge, practice and bodily discipline."

"Salvation is accomplished through the efforts of the individual. There is no mediator between man and his / her salvation."

"Salvation is the freeing of the soul from its bodily fetters, becoming a God through knowledge and wisdom, controlling the forces of the cosmos instead of being a slave to them, subduing the lower nature and through awakening the Higher Self, ending the cycle of rebirth and dwelling with the Neters who direct and control the Great Plan."

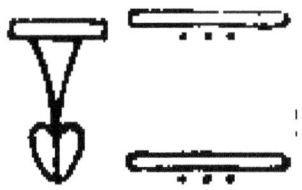

Smai Tawi
(From Chapter 4 of
the *Prt m Hru*)

EGYPTIAN TANTRIC YOGA

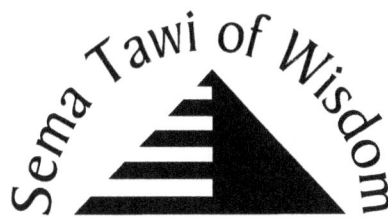

One discipline of Yoga requires special mention here. It is called Wisdom Yoga or the Yoga of Wisdom. In the Temple of Aset (Aset) in Ancient Egypt the Discipline of the Yoga of Wisdom is imparted in three stages:

1-<u>Listening</u> to the wisdom teachings on the nature of reality (creation) and the nature of the Self.
2-<u>Reflecting</u> on those teachings and incorporating them into daily life.
3-<u>Meditating</u> on the meaning of the teachings.

Aset (Aset) was and is recognized as the goddess of wisdom and her temple strongly emphasized and espoused the philosophy of wisdom teaching in order to achieve higher spiritual consciousness. It is important to note here that the teaching which was practiced in the Ancient Egyptian Temple of Aset[8] of **Listening** to, **Reflecting** upon, and **Meditating** upon the teachings is the same process used in Vedanta-Jnana Yoga of India of today. **The Yoga of Wisdom** is a form of Yoga based on insight into the nature of worldly existence and the transcendental Self, thereby transforming one's consciousness through development of the wisdom faculty. Thus, we have here a correlation between Ancient Egypt that matches exactly in its basic factor respects.

THE THREE-FOLD PROCESS OF WISDOM YOGA IN EGYPT:

According to the teachings of *the Ancient Temple of Aset* the Yoga of Wisdom, entails the process of three steps:

Discipline of Wisdom Yoga in Ancient Egypt
1-<u>Listening</u> to the wisdom teachings on the nature of reality (creation) and the nature of the Self.
2-<u>Reflecting</u> on those teachings and incorporating them into daily life.
3-<u>Meditating</u> on the meaning of the teachings.

---

[8] See the book *The Wisdom of Aset* by Dr. Muata Ashby

Mystical Philosophy of Universal Consciousness

Figure 1: The image of goddess Aset (Aset) suckling the young king is the quintecential symbol of initiation in Ancient Egypt.

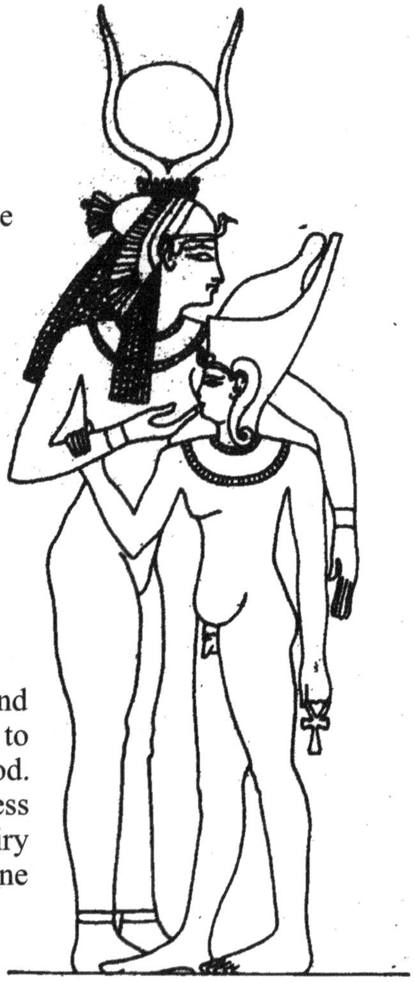

Temple of Aset
GENERAL DISCIPLINE

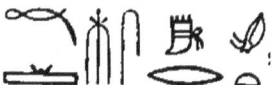

Fill the ears, listen attentively- Meh mestchert.

Listening

1- Listening to Wisdom teachings. Having achieved the qualifications of an aspirant, there is a desire to listen to the teachings from a Spiritual Preceptor. There is increasing intellectual understanding of the scriptures and the meaning of truth versus untruth, real versus unreal, temporal versus eternal. The glories of God are expounded and the mystical philosophy behind the myth is given at this stage.

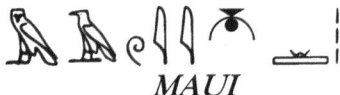
MAUI
"to think, to ponder, to fix attention, concentration"

Reflection

2- Reflection on those teachings that have been listened to and living according to the disciplines enjoined by the teachings is to be practiced until the wisdom teaching is fully understood. Reflection implies discovering, intellectually at first, the oneness behind the multiplicity of the world by engaging in intense inquiry into the nature of one's true Self. Chanting the hekau and divine singing *Hesi,* are also used here.

"Devote yourself to adore God's name."
—Ancient Egyptian Proverb

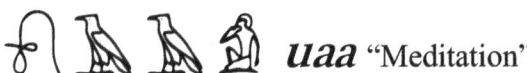 *uaa* "Meditation"

Meditation

3- Meditation in Wisdom Yoga is the process of reflection that leads to a state in which the mind is continuously introspective. It means expansion of consciousness culminating in revelation of and identification with the Absolute Self.

Note: It is important to note here that the same teaching which was practiced in ancient Egypt of **Listening** to, **Reflecting** upon, and **Meditating** upon the teachings is the same process used in Vedanta-Jnana Yoga (from India) of today.

EGYPTIAN TANTRIC YOGA

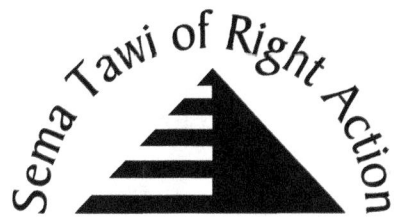

**GENERAL DISCIPLINE
In all Temples especially
The Temple of Heru and Edfu**

Scripture: Prt M Hru and special scriptures including the Berlin Papyrus and other papyri.

1- Learn Ethics and Law of Cause and Effect-Practice right action
(42 Precepts of Maat)
to purify gross impurities of the personality
Control Body, Speech, Thoughts

2- Practice cultivation of the higher virtues
(selfless-service)
to purify mind and intellect from subtle impurities

3- Devotion to the Divine
See maatian actions as offerings to the Divine

4- Meditation
See oneself as one with Maat, i.e. United with the cosmic order which is the Transcendental Supreme Self.

Plate: The Offering of Maat-Symbolizing the Ultimate act of Righteousness (Temple of Seti I)

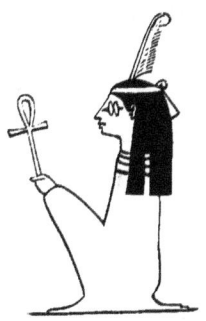
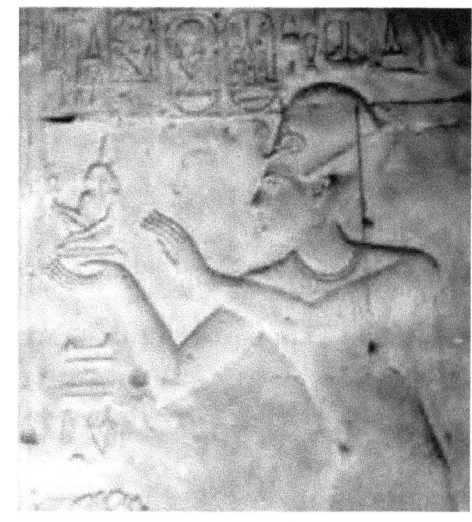

Mystical Philosophy of Universal Consciousness

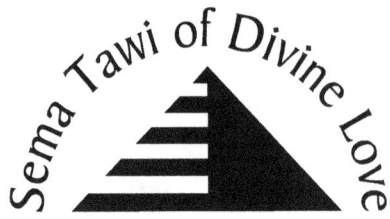

GENERAL DISCIPLINE
In all Temples

Scripture: Prt M Hru and Temple Inscriptions.

<u>Discipline of Devotion</u>

1– Listening to the myth
- Get to know the Divinity
- Empathize
- Romantisize

2- Ritual about the myth
- Offerings to Divinity – propitiation
- act like divinity
- Chant the name of the Divinity
- Sing praises of the Divinity
- COMMUNE with the Divinity

3– Mysticism
- Melting of the heart
- Dissolve into Divinity

IDENTIFY-with the Divinity

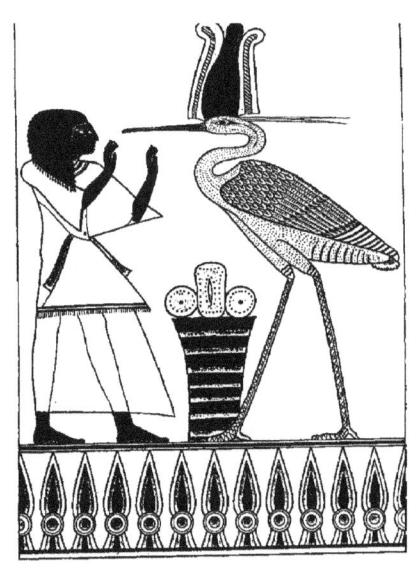

In the Kamitan teaching of Devotional love:

God is termed *Merri,* "Beloved One"

Love and Be Loved
"That person is beloved by the Lord." PMH, Ch 4

Offering Oneself to God-Surrender to God- Become One with God

Figure 2: The Dua Pose- Upraised arms with palms facing out towards the Divine Image

EGYPTIAN TANTRIC YOGA

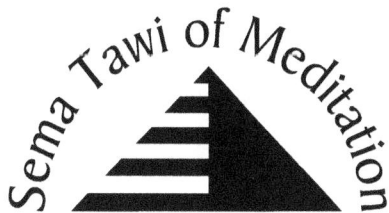

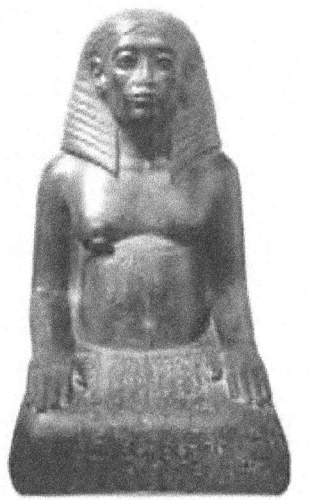

Posture-Sitting With Hands on Thighs

It is well known and commonly accepted that meditation has been practiced in India from ancient times. Therefore, there is no need to site specific references to support that contention. Here we will concentrate on the evidence supporting the existence of the philosophy of meditation in Ancient Egypt.

The Paths of Meditation Practiced in Ancient Egypt

System of Meditation: **Glorious Light System**
Location where it was practiced in ancient times: **Temple of Seti I, City of Waset (Thebes)** [9]

System of Meditation: **Wisdom System**
Location where it was practiced in ancient times: **Temple of Aset – Philae Island, Aswan**

System of Meditation: **Serpent Power System**
Location where it was practiced in ancient times: **Temple of Asar- City of Abdu**

System of Meditation: **Devotional Meditation**
Location where it was practiced in ancient times: **IN ALL TEMPLES- GENERAL DISCIPLINE**

Basic Instructions for the Glorious Light Meditation System- Given in the Tomb of Seti I. (1350 B.C.E.)

Formal meditation in Yoga consists of four basic elements: Posture, Sound (chant-words of power), Visualization, Rhythmic Breathing (calm, steady breath). The instructions, translated from the original hieroglyphic text contain the basic elements for formal meditation.

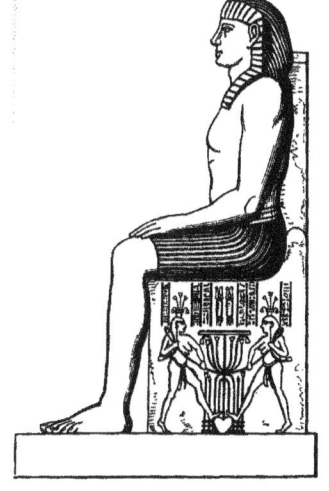

---

[9] For More details see the book *The Glorious Light Meditation System of Ancient Egypt* by Dr. Muata Ashby.

Mystical Philosophy of Universal Consciousness

(1)-Posture and Focus of Attention

iuf iri-f ahau maq b-phr nty   hau iu
body do   make stand, within the Sundisk (circle of Ra)

This means that the aspirant should remain established as if in the center of a circle with a dot in the middle.

(2)- Words of power-chant[10]

Nuk Hekau (I am the word* itself)
Nuk Ra Akhu (I am Ra's Glorious Shinning** Spirit)
Nuk Ba Ra (I am the soul of Ra)
Nuk Hekau (I am the God who creates*** through sound)

(3)- Visualization

Iuf mi Ra heru mestu-f n-shry chet
"My body is like Ra's on the day of his birth

This teaching is what in Indian Vedanta Philosophy is referred to as Ahamgraha Upashama – or visualizing and meditating upon oneself as being one with God. This teaching is the main focus of the Prt m Hru (Book of Enlightenment) text of Ancient Egypt. It is considered as the highest form of meditation practice amongst Indian mystics.[11]

---

[10] The term "Words of Power" relates to chants and or recitations given for meditation practice. They were used in a similar way to the Hindu "Mantras."
[11] Statement made by Swami Jyotirmayananda in class with his disciples.

EGYPTIAN TANTRIC YOGA

Plate: Basic Instructions for the Glorious Light Meditation System- Given in the Tomb of Seti I. (c. 1350 B.C.E.)

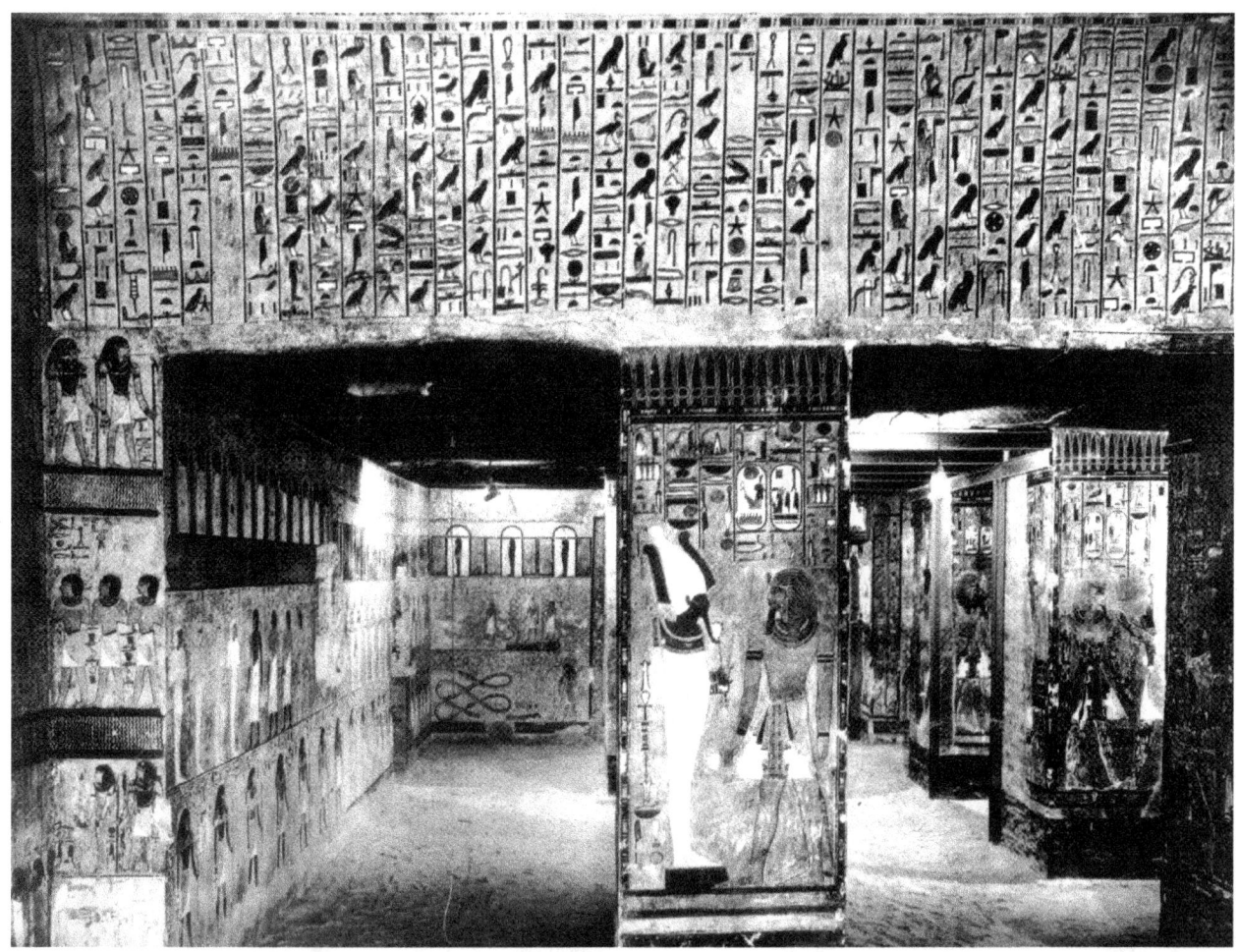

As we have seen, the practice of meditation in Ancient Egypt and its instruction to the masses and not just to the priests and priestesses, can be traced to at least 800 years earlier. If the instructions given by sage Seti I and those given by sage Patanjali are compared, many similarities appear.

Mystical Philosophy of Universal Consciousness

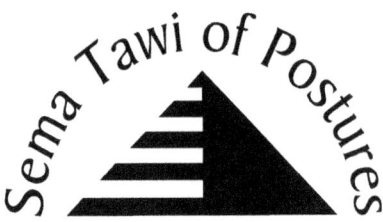

The Yogic Postures in Ancient Egypt

Since their introduction to the West, the exercise system of India known as "Hatha Yoga" has gained much popularity. The disciplines related to the yogic postures and movements were developed in India around the 10th century A.C.E. by a sage named Goraksha.[12] Up to this time, the main practice was simply to adopt the cross-legged meditation posture known as the lotus for the purpose of practicing meditation. The most popular manual on Hatha Yoga is the *Hatha Yoga-Pradipika ("Light on the Forceful Yoga)*. It was authored by Svatmarama Yogin in mid. 14th century A.C.E.[13]

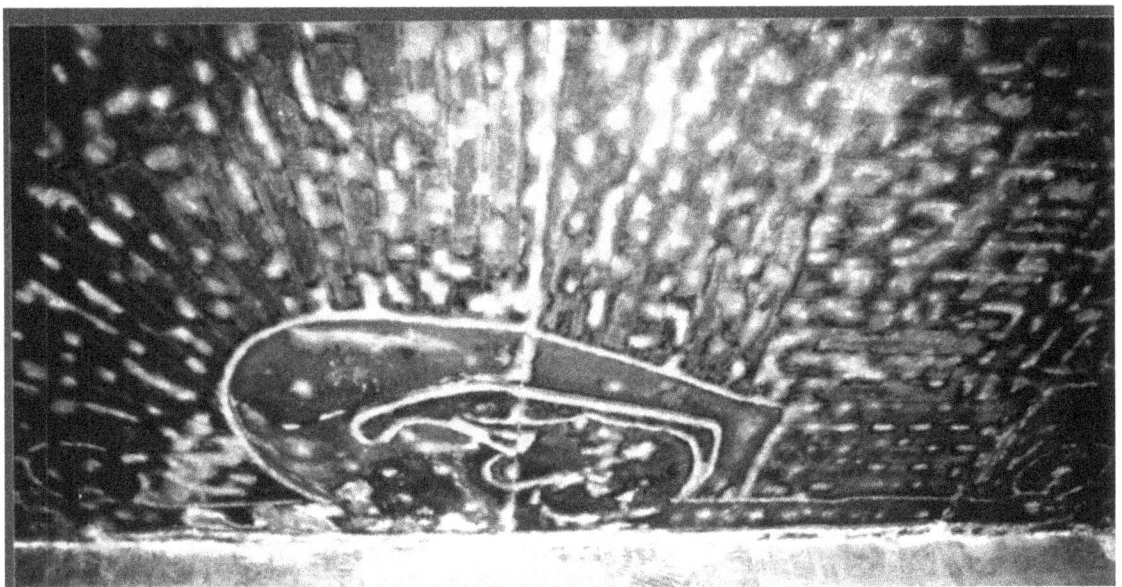

Plate: Above- The god Geb in the plough posture engraved on the ceiling of the antechamber to the Asarian Resurrection room of the Temple of Hetheru in Egypt. (photo taken by Ashby). Below: Illustration of the posture engraved on the ceiling.

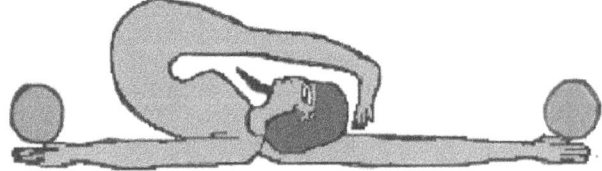

---

[12] Yoga Journal, {The New Yoga} January/February 2000
[13] **Hatha-Yoga-Pradipika,** *The Shambhala Encyclopedia of Yoga* by Georg Feuerstein, Ph. D.

EGYPTIAN TANTRIC YOGA

Prior to the emergence of the discipline of the physical movements in India just before 1000 A.C.E.,[14] a series of virtually identical postures to those which were practiced in India can be found in various Ancient Egyptian papyruses and inscribed on the walls and ceilings of the temples. The Ancient Egyptian practice can be dated from 10,000 B.C.E to 300 B.C.E and earlier. Examples: Temple of Hetheru (800-300 B.C.E.), Temple of Heru (800-300 B.C.E.), Tomb of Queen Nefertari (reigned 1,279-1,212 B.C.E.), and various other temples and papyruses from the New Kingdom Era (c. 1,580 B.C.E). In Ancient Egypt the practice of the postures, called *Tjef Sema Paut Neteru* which means "Movements to promote union with the gods and goddesses" or simply *Sema Paut* (Union with the gods and goddesses), were part of the ritual aspect of the spiritual myth, which when practiced, served to harmonize the energies and promote the physical health of the body and direct the mind in a meditative capacity to discover and cultivate divine consciousness. These disciplines are part of a larger process called Sema or *Smai Tawi* (Egyptian Yoga). By acting and moving like the gods and goddesses one can essentially discover their character, energy and divine agency within one's consciousness, and thereby also become one of their retinue, that is, one with the Divine Self. In modern times, most practitioners of Indian Hatha Yoga see it primarily as a means to attain physical health only. However, even the practice in India had an origin in myth and a mythic component which is today largely ignored by modern practitioners.

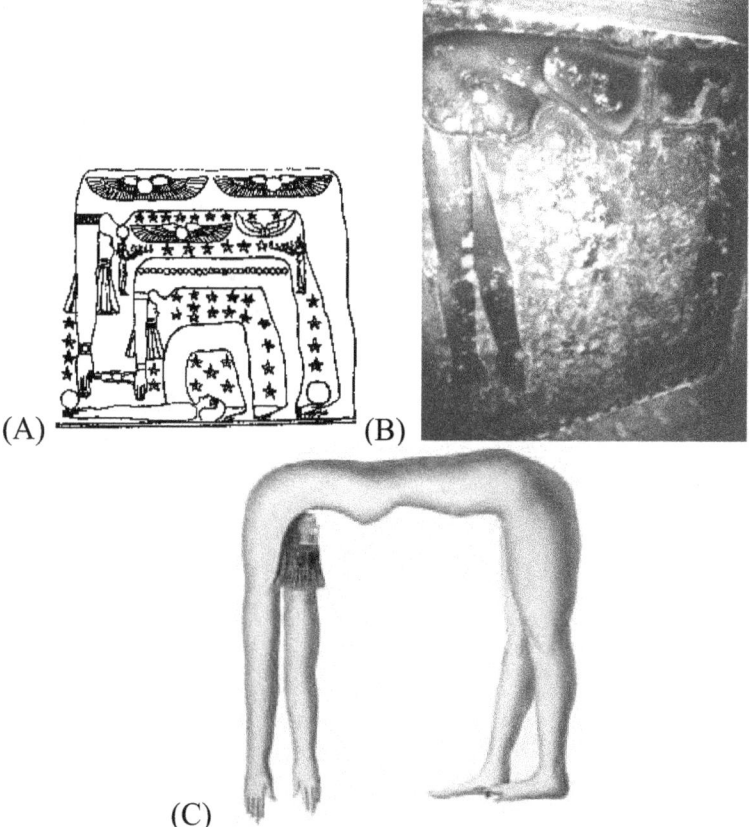

Figure: Above left: The Kamitan goddess Nut and god Geb and the higher planes of existence. Above center and right: The goddess Nut performs the forward bend posture.

---

[14] *The Shambhala Encyclopedia of Yoga* by Georg Feuerstein, Ph. D.

Mystical Philosophy of Universal Consciousness

The figure above (left) depicts another conceptualization of the Netherworld, which is at the same time the body of Nut in a forward bend yoga exercise posture. The innermost goddess symbolizes the lower heaven where the moon traverses, the physical realm. The middle one symbolizes the course of the sun in its Astral journey. This shows a differentiation between the physical heavens and the Astral plane, as well as time and physical space and Astral time and space, i.e., the concept of different dimensions and levels of consciousness. The outermost symbolizes the causal plane.

Plate: Below- The Egyptian Gods and Goddesses act out the Creation through their movements: Forward bend -Nut, Spinal twist -Geb, Journey of Ra – Ra in his boat, and the squatting and standing motions of Nun and Shu.

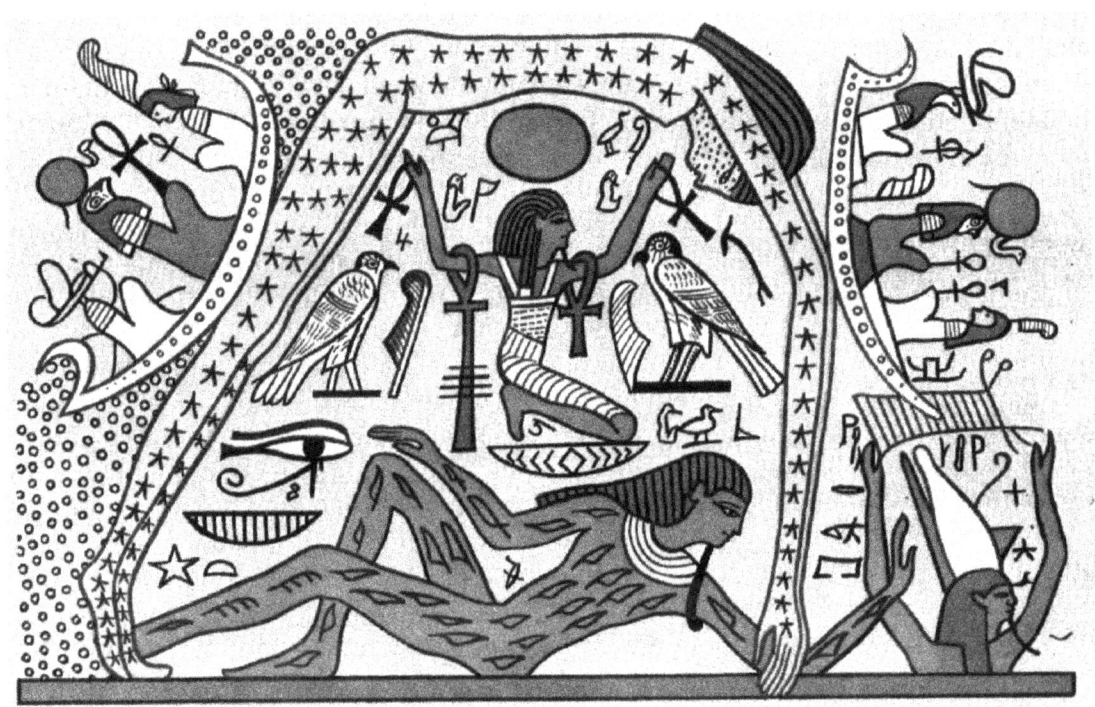

EGYPTIAN TANTRIC YOGA

The varied postures found in the Kamitan papyruses and temple inscriptions.

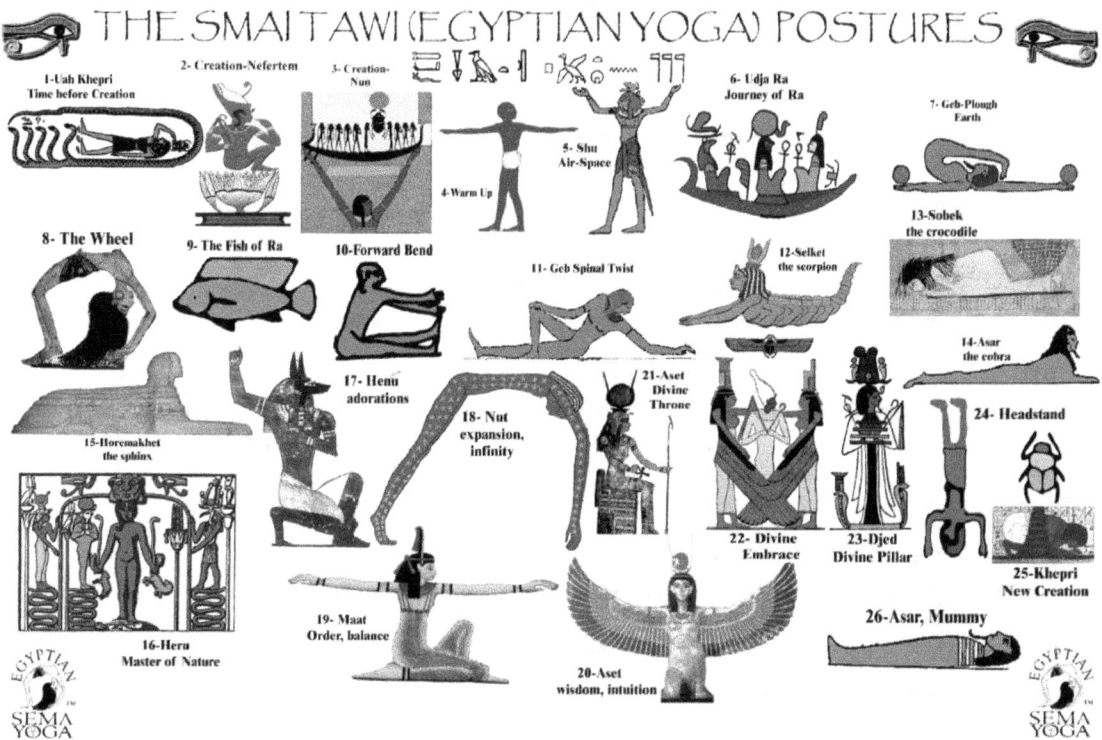

The practice of the postures is shown in the sequence below.

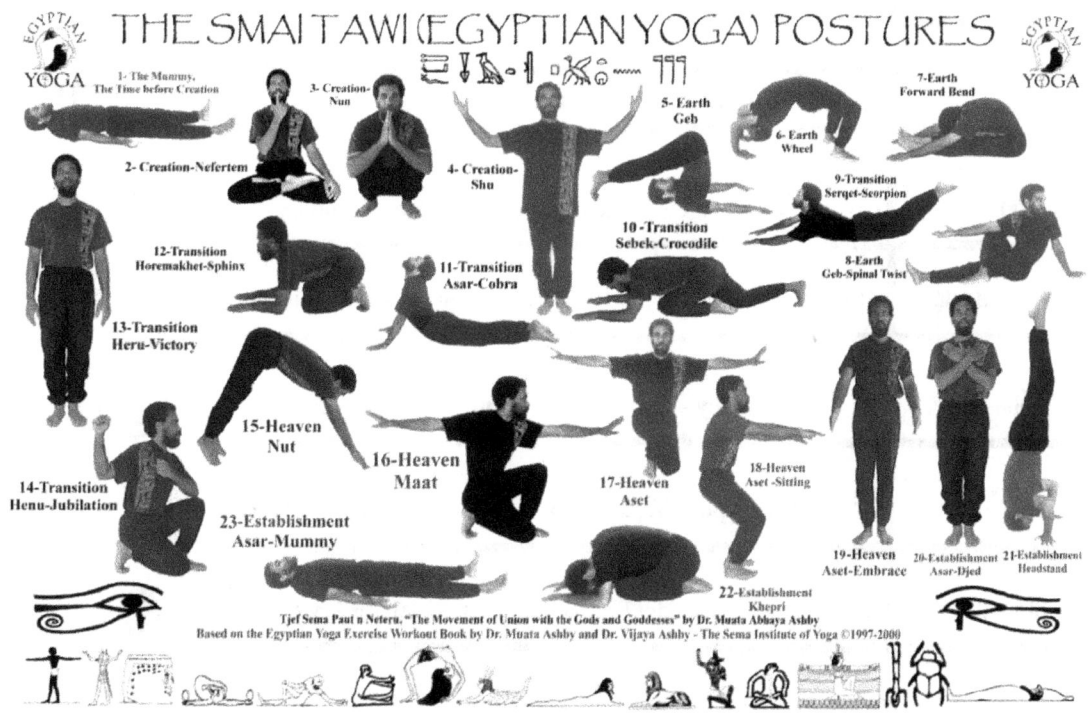

Mystical Philosophy of Universal Consciousness

20th Century A.C.E.
1. **Ananda Yoga** (Swami Kriyananda)
2. **Anusara Yoga** (John Friend)
3. **Ashtanga Yoga** (K. Pattabhi)
4. **Ashtanga Yoga** (Pattabhi Jois)
5. **Bikram Yoga** (Bikram Choudhury)
6. **Integral Yoga** (Swami Satchidananda b.
7. **Iyengar Yoga** (B.K.S. Iyengar)
8. **Kripalu Yoga** (Amrit Desai)
9. **Kundalini Yoga** (Yogi Bhajan)
10. **Sivananda Yoga** (Swami Vishnu-devananda)
11. **Svaroopa Yoga** (Rama Berch)

Women first admitted to Hatha Yoga practice

1893 A.C.E.	World Parliament of Religions – Vedanta Introduced to the West
1750 A.C.E.	Shiva Samhita – Hatha Yoga text – melds Vedanta with Hatha
1539 A.C.E.	Birth of Sikhism
1350 A.C.E.	Hatha Yoga Pradipika text – India
1000 A.C.E.	Goraksha – Siddha Yogis First Indian Hatha Yoga Practice
600 A.C.E.	Birth of Islam
Year 0	Birth of Jesus – Christianity
300 B.C.E.	Arat, Geb, Nut Egyptian Yoga Postures – Late Period
1,680 B.C.E.	Geb, Nut, Ra, Asar, Aset, Sobek Egyptian Yoga Postures – New Kingdom
2,000 B.C.E.	Indus Valley – Kundalini – Serpent Power-Lotus Pose
3,600 B.C.E.	Nefertem Egyptian Yoga Posture – Old-Middle Kingdom Period
10,000 B.C.E.	Serpent Power-Horemakhet Egyptian Yoga Posture – Ancient Egyptian

Part 3: The Philosophy of Tantra in World Spirituality

Sexual Energy and The Evolution of Human Consciousness

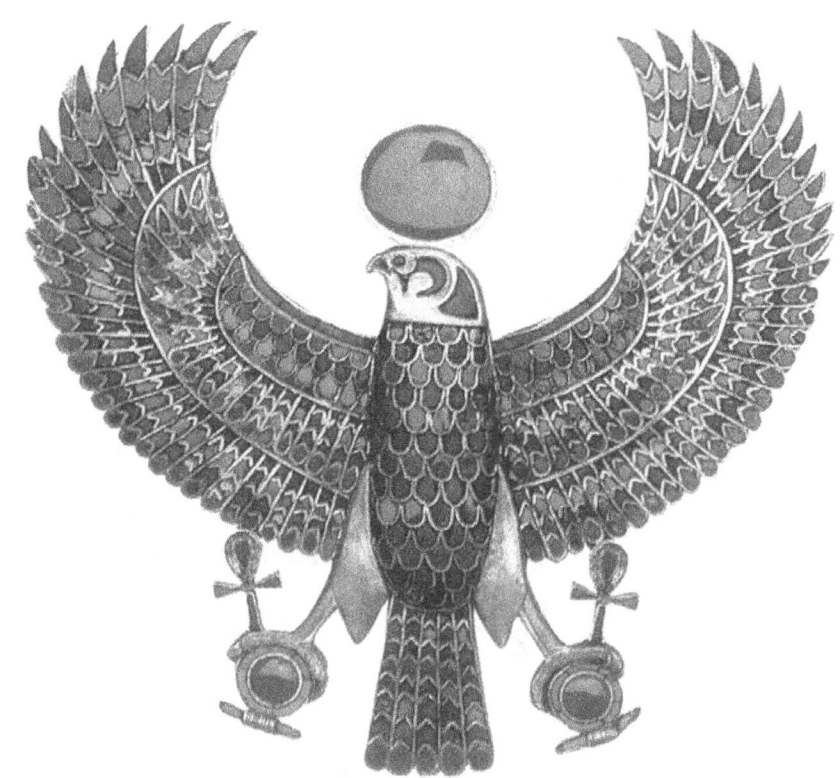

Mystical Philosophy of Universal Consciousness

Tantrism in Ancient Egypt and India

Tantra Yoga is purported to be the oldest system of Yoga. Tantra Yoga is a system of Yoga which seeks to promote the re-union between the individual and the Absolute Reality, through the worship of nature and ultimately the Cosmos as an expression of the Absolute. Since nature is an expression of GOD, it gives clues as to the underlying reality that sustains it and the way to achieve wisdom, i.e. transcendence of it. The most obvious and important teaching that nature holds is the idea that creation is made up of pairs of opposites: Up-down, here-there, you-me, us-them, hot-cold, male-female, Ying-Yang, etc. The interaction of these two complementary opposites we call life and movement.

Insight (wisdom) into the true nature of reality gives us a clue as to the way to realize the oneness of creation within ourselves. Tantra is a recognition of the male and female nature of Creation as a reflection of the male and female nature of the Divine which were brought together to create the universe. By re-uniting the male and female principles in our own bodies and minds, we may reach the oneness that underlies our apparent manifestation as a man or woman. Thus, the term Tantra means to create a bridge between the opposites and in so doing, the opposites dissolve, leaving unitary and transcendental consciousness. The union of the male and female principles may be effected by two individuals who worship GOD through GOD's manifestation in each other or by an individual who seeks union with GOD through uniting with his or her female or male spiritual principles, respectively, within themselves. All men and women have both female and male principles within themselves.

In the Egyptian philosophical system, all Neteru or God principles emanate from the one GOD. When these principles are created, they are depicted as having a **_male and female_** principle. All objects and life forms appear in creation as either male or female, but underlying this apparent duality, there is a unity which is rooted in the pure consciousness of oneness, the consciousness of the Transcendental Divine, which underlies and supports all things. To realize this oneness consciously deep inside is the supreme goal.

In Tantrism, sexual symbolism is used frequently because these are the most powerful images denoting the opposites of Creation and the urge to unify and become whole, for sexuality is the urge for unity and self-discovery, albeit limited to physical intercourse by most people. If this force is understood, harnessed and sublimated it will lead to unity of the highest order that is unity with the Divine Self.

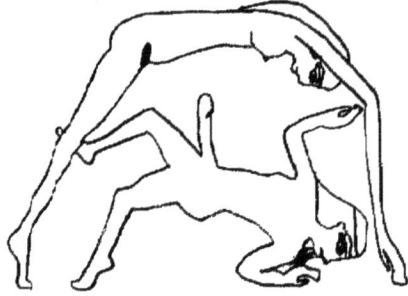

Above- The Kamitan God Geb and the Kamitan Goddess Nut separate after the sexual union that gave birth to the gods and goddesses and Creation. Figure 3: Below: Three depictions of the god Asar in tantric union with Aset.

EGYPTIAN TANTRIC YOGA

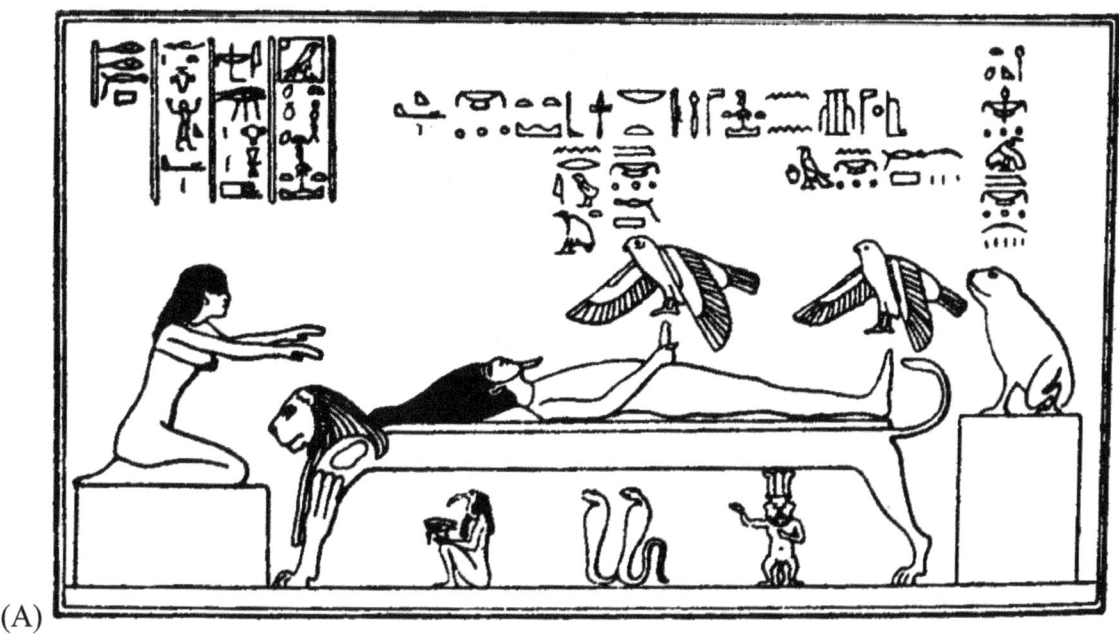

(A)

Above-(A) Reliefs from Ancient Egyptian Temples of the virgin birth of Heru (Horus) - The resurrection of Asar (Asar) - Higher Self, Heru consciousness). Aset in the winged form hovers over the reconstructed penis of the dead Asar.

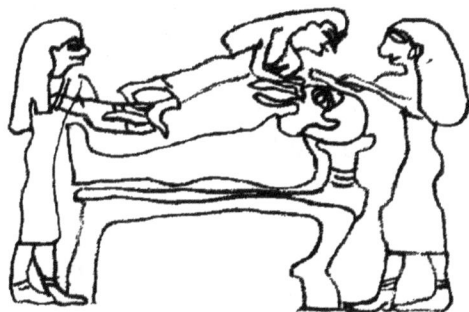

Drawing found in an Ancient Egyptian Building of The Conception of Heru[15]-*From a Stele at the British Museum 1372. 13th Dyn.*

Above: Aset (representing the physical body-creation) and the dead body of Asar (representing the spirit, that essence which vivifies matter) are shown in symbolic immaculate union (compare to the "Kali Position" on the following page) begetting Heru, symbolizing to the immaculate conception which takes place at the birth of the spiritual life in every human: the birth of the soul (Ba) in a human is the birth of Horus.

---

[15] *Sexual Life in Ancient Egypt* by Lise Manniche

Mystical Philosophy of Universal Consciousness

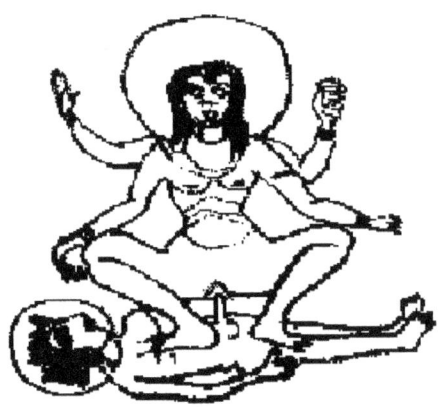

Above- the god Shiva and his consort Shakti

The "Kali position" (above) features **Shiva and Shakti (Kundalini-Prakriti)** in divine union (India). As with Aset and Asar of Egypt, Shiva is the passive, male aspect who "gives" the life essence (Spirit) and creative impetus and Shakti is energy, creation, the active aspect of the Divine. Thus Creation is akin to the idea of the Divine making love with him/herself. Shiva and Shakti are the true essence of the human being, composed of spirit and matter (body). In the active aspect, the female is in the "active" position while the male is in the "passive" position. Notice in the pictures above and below that the females are in the top position and the males are on the bottom. In Kamitan philosophy, the god Geb is the earth and the goddess Nut is the sky. Just as the earth is sedentary and the sky is dynamic, so too are the divinities depicted in this way in Southern (African) and Eastern (India) iconography. Notice that the female divinities are always on the top position. This is classic in Eastern and Kamitan mysticism. It is a recognition that the spirit (male aspect) is sedentary while matter, the female aspect, is in perpetual motion, and the two complement and complete each other.

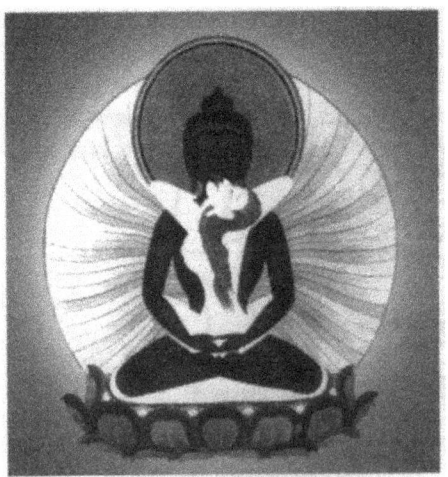

Above- Buddha and his consort. Tibetan Buddhist representation of The Dharmakaya, the cosmic father-mother, expressing the idea of the Supreme Being as a union of both male and female principals.

EGYPTIAN TANTRIC YOGA

Tantric philosophy makes use of sexual imagery to convey the teaching of the principle of the opposites in creation as well as the principle of all encompassing divinity. Sexuality encompasses the entire creation and any symbol that denotes all-encompassing divinity is a tantric symbol. The phallic symbols as well as the winged disk and the multi-armed divinity all symbolize all-encompassing divinity.

Below left- The Triune ithyphallic form of Asar.[16]

Below right- the Trilinga (Triune ithyphallic form) of Shiva.[17]

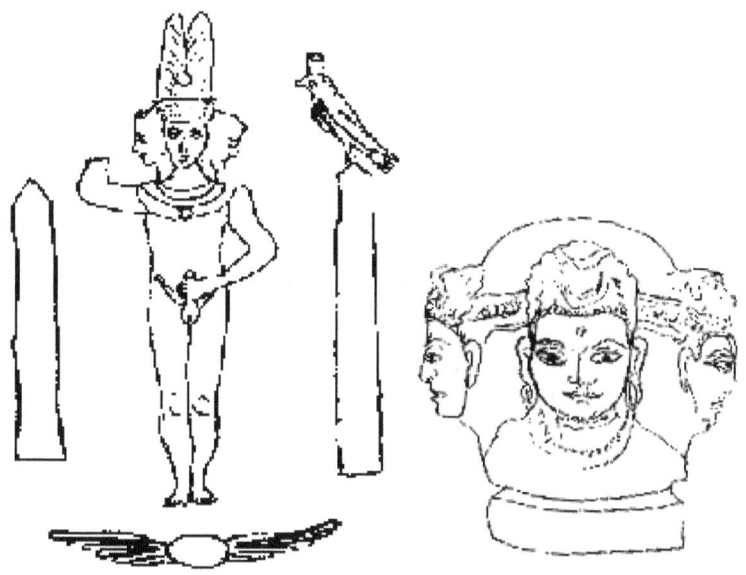

The Winged Sundisk of Heru – Kamitan.

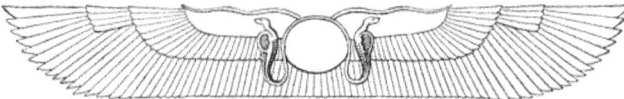

Below - the multi-armed (all-pervasive) dancing Shiva-whose dance sustains the Creation.

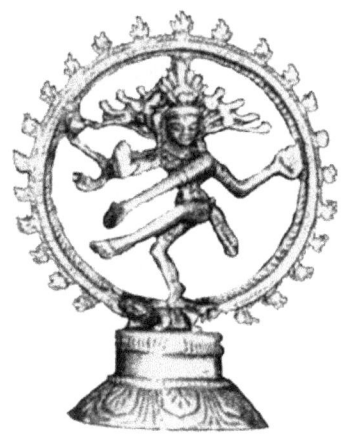

---

[16] For more details see the book *Egyptian Yoga Volume 1*
[17] For more details see the book *Egyptian Yoga Volume 1*

Mystical Philosophy of Universal Consciousness

Below- left Ashokan[18] pillar with lion capital-Kamitan pillar with lion capitals. Center: Ancient Egyptian pillar with lion capitals. Far right: the Ethiopian divinity Apedemak, displaying the same leonine trinity concept and the multi-armed motif.

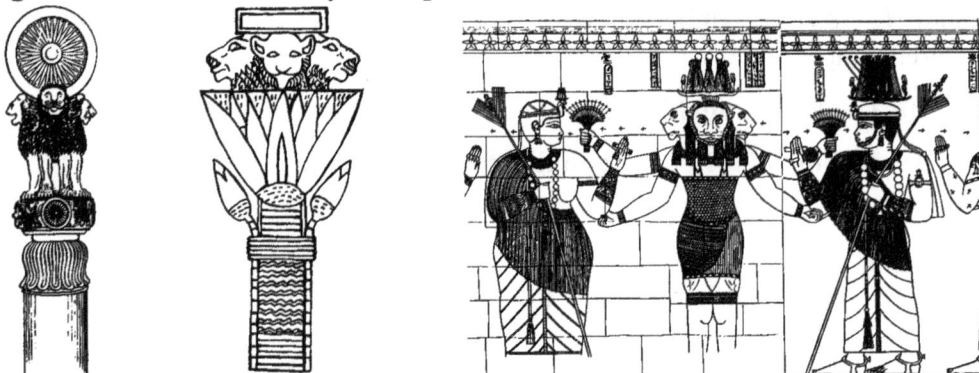

The trinity symbolically relates the nature of the Divine, who is the source and sustenance of the three worlds (physical, astral and causal), the three states of consciousness (conscious, subconscious and unconscious), the three modes of nature (dull, agitated and lucid), the three aspects of human experience (seer, seen and sight), as well as the three stages of initiation (ignorance, aspiration and enlightenment). This triad idea is common to Neterianism, Hinduism and Christianity.

The idea of the multi-armed divinity is common in Indian Iconography. However, the depiction above from Ethiopia spiritual iconography shows that it was present in Africa as well.

---

[18] Constructed in the period of the Indian King Asoka (Ashoka) who adopted Buddhism.

EGYPTIAN TANTRIC YOGA
INTRODUCTION TO TANTRIC PHILOSOPHY

Sexual Energy and Yoga

Tantric Yoga is not "Sex Yoga"

Sexual energy is the most potent force in human consciousness. Sexual energy is the mover and motivator which causes each human being to search for objects or relationships in the world which will satisfy the urge of the soul. Therefore, the understanding of sexual energy and the method for its control and sublimation must form an integral part of every spiritual discipline.

No spiritual progress is possible if the sexual energies are not controlled. If out of control, the subject moves in the world seeking relationships and other situations in which to express the sexual feeling. Sometimes the feeling will be confused with love. At other times the feeling will be confused with fulfillment and happiness. This fulfillment is illusory, however, because it is fleeting and it breeds a need for more activity in the search for more fulfillment in much the same way an addict needs to find more activities which will bring back the "feeling". This is the predicament of all human beings who are not in control of the sexual energy which is operating in their body.

This energy is a Divine force whose purpose is to drive the soul toward situations which will provide the possibility for evolution. These sexual impulses cannot always be fulfilled through an expression of sexual activity with another human being. Therefore, feelings of frustration and disappointment arise. If these feelings of frustration evolve, they do not find expression downward through the sexual organs. Instead, they move up through the psycho-spiritual energy centers and the subtle spiritual body. When this occurs, human consciousness moves with the energy and discovers higher forms of fulfillment which are more internal rather than external. This is known as spiritual evolution.

Myths and mystical philosophies have expressed the teachings of yoga through sexual motifs and myths from the earliest times. One of the reasons is that sexual energy is an integral part of human existence that needs to be treated openly and with understanding. Another reason is that sexual motifs and symbols are powerful ways to convey the basic teachings of yoga related to the singularity of the Supreme Being and the duality or multiplicity of the relative world of time and space.

In ancient Egyptian mythology, God in the primordial form before creation, is presented as an androgynous being (composed of male and female halves). Then after the creation, Divinity was presented as a separation of that original essence into the male and female principle and all of the other qualities of nature. However, the understanding is always present that even though the world appears to be filled with opposites (up-down, good-bad, here-there, male-female, etc.), in reality, all objects within creation are composed of the same underlying essence. Therefore, this apparent multiplicity is some kind of an illusion and the primeval ocean which existed before the multiplicity, in reality, never ceased to exist. This world of apparent dualities is, in reality, the expression of the one singular Supreme Being. This is the profound declaration presented by Tantric Yoga.

Mystical Philosophy of Universal Consciousness

But how is this all possible? Also, what are the implications for human existence? In order to answer these questions we will begin by tracing the development of Tantrism in Indian philosophy and then move back in time to discover the practice of Tantrism in Ancient Egypt.

TANTRA YOGA

Tantrism is a philosophy and culture expounded in the **Hieroglyphic** writings of ancient Egypt and in the Indian scriptures called **Tantras.** *Tantra* means *to extend.* Extension here refers to extending one's understanding from the limited ego self, to encompass the entire creation.

Having originated in pre-dynastic times, Tantrism is found in the earliest hieroglyphic texts (c.5,000 B.C.E.) and in all phases of Ancient Egyptian religion thereafter. Tantrism existed in India in pre-Vedic times (before 1,500 B.C.E.) and it developed as a distinct tradition within Hinduism, Buddhism and Jainism.

According to Indian tantric philosophy the cosmos is seen as the **Shakti** of feminine principle of the Divine Self **Shiva**. Unlike other forms of philosophy which advocate masculine primacy, asceticism, world denial and self-denial, Tantrism affirms the human body and nature itself as a vehicle of liberation. Tantrism also affirms the female aspect of creation equally with the male.

Tantra means *"loom"* which is derived from the root *"tan"* which means *"to extend or expand"*. Tantra in India is the name of the practices which were given literary form in the first millennium of the common era but which had existed since the Indus Valley times of Indian civilization. While Tantrism includes a wide variety of yogic techniques for self-transformation, it has traditionally been equated by many people with sexuality. Perhaps because there have been many who under the pretext of practicing Tantra have used the art to engage in orgiastic affairs. The original idea of Tantrism as we will see, is to promote transcendence in consciousness, to *"extend"* it from it's constricted, confined state (the ordinary mortal human being) to encompass all of creation (cosmic consciousness). In effect to extend to infinity. For this purpose, many yogic techniques have been devised. Having realized that the whole world is a divine stage, the Tantric Sages realized that any activity in human experience may be used for transcendence if they are practiced with the correct understanding and guidance. Tantrism may be practiced through seeking union with God as the male element, known in India as *Shaivism* or seeking union with God as the female element, known in India as *Shaktism* or as a combination of the two (Androgynous and with or without name or form -(*Saguna-Nirguna, Ardhanari-Ishwara*). Of the various Tantric disciplines, two of the most powerful have been found to be the development of the dormant Life Force (Serpent Power-Kundalini Yoga) and the sublimation of sexual energy (Brahmacharya). Another notable feature of Tantrism is that in contrast to other forms of Yoga, it affirms the experience aspect of life rather than advocating self-mortification or deprivation. Tantrism is thought to be a form of Yoga specially designed for the current age of mankind because it makes use of the physical forces which characterize the current cycle of cosmic time which predominated in gross forms of energy rather than the more subtle forms of past ages. During their height around 460 A.C.E., the Shakta and Tantra cults became important in India. They emphasized mystical speculation on divine fertility and energy. These doctrines were regarded as unorthodox by other religious teachers, but Tantrism had a strong secret

EGYPTIAN TANTRIC YOGA

following as well as those who followed the teachings openly. Tantrism also became an important trend in the Buddhist tradition, especially in Tibet.

Three main paths of Tantrism include:

<table>
<tr><td>1</td><td>2</td><td>3</td></tr>
<tr><td colspan="3">Dakshina-marga - Vama-marga - Kula-marga</td></tr>
<tr><td>(right-hand path)</td><td>(left-hand path)</td><td>(Kundalini path)</td></tr>
</table>

The first path is the conservative mainline of Tantrism including mandala meditations and worship of the Divine in the form of the Mother Goddess. The second includes traditionally forbidden elements, especially sexual intercourse (with detachment and non-ejaculation). The third is practiced by the Kula sect and is equivalent to Kundalini Yoga (Serpent Power). The following features commonly associated with Hinduism, Yoga and Vajrayana Buddhism originated in the Tantric disciplines:

Mantras (words of power-hekau), mudras (seals-manipulation of psychic energy), mandalas (circular designs for meditation), Yantras (special designs for meditation), and Chakra/nadi physiology (subtle energy channels).

KUNDALINI YOGA

Kundalini yoga is the Tantric discipline involving the deliberate arousal of Kundalini energy in order to effect a union of individual consciousness with the universal. The first stage of Kundalini yoga is known as **Bhuta-shudhi** or purification of the elements. The elements are gradually dissolved and a **Divia-deha** (quasi-divine body) is formed. The body's energy (**Kundalini-Shakti**) and consciousness (**Buddhi**) becomes one with the energy and consciousness of God (**Shiva**).

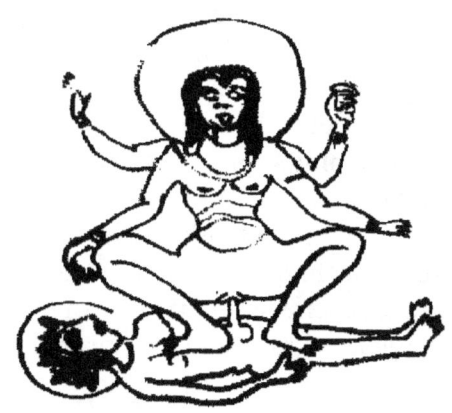

Above: *The "Kali position":* **Shiva and Shakti (Kundalini-Prakriti)** *in divine union (India). As with Asar and Aset of Egypt,*

Mystical Philosophy of Universal Consciousness

Shiva is the passive aspect who "gives" the life essence (spirit) and creative impetus and Shakti is energy, creation, the active aspect of GOD. Thus Creation is akin to the idea of GOD making love with him/herself. Shiva and Shakti are the true essence of the human being, composed of spirit and matter (body). In the active aspect, the female is in the "active" position while the male is in the "passive" position.

LAYA YOGA

Laya yoga is a form of Tantric discipline based on the dissolution of the individual consciousness into the divine through special meditations.

The Tantric Origins of Christian Gnosticism in Ancient Egypt and Africa

Hexapla is an Old Testament edition compiled in six columns by the Alexandrian Philosopher Origen (c. 185- c. 254) about 231-245. Each page of the work has six versions of text: Greek translation of the Hebrew, Hebrew, and the four Greek versions--Symmachus, Aquila, Theodotion, and Septuagint. Origen introduced a concept through an allegorical interpretation of the *Song of Songs* book of the Old Testament. This interpretation gave impetus to the love-mysticism which talks about a "marriage" between Christ or God and the "soul bride" (soul of the individual human being). The love mystics speak of *kisses* and secret embraces between the bridegroom (God) and the soul bride. Herein lies the flowering of Tantrism, which is evident in even earlier Christian Gnosticism in the Gospel of Phillip and other Christian Gospels which originated in Alexandria (Egypt). Here again, Egypt figures prominently in Tantrism and the development of Gnostic Christianity.

Tantrism, especially in the doctrines concerning the wisdom of sexuality and the Life Force energy existed much earlier in Africa. In the book *Egyptian Yoga: The Philosophy of Enlightenment*, the focus was on defining yoga and tracing its roots in Africa and its development in India. In this volume, we will go deeper into the Yogic teachings of Egypt, focusing on a profound study of the esoteric aspects of Tantric yoga. From here, the goal will be to explore the teachings the Tantric forms of thought and leading into two specific forms of Tantrism: Yoga of Sexual energy sublimation and Yoga of Life Force energy development, commonly known as Kundalini Yoga. Since both Indian and Gnostic mystical philosophies are directly linked to Egyptian religion, philosophy and Yoga, we will be using both Gnostic (Coptic) Christian and Sanskrit terminology along with the Egyptian through the course of this work. This will help those who are familiar with other mystical philosophies and those who have a working knowledge of world religions to better comprehend the Ancient Egyptian teachings in the context of the individual's own experience. It is our hope that the Egyptian teachings will shed light on other Yogas and Religions so as to add to their understanding and practice.

One of the most important Tantric-Buddhist doctrines is *"Samsara equals Nirvana"*. When viewed from the standpoint of the individual ego, one's personality looks on the world as separate, filled with separate objects and people from oneself. From the standpoint of the enlightened mind, however, all things including one's ego are "known" to be rooted in the same reality (absolute reality) and therefore, not separate and distinct.

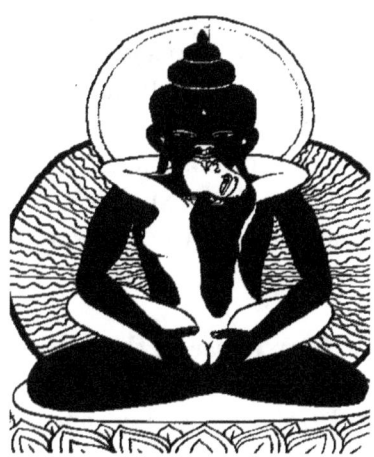

Above: Tibetan Buddhist representation of The Dharmakaya, the cosmic father-mother. expressing the idea of the Supreme Being as a union of both male and female principals.

When Jesus states *"The Kingdom of the Father is spread upon the earth and men do not see it!"*, he is expressing the Tantric idea that the Kingdom (Heaven) is equal to the world we perceive. The difference is in the perception as either unified and holistic where one sees oneself as one with all things or dualistic and separate, where one sees oneself as a separate individual among many individuals in a world of countless objects. Once we are able to transcend our mistaken belief that our ego exists as an entity separate from creation, we are able to realize that the phenomenal world and God are one and the same: Creation and the Kingdom of Heaven are one and the same.

If we understand the Tantric idea of *extension* or *continuity* between heaven and earth, the logical assumption then is that sexuality may be used for achieving knowledge or realization of the absolute if it is carried out in a way which directs the mind toward understanding that all objects and activities are rooted in the absolute. The Tantric systems of Egypt and India developed the understanding of the subtle bodies beyond the physical and of the subtle energy channels (nadis) through which life force energy travels in all human beings. Tantrism also developed the technology or yoga technique (*Kundalini Yoga*) for purifying these channels in order to allow the mind to perceive the more subtle realms of existence and its own nature.

Due to conditioning, most people are inculcated with preconceived notions about what a spiritual preceptor (Hierophant, guru) should be like. Most would find the idea of a sexually active spiritual teacher objectionable. In modern day India, Tantrism is not viewed with favor by the government. Attempts are made to suppress rituals involving sexuality. It is therefore, to be expected that the idea of a sexually active Jesus would be abhorrent to modern day Christians since most evidence of Tantrism in Christianity was destroyed or suppressed by the orthodox church. After two thousand years of Christian doctrines espoused by the Roman Catholic view which tended to view sexuality as inherently evil, a negative view of sexuality and women in general among the priesthood and in society is to be expected. However, in the early, formative years of the Roman Catholic church, the attitudes were radically different among the varying Christian sects alongside the orthodox church.

In the early Christian period (0-300 A.C.E.) no such repudiation of sexuality or of the female gender occurred in certain Christian sects. In much the same way as other rituals and customs such as the birthday of Jesus and the Cross were adopted and assimilated into Christianity, spiritual rites involving sexuality were also assimilated. It was not until the orthodox catholic sect assumed control of the Roman Empire that sexuality, equal rights between the sexes, and the doctrine of self-salvation through acquiring wisdom, were systematically excluded from the Christian cannon.

The Gnostic Jesus and Mary: The New Phase of the Min and Hathor Tantrism

The tantric relationship between Horus and Hathor, and Asar and Aset, and Geb and Nut in ancient Egypt had a profound effect on the development of the Christian and Hindu mythologies. These principles became embodied in the characters of Jesus and Mary Magdalene in the Christian myth and Krishna and Radha - Shiva and Parvati/Kali of Hinduism.

Mary Magdalene was the most ardent female follower of Jesus. She has been canonized by the catholic church as a Saint. A saint is usually described as: A person considered holy and worthy of public veneration, especially one who has been canonized; or a very virtuous person. In the capacity as saint, Mary's position in Christianity has been only half expressed. In the Gnostic Christian texts her position emerges as a teacher to common people and to the Apostles as well. In the following text from the *Gospel of Philip,* we see a new interpretation of the New Testament relationship between Jesus and Mary Magdalene. It may be compared in one aspect to the relationship between *Krishna and Radha* of India or that of Horus and Hathor in Ancient Egypt in that it implies a complementation of each other. The Gnostic Christian text depicts a relationship between Jesus and Mary that is above and beyond the ordinary conjugal that experience. In this sense, the sum of the two is greater than the parts.

The fact that Mary Magdalene was the first to witness the resurrection of Jesus and to report this to the Apostles bestows her figure with great importance. It was not until Pope Gregory combined her image with a repentant prostitute who anointed Christ's feet that she came to be known as "Mary the repentant prostitute". While some believe that this combination was an intentional effort to denigrate the position of women in the Bible, it also gave impetus to the idea that even a person who committed the "worst sins" could be absolved and hope to achieve sainthood. Even today, long after the Vatican has issued edicts (1969) correcting the error, the image of Mary Magdalene as a reformed prostitute or her portrayals as a "sexual saint" persists among misguided individuals in the case of the former and among certain feminist groups in the case of the latter. While the openness of modern society is allowing the expression of many points of view with respect to the image of women, there are some significant psychological aspects to the continued development of the image of Mary Magdalene as a sexual saint. The continued use of an avowed erroneous interpretation may signify a need by some to validate their status as legitimate sexual outsiders while still identifying with the religious aspect within themselves. In exploring these aspects of themselves some women view themselves as holy temptresses, as a combination of the whore and the saint, while others may simply seek to honor the two impulses (sexual desire and spiritual devotion) within themselves in an effort to find a balance or resolution.

When we turn to the Gnostic gospels and other Gnostic Christian texts, a deeper mythology surrounding the relationship of Jesus and Mary Magdalene emerges. A very important similarity should be noted here. In one episode of the battle between Horus and Set, Set injured Horus. At this time Horus was in pain and spiritually disheartened since Set had gouged out his eyes which represented intuitional vision and divine awareness. In one version of the story it is Hathor, his consort, who comes to him first and heals his wounds enabling him to do battle against Set and to be victorious against Evil.

Part 4: The Tantra of Ancient Egypt

SUMMARY OF ANCIENT KEMETIC (ANCIENT EGYPTIAN) TANTRIC YOGA PHILOSOPHY

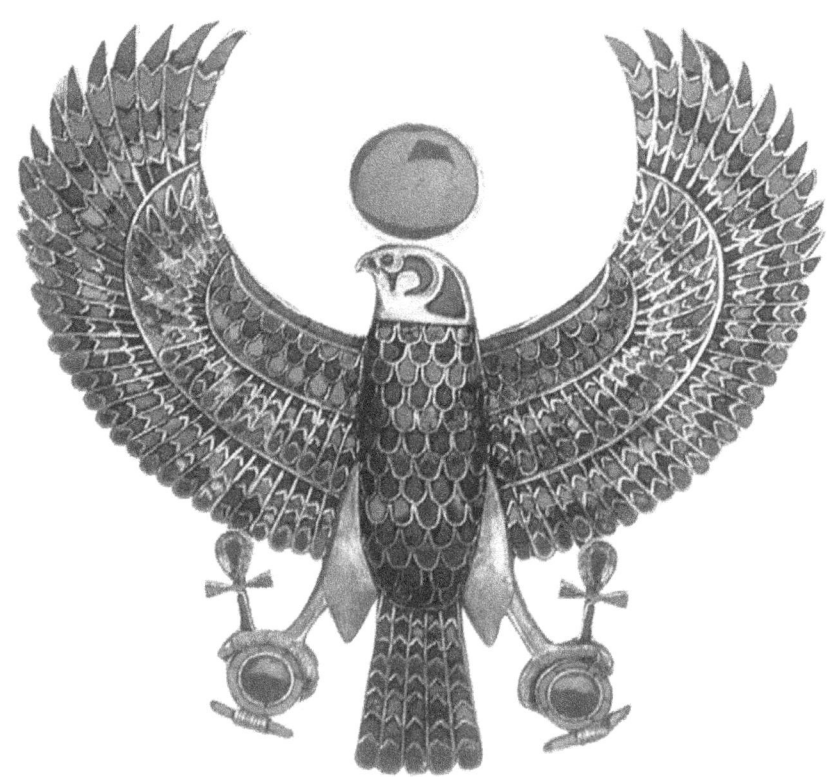

EGYPTIAN TANTRIC YOGA

The component disciplines of Ancient Egyptian Tantrism may be summarized as follows:

1. **Myth:** legendary-mythic story of the Divine
   a. creating the cosmos in the beginning
   b. creating the cosmos continually
      i. sexual symbolism as metaphor of creation act

2. **Philosophy:** based on myths- Tantric Union with the Divine

3. **Ritual:**
   a. reenactment of the acts of creation
   b. reenactment of the acts of reunion with the Divine

4. **Meditation:** in Egyptian Tantra Yoga the Meditative movement is composed of a culmination of myth, philosophy and ritual in the absorption into the higher, underlying nature of Self through in-depth understanding of the mythic teaching and experiencing it by assuming the characters being united in the teaching.
   a. **Visualization:** based on philosophy: seeing the underlying unity of Creation: Amun-Mut, Asar-Aset, Ptah, Hetheru-Heru, etc. who represent heaven and earth not separated but as aspects of one being.
   b. **Visualization:** based on philosophy: seeing the individual self as becoming one with the Universal Self underlying all.
   c. **Visualization:** sexual symbolism as metaphor of the reunion act of individual initiate and the Universal Self.

In order to comprehend the depth of tantric philosophy in ancient Egypt it will be necessary to have a basic understanding of the myth upon which ancient Egyptian spirituality is based. The most powerful myth in ancient Egypt was the Ausarian Resurrection. Therefore, a summary of the myth has been included as the introduction to this section.

Mystical Philosophy of Universal Consciousness
A COMPENDIUM OF THE AUSARIAN RESURRECTION MYTH

THE CREATION

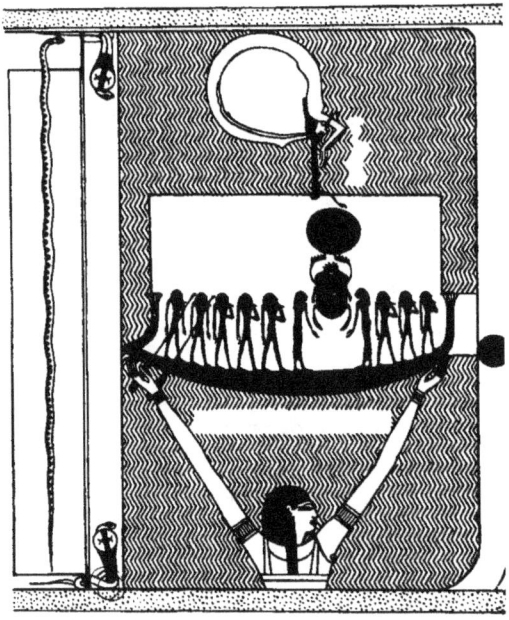

Above: The Ancient Egyptian Creation scene. The Supreme Being emerges out of the primeval waters which were previously without form, gender or name.

Ra (Supreme Being) establishes order in the form of gods and goddesses, the opposites of creation.

The process of creation is explained in the form of a cosmological system for better understanding. Cosmology is a branch of philosophy dealing with the origin, processes, and structure of the universe. Cosmogony is the astrophysical study of the creation and evolution of the universe. Both of these disciplines are inherent facets of Egyptian philosophy through the main religious systems or Companies of the Gods and Goddesses. A company of gods and goddesses is a group of deities which symbolize a particular cosmic force or principle which emanates from the all-encompassing Supreme Being, from which they have emerged. The Self or Supreme Being manifests creation through the properties and principles represented by the *Pautti* Company of gods and goddesses-cosmic laws of nature. The system or company of gods and goddesses of Anu is regarded as the oldest, and forms the basis of the Osirian Trinity. It is expressed in the diagram below.

EGYPTIAN TANTRIC YOGA

```
              Ra-Tem
                ⇩
              Hathor
              Djehuti
               Maat
                ⇩
          Shu ⇔ Tefnut
                ⇩
           Geb ⇔ Nut
              ⇙ ⇩ ⇘
Set — Nebethet   Asar ⇔ Aset   Asar ⇔ Nebethet
                   ⇩                ⇩
                 Horus            Anubis
```

The diagram above shows that *Psedjet* (Ennead), or the creative principles which are embodied in the primordial gods and goddesses of creation, emanated from the Supreme Being. Ra or Ra-Tem arose out of the *"Nu"*, the Primeval waters, the hidden essence, and began sailing the *"Boat of Millions of Years"* which included the company of gods and goddesses. On his boat emerged the "Neters" or cosmic principles of creation. The Neters of the Ennead are Ra-Atum, Shu, Tefnut, Geb, Nut, Asar, Aset, Set, and Nebethet. Hathor, Djehuti and Maat represent attributes of the Supreme Being as the very *stuff* or *substratum* which makes up creation. Shu, Tefnut, Geb, Nut, Asar, Aset, Set, and Nebethet represent the principles upon which creation manifests. Anpu (Anubis) is not part of the Ennead. He represents the feature of intellectual discrimination in the Osirian myth. "Sailing" signifies the beginning of motion in creation. Motion implies that events occur in the realm of time and space, thus, the phenomenal universe comes into existence as a mass of moving essence we call the elements. Prior to this motion, there was the primeval state of being without any form and without existence in time or space.

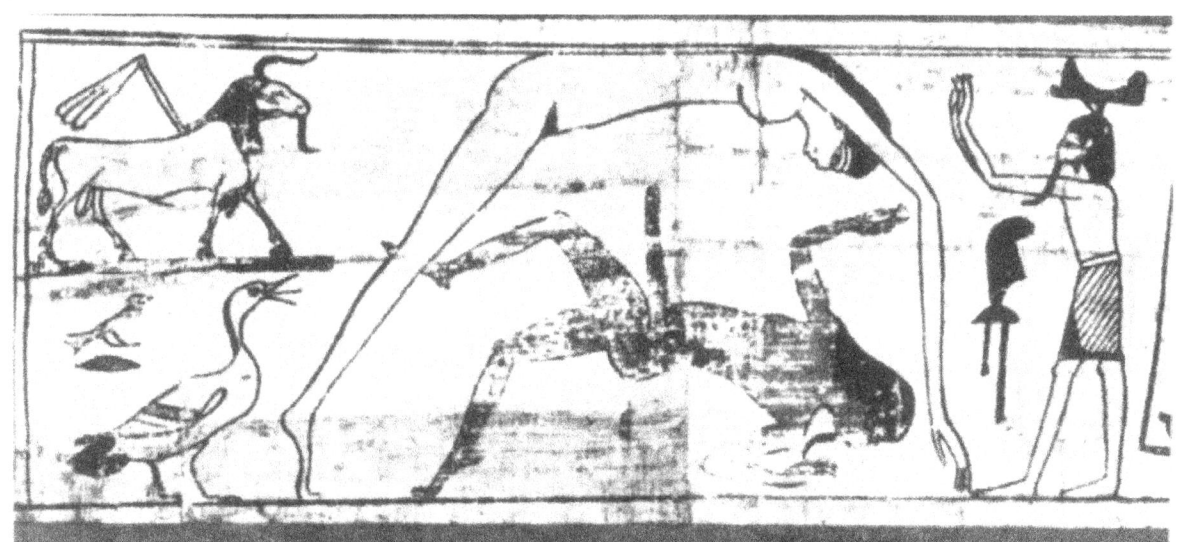

The union of Geb and Nut

Mystical Philosophy of Universal Consciousness

The Main Characters from the Ausarian Resurrection

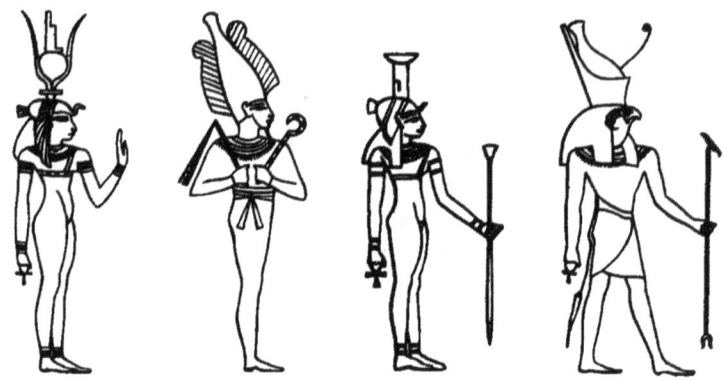

Above from left to right: Isis, Osiris, Nephthys, Horus.

Below from left to right: Anubis, Ra, Djehuti, Hathor.

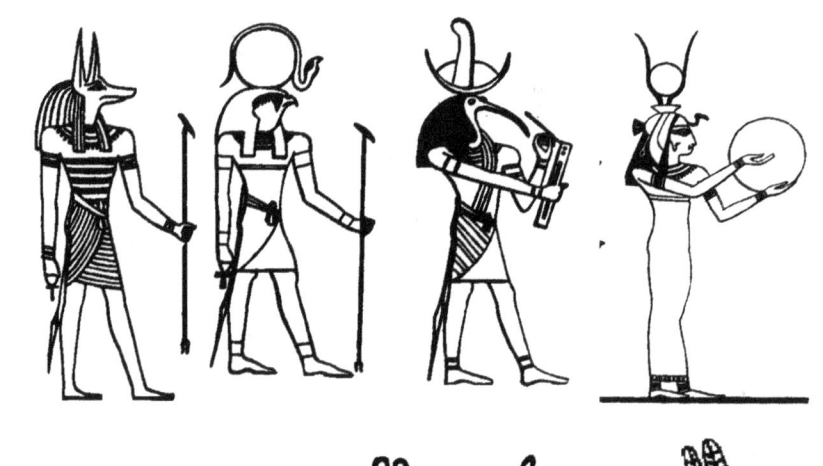

From left to right:

Set and Min.

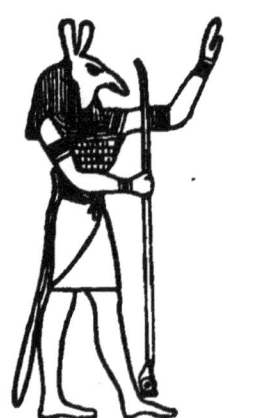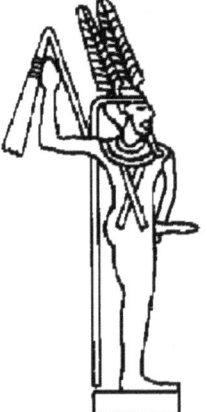

EGYPTIAN TANTRIC YOGA

Asar, Aset and Horus

Asar and Aset dedicated themselves to the welfare of humanity and sought to spread civilization throughout the earth, even as far as India and China.

During the absence of Asar from his kingdom, his brother Set had no opportunity to make innovations in the state, because Aset was extremely vigilant in governing the country, and always upon her guard and watchful for any irregularity or unrighteousness.

Upon Asar' return from touring the world and carrying the teachings of wisdom abroad, there was merriment and rejoicing throughout the land. However, one day after Asar' return, through his lack of vigilance, became intoxicated and slept with Set's wife, Nebethet. Nebethet, as a result of the union with Asar, begot Anubis.

Set, who represents the personification of evil forces, plotted in jealousy and anger (the blinding passion that prevents forgiveness and understanding) to usurp the throne and conspired to kill Asar. Set secretly got the measurements of Asar and constructed a coffin. Through trickery, Set was able to get Asar to "try on" the coffin for size. While Asar was resting in the coffin, Set and his assistants locked it and then dumped it into the Nile river.

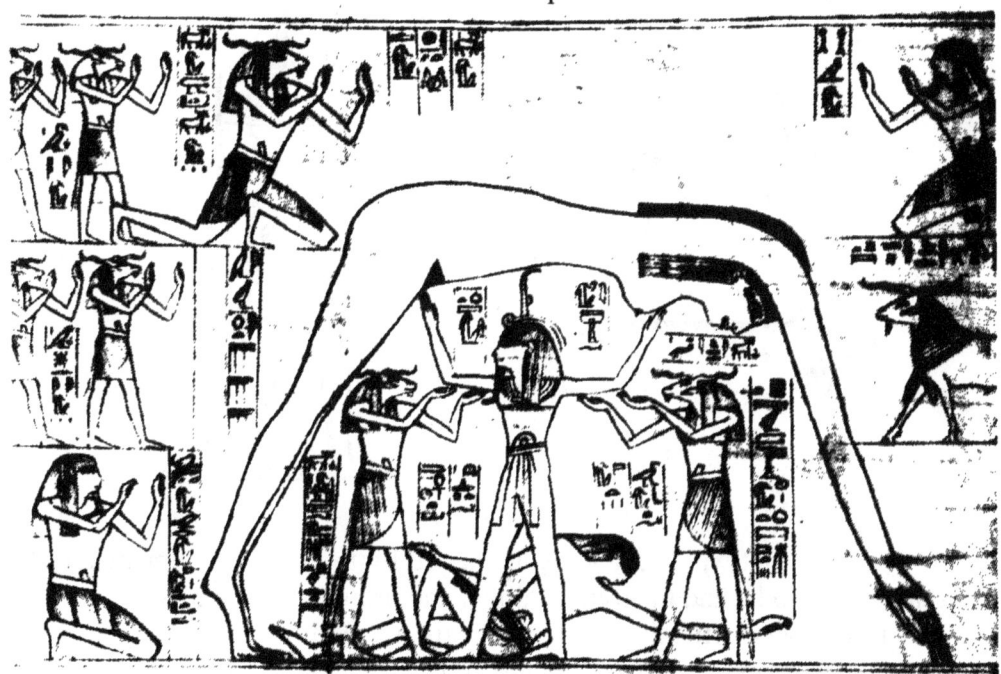

Nut and Geb being separated by Shu by the command of Ra.

The coffin made its way to the coast of Syria where it became embedded in the earth and from it grew a tree with the most pleasant aroma in the form of a DJED. The pillar is the symbol of Asar' BACK. It has four horizontal lines in relation to a firmly established, straight column. The DJED column is symbolic of the upper energy centers (chakras) that relate to the levels of consciousness of the spirit.

Mystical Philosophy of Universal Consciousness

Images From The Ausarian Resurrection

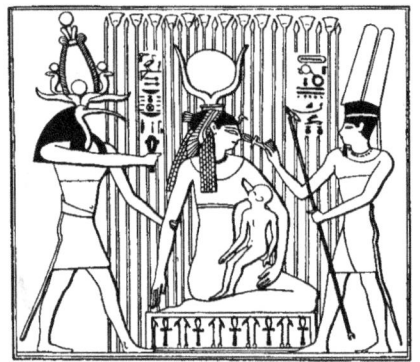

The birth of Horus

Horus and Set in one personality.

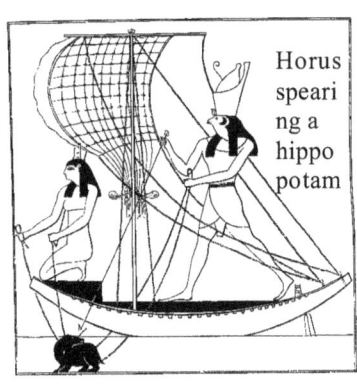

Horus spearing a hippopotam

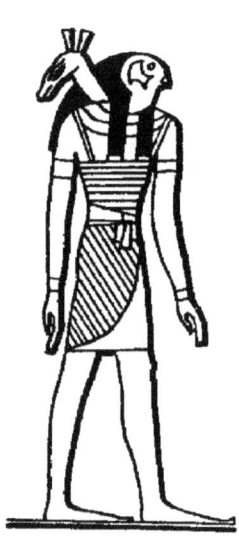

The King of Syria was out walking and as he passed by the tree, he immediately fell in love with the pleasant aroma, so he had the tree cut down and brought to his palace. Aset (Auset, Ast), Asar' wife, who is the personification of the life giving, mother force in creation and in all humans, went to Syria in search of Asar. Her search led her to the palace of the Syrian King where she took a job as the nurse of the King's son. Every evening, Aset would put the boy into the "fire" to consume his mortal parts, thereby transforming him to immortality. Fire is symbolic of both physical and mental purification. Most importantly, fire implies wisdom, the light of truth, illumination and energy. Aset, by virtue of her qualities, has the power to bestow immortality through the transformative power of her symbolic essence. Aset then told the king that Asar, her husband, is inside the pillar he made from the tree. He graciously gave her the pillar (DJED) and she returned with it to Kamit (Kmt, Egypt).

EGYPTIAN TANTRIC YOGA

Upon her return to Kmt, Aset went to the papyrus swamps where she lay over Asar' dead body and fanned him with her wings, infusing him with new life. In this manner Aset revived Asar through her power of love and wisdom, and then they united once more. From their union was conceived a son, Heru (Horus), with the assistance of the Gods Thoth (Djehuti) and Amon.

One evening, as Set was hunting in the papyrus swamps, he came upon Aset and Asar. In a rage of passion, he dismembered the body of Asar into several pieces and scattered the pieces throughout the land. In this way, it is Set, the brute force of our bodily impulses and desires that "dismembers" our higher intellect. Instead of oneness and unity, we see multiplicity and separateness which give rise to egoistic (selfish) and violent behavior. The Great Mother, Aset, once again set out to search, now for the pieces of Asar, with the help of Anubis and Nebethet.

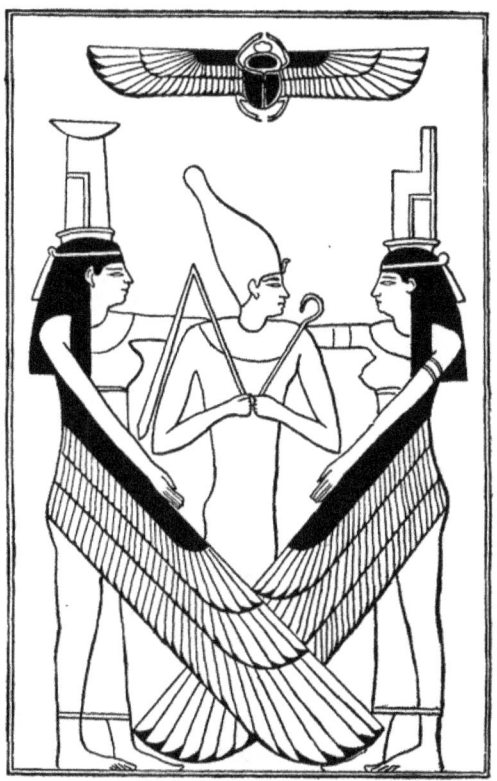

The Kemetic Caduceus:
Nebethet, Asar and Aset.

After searching all over the world, they found all the pieces of Asar' body, except for his phallus which was eaten by a fish. In Eastern Hindu-Tantra mythology, the God Shiva, who is the equivalent of Asar, also lost his phallus in one story. In Egyptian and Hindu-Tantra mythology, this loss represents seminal retention in order to channel the sexual energy to the higher spiritual centers, thereby transforming it into spiritual energy. Aset, Anubis, and Nebethet re-membered the pieces, all except the phallus which was eaten by a fish. Asar thus regained life in the realm of the dead.

Mystical Philosophy of Universal Consciousness

Horus, therefore, was born from the union of the spirit of Asar and the life giving power of Aset (physical nature). Thus, Horus represents the union of spirit and matter, and the renewed life of Asar, his rebirth. When Horus became a young man, Asar returned from the realm of the dead and encouraged him to take up arms (vitality, wisdom, courage, strength of will) and establish truth, justice and righteousness in the world by challenging Set, its current ruler.

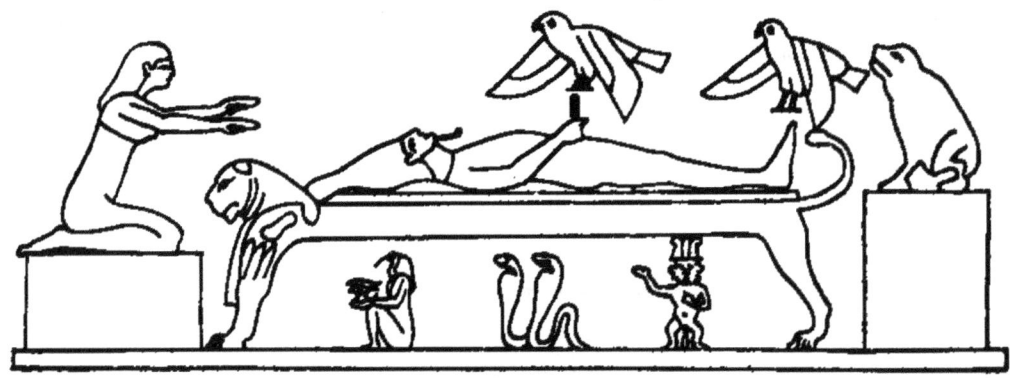

The virgin birth of Horus (The resurrection of Asar - higher, Horian consciousness). Aset in the winged form hovers over the reconstructed penis of dead Asar. Note: Asar uses right hand.

> I am your sister Aset. There is no other god or goddess who has done what I have done. I played the part of a man, although I am a woman, to let your name live on earth, for your divine seed was in my body."

A Hymn of Aset from the Ancient Egyptian Ausarian Resurrection

The Battle of Horus (Heru) and Set

The battle between Horus and Set took many twists, sometimes one seeming to get the upper hand and sometimes the other, yet neither one gaining a clear advantage in order to decisively win. At one point, Aset tried to help Horus by catching Set, but due to the pity and compassion she felt towards him, she set him free. In a passionate rage, Horus cut off her head and went off by himself in a frustrated state. Even Horus is susceptible to passion which leads to performing deeds that one later regrets. Set found Horus and gouged out Horus' eyes. During this time, Horus was overpowered by the evil of Set. He became blinded to truth (as signified by the loss of his eyes) and thus, was unable to do battle (act with MAAT) with Set. His power of sight was later restored by Hathor (Goddess of passionate love, desire and fierce power), who also represents the left Eye of Ra. She is the fire spitting, destructive power of light, which dispels the darkness (blindness) of ignorance.

When the conflict resumed, the two contendants went before the court of the Ennead Gods (company of the nine Gods who ruled over creation, headed by Ra). Set, promising to end the fight and restore Horus to the throne, invited Horus to spend the night at his house, but Horus soon found out that Set had evil intentions when he tried to have intercourse with him. The uncontrolled Set also symbolizes unrestricted sexual activity. Therefore, all sexual desires should be pursued in accordance with moral and intellectual principles which dictate rules of propriety that lead to health, and personal, societal and spiritual order (MAAT). Juxtaposed against this aspect of Set (uncontrolled sexual potency and desire) is Horus in the form of ithyphallic (erect phallus) MIN, who represents not only control of sexual desire, but its sublimation as well (see Min and Hathor). Min symbolizes the power which comes from the sublimation of the sexual energy.

Through more treachery and deceit, Set attempted to destroy Horus with the help of the Ennead, by tricking them into believing that Horus was not worthy of the throne. Asar sent a letter pleading with the Ennead to do what is correct. Horus, as the son of Asar, should be the rightful heir to the throne. All but two of them (the Ennead) agreed because Horus, they said, was too young to rule. Asar then sent them a second letter (scroll of papyrus with a message) reminding them that even they cannot escape judgment for their deeds; they will be judged in the end when they have to finally go to the West (abode of the dead).

This signifies that even the Gods cannot escape judgment for their deeds. Since all that exists is only a manifestation of the absolute reality which goes beyond time and space, that which is in the realm of time and space (humans, spirits, Gods, Angels, Neters) are all bound by its laws.

Following the receipt of Asar' scroll (letter), Horus was crowned King of Egypt. Set accepted the decision and made peace with Horus. All the Gods rejoiced. Thus ends the legend of Asar, Aset, and Horus. The Resurrection of Asar and his reincarnation in the form of Horus is a symbol for the resurrection which must occur in the life of every human being. In this manner, the story of the Osirian Trinity, Asar, Aset and Horus, and the Egyptian Ennead holds hidden teachings, which when understood and properly practiced, will lead to spiritual enlightenment.

Egyptian (Kemetic) Tantra Yoga In the Ancient Creation Myths

The tantric teachings of Egypt are embodied in the creation stories which involve the emanation of the *neters* from *The Neter*. As soon as the pairs of neters (*Shu and Tefnut, Geb and Nut, Asar and Aset, Horus and Hathor, Set and Nebethet, etc.*) arise out of the Supreme, Androgynous Being, there is a tantric relationship being described. The next teaching of Tantrism appear in the relationships between the neters which comprise the companies of the major theological systems.

One of the most ancient creation myths of Egypt tells of how Ra (Supreme Being) emerged out of the primeval waters and from Ra emanated Geb and Nut in this cosmological system. Geb represents the earth or physical nature, and Nut represents the heavens or the subtle nature of creation. In the beginning creation consisted of Heaven and Earth and nothing else because they held each other in such a tight embrace that it did not allow anything to exist. So creation consisted of the separation of heaven and earth through the medium of space and time (Shu). Thus, Ra separated Geb and Nut with Shu or space-ether. There are many depictions of Geb and Nut after their separation by Shu. Geb is laying on his back or sitting on the ground and sometimes he is depicted with an erect penis, pointing up toward Nut, whom he has just been separated from.

Mystical Philosophy of Universal Consciousness

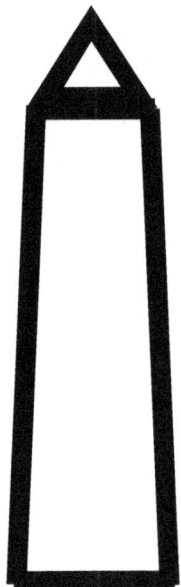

At left: The Obelisk represents the penis of Geb (earth). The skyline around it is Nut (heavens-cosmos). Thus, by directing sexual energy toward heaven, the unification of heaven and earth within oneself may be effected.

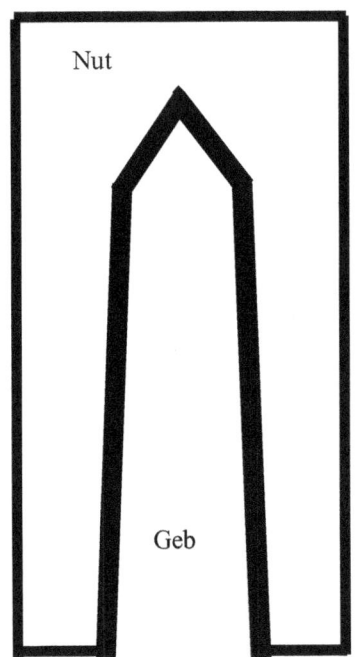

At right: Nut, that which surrounds and encompassed the Obelisk. Nut is everything adjacent to the Geb (earth) and therefore symbolizes the unity of creation.

As a polar principle, Nut represents the female aspect of creation and Geb represents the male. However, the two together are seen as complementary symbolic elements of the original matrices, The Supreme Self.

One of the most important tantric symbols related to Geb and Nut is the Obelisk. The obelisk is a tall structure which tapers toward the top wherein there is a small pyramid structure. It may be inscribed with hieroglyphic writing. The obelisk is a symbol of the penis of Geb. It rises out of the earth and reaches up toward the sky, reminding us of the original separation which caused heaven and earth to come into being. The deeper mystical symbolism of the obelisk can be seen when it is viewed from a distance. The space around it symbolizes heaven. Therefore, heaven and earth, though appearing to be separate, are in reality always one if the earth itself is viewed from outer space it is surrounded and enfolded by the heavens. This is exactly what is being conveyed through the depiction of Nut enveloping Geb from east to west (see pages 50, 53 and

93). This is the underlying oneness of creation and it is the same oneness which must be realized in the human heart.

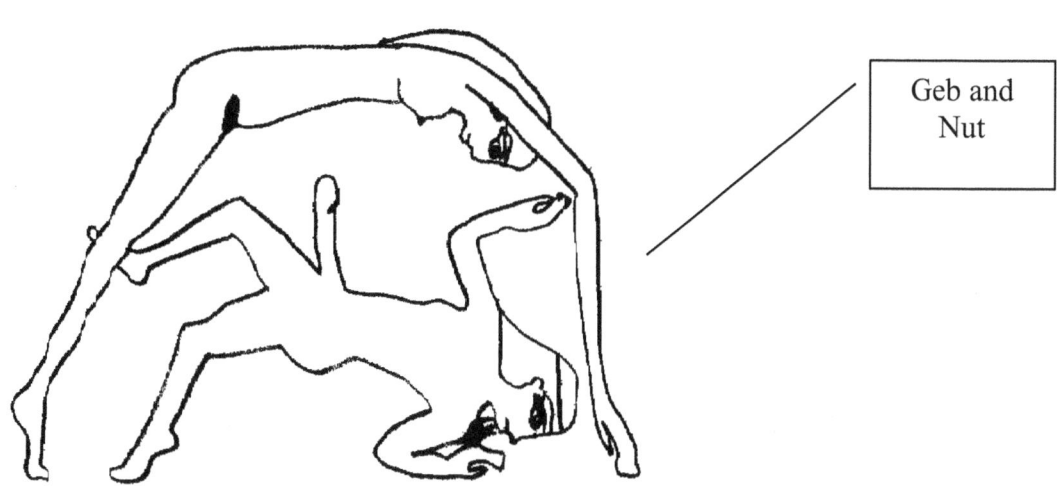

Geb and Nut

Though appearing to be separate from creation, in reality, every human being is enfolded by and indeed one with creation. Therefore, rituals developed wherein the symbolic raising of the obelisk were equated with the raising of the human soul to discovering its oneness with creation to be established (Tettu) in a vertical movement which is rooted in physical nature (Geb), while at the same time being in touch with the spirit (Nut). As long as there is separateness from creation, the feeling that one is a separate and finite individual, then there can be no true peace, contentment or happiness. The supreme Being and creation are one and the same. Also the Soul of every individual and the Supreme Being are one and the same. Therefore, uniting with the universe is the natural progression of self-discovery. The separation and individuality experienced by most people and reinforced by society is an expression of ignorance of the truth.

Mystical Philosophy of Universal Consciousness
Egyptian (Kemetic) Tantra Yoga

Tantra Yoga is purported to be the oldest system of Yoga as stated previously. Tantra Yoga is a system of Yoga which seeks to promote the re-union between the individual and the Absolute Reality, *"NETER"* (GOD), through the worship of nature (NETERU) as an expression of the Divine. Since nature is an expression of GOD, it gives clues as to the underlying reality that sustains it and the way to achieve wisdom. The most obvious and important teaching that nature holds is the idea that creation is made up of pairs of opposites: Up-down, here-there, you-me, us-them, hot-cold, male-female, Ying-Yang, etc. The interaction, of these two complementary opposites is what we call life and movement.

Insight (wisdom) into the true nature of reality gives us a clue as to the way to realize the oneness of creation within ourselves. By re-uniting the male and female principles in our own bodies and minds, we may reach the oneness that underlies our apparent manifestation as a man or woman. The union of the male and female principles may be effected by two individuals who worship GOD through GOD's manifestation in each other or by an individual who seeks union with GOD through uniting with his or her male or female spiritual half. All men and women have both female and male principles within themselves.

In the Egyptian philosophical system, all Neters or God principles emanate from the one Supreme GOD, Pa Neter. When these principles are created, they are depicted as having a ***male and female*** principle i.e. a god or goddess. All objects and life forms appear in creation as either male or female, but underlying this apparent duality, there is a unity which is rooted in the pure consciousness of oneness, the consciousness of GOD, which underlies and supports all things. To realize this oneness consciously deep inside is the supreme goal of Tantrism.

"PA-NETER" (Supreme Being) created the Goddess *NUT* (Sky-Heaven-Fire) and the God *GEB* (Earth-Solid). The God *GEB* and the Goddess *NUT* represent the male and female principles of creation, respectively. Then the Supreme "nameless" GOD created *SHU* (air) to separate heaven and earth, making a physical world and a heavenly world. Thus it is through the separation of Heaven and Earth by the god *SHU* that the universe was created.

The *"Obelisk"*, a tall tapering tower with a pyramid at the top, represents the erectile power of the physical human body as personified by the god of the earth principle, Geb. Our physical nature, though susceptible to the temptations of the flesh, is capable of great energy. In viewing any Obelisk, it should be noted that it represents a phallus uniting "Heaven and Earth" as it reaches up out of the earth *(Geb)*, through the air *(Shu)*, towards Heaven *(Nut)*, just as an erect phallus on a man's body projects up out and away from his body. As it projects it is unifying with space. Thus, symbolically, an obelisk represents the unity of the female and male powers (Heaven and Earth).

Geb and Nut symbolize an extention of the tantric symbolism of Creation. They are personifications in "dual" of what the supreme God or Goddess does him/her self, by him/her self "alone," i.e. androgynously.

EGYPTIAN TANTRIC YOGA

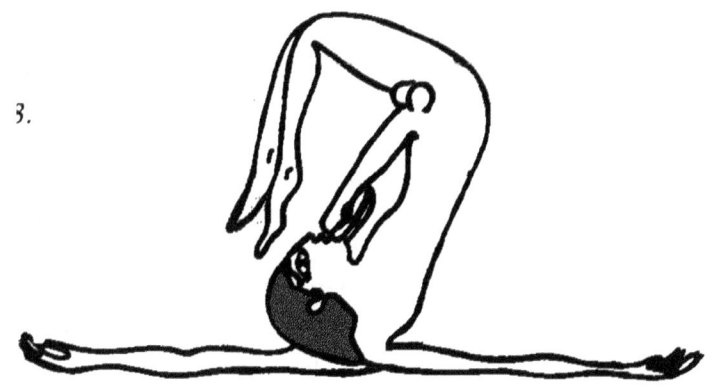

3.

The Tantric Symbolism of Creation in Neterian Spirituality

As you have seen many Ancient Egyptian symbols make use of sexual symbols in order to teach the mysteries of creation because creation manifests as both male and female. However, the idea of opposites or duality originates in nonduality. So this mystical symbolism is portrayed both as mystical teaching as well as in picture form. The picture above is of God engendering creation by consuming his own seed (seminal fluid) and becoming pregnant with the world. This teaching is also embodied in the following verse. In the creation story involving the Ausarian Mysteries, Asar (Asar) assumes the role of Khepera and Tem:

"Neb-er-tcher saith, I am the creator of what hath come into being, and I myself came into being under the form of the god Khepera, and I came into being in primeval time. ***I had union with my hand,*** and I embraced my shadow in a love embrace; ***I poured seed into my own mouth,*** and I sent forth from myself issue in the form of the gods Shu and Tefnut." "I came into being in the form of Khepera, and I was the creator of what came into being, I formed myself out of the primeval matter, and I formed myself in the primeval matter. My name is Ausares (Asar).

I was alone, for the Gods and Goddesses were not yet born, and I had emitted from myself neither Shu nor Tefnut. I brought into my own mouth, *hekau*, and I forthwith came into being under the form of things which were created under the form of Khepera."

The important passage and iconography above explain and illustrate the majestic vision of tantric philosophy in Neterian spirituality. Far from sexual vulgarity, the teaching reveales secrets about the nature of the Divine Self. It means that Neberdjer impregnated "himself," at once making him an androgynous being as well as the source matter of "her" own creation. So from the All comes the All. Everything comes from God and is composed of God, so too all is Divine, exists in the Divine and is rooted in the Divine.

The idea of creation above is portrayed as a masturbation but in reality it is an idea of androgynous conception which is being given. The idea is that while the world appears to be dual in reality it is non-dual. God has created the world within himself just as a person creates a dream world within him or herself when they have a dream or when using the imagination. The dream arises from, occurs in and dissolves back into your mind. It is within you so to speak. This

Mystical Philosophy of Universal Consciousness

is the kind of creation we are talking about. The Self creating within the very same Self. Thus there is nothing other than the Self and indeed nothing has in reality been created. There is only the Self, God and all things within the Self are the very same Self.

This utterance is the progenitor of the Christian and Hebrew idea of creation described in the book of Genesis where God or the Spirit hovers over and stirs the primeval waters. The original Biblical texts express the creation more in terms of an act of sexual union: *Elohim* (Ancient Hebrew for gods/goddesses) impregnates the primeval waters with *ruach*, a Hebrew word which means *spirit, wind* or the verb *to hover*. The same word means *to brood* in Syriac. Thus, as the book of Genesis explains, creation began as the spirit of God moved over the waters and agitated those waters into a state of movement. In Western traditions, the active role of Divinity has been assigned to the male gender while the passive (receiving) role has been assigned to the female gender. This movement constitutes the dynamic *female* aspect of the Divine in Tantric (Eastern and African) terms while the potential-passive aspect is male. Creation is therefore understood to be a product of the interaction between these two aspects of the same reality: spirit (male) and primeval waters (female).

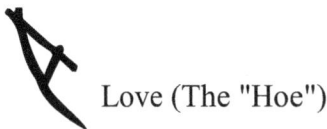 Love (The "Hoe")

The ritual of *"Hoeing of the Earth"*, relates to the preparation of the human mind and body, cultivating physical health in order to allow higher spiritual growth. The "Hoe" is the symbol of *"Love,"* therefore, the earth (Geb-physical human body) must be carefully "cultivated" (prepared to receive spirituality), through the practice of selfless love of others and developing devotion to God (Divine Love).

As it is the God Shu (air) who is responsible for keeping Geb and Nut (earth-male and heaven-female) apart, it is also Shu (air) who perpetuates the appearance of a world of duality, separation, with many male and female forms. Therefore, it is Shu (air) to whom we must turn to reunite the illusion of separation in our consciousness in order to end the appearance of duality.

The study of Shu (Ether, Air, Space) implies the discovery of what is subtle in Creation. The study of mystical philosophy and the practice of meditation reveal that space is only a projection of the mind just as a dream world is a projection of consciousness during sleep. Having discovered the subtle matter which pervades all, there must be a movement to discover what sustains the mind - The Self.

SHU: The breathing process is the only autonomic body system that can be consciously controlled by most people. Therefore, through breath control (control of air which contains within it the Life Force, Sekhem, Prana that sustains all life), we have an effect on our own consciousness and thereby a reunification of *NUT* and *GEB* (the opposites) within our own consciousness. That is to say, we may unite our human consciousness, female principle-receiver of life, with the cosmic consciousness GOD, male principle-giver of life and they discover the transcendental oneness underlying the opposite of creation.

EGYPTIAN TANTRIC YOGA

During Tantric training, each individual is instructed to regard the other as a divinity (which all humans are innately) and to worship each other as such and to alternate roles (each partner sees themselves as male or female) as they visualize the Life Force growing. During "physical" sexual intercourse between a man and a woman, it is the male who "gives" and the female who "receives". Sexual intercourse is used to heighten the ecstatic feelings and to develop psychic energy for spiritual attainment. Due to the power of the sexual force and the danger of one's inability to control one's mind and direct it to GOD while in practice, Tantra Yoga involving sexual intercourse is not advised except for those aspirants who undergo the rigorous psychological training which may take months or years. It is possible that a misdirected practitioner may fall deeper into the earthly desires rather than using them to transcend the earth bound existence. Breathing exercises, physical and mental purification are necessary before pursuing Tantra Yoga.

Thus, the participants are not allowed to reach climax (physical sexual orgasm) in order to channel all energies towards concentrating on the goal: development of their Life Force and its union with the Transcendental - Absolute divine through ever increasing ecstasy and devotion (Uraeus). Through repeated stimulation and concentration of the energies to the higher energy centers, the sublimation of the primal sexual and mental energy is possible. Apophis (lower self) is thus transformed into the divine eye symbolized by Goddess Arat (Uraeus).

The Indian Kundalini Yoga system which teaches the development of sexual energy through the development of the seven energy-consciousness centers in the spiritual body is viewed as an outgrowth of the Tantra Yoga system. Kundalini Yoga seeks to unite the Life Force energy, Goddess Kundalini Shakti (Egyptian Goddess Buto-ASET-Nut), the female principle, with the male God principle, Shiva (Egyptian Ra-ASAR-Geb).

The Life Force energy (Ra-Sekhem, Prana, Chi) is increased normally as one progresses along any path of spiritual development, regardless of whether a spiritual aspirant practices specific exercises or whether he or she is consciously or unconsciously trying to affect it. It might be said that no undertaking is possible without this force (The Sexual Life Force Energy). Indeed, life would not exist without it. It is the same energy that allows a person to walk, think, talk, etc.

It is important to understand that nothing is to be "given up." That is to say, when it is stated that one refrains from physical orgasm, it is meant that this is not practiced in order to experience "orgasm" on a higher level of consciousness. If there is a feeling of "giving anything up", then the subject is not ready to practice this discipline. There are many roads to spiritual evolution, however, some control of the bodily urges and desires must be exerted to channel energies to any desired goal in life. There have been many married and fully active people (male and female) throughout history who became enlightened human beings. Since all souls have accumulated different experiences and are at different levels of evolution, each must choose their own method of spiritual discipline. Total or partial celibacy can only be effective if the subject is ready to willingly and freely choose that path, otherwise the discipline would not work and might even be harmful since the subject's consciousness is still very much attached to his/her physical nature. Depriving oneself from needs and desires is neither wise nor healthy if there is deficiency of

Mystical Philosophy of Universal Consciousness

understanding and a lack of a higher outlet or higher need to be pursued. However, "natural needs and desires" change according to one's level of evolution. All the philosophical and religious systems now in existence are at best merely guidelines or general outlines of the way. A map is not the land.

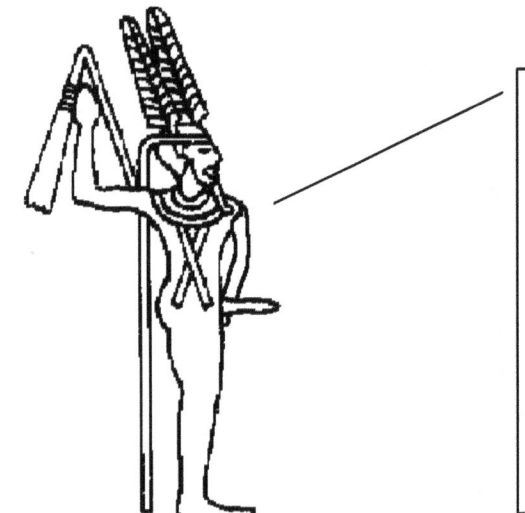

At left: the god Amsu-Min (Horus)

Min is known as the aspect of Horus called "the avenger of his father". His two plumes represent "Isis and Nephthys" or the Serpent Power which operates as pairs of opposites. The erect phallus represents the unification of the opposite forces. The left hand holding the phallus represents the harnessing of the forces. The right hand, holding the flail represents the control and mastery over the forces.

The statues and depictions of the god Min suggest to the initiate that the way to achieve higher mental and spiritual power is by sublimating one's sexual energy. In one statue, Min is shown holding his erect penis with his left (magnetic) hand signifying that the sexual energy is being drawn back into the body and up to the higher energy centers instead of being allowed to go out of the body. In this manner, the human body becomes a crucible for the creation of a higher physical, mental and spiritual state of being and consciousness.

In the Ausarian Resurrection, after the dismemberment of Asar (Ausar) by Set, Aset, Nebethet and Anubis searched all over the world for the pieces. They found all the pieces of Asar' body, except for his phallus which was eaten by a fish. In Eastern Hindu-Tantra mythology, the God Shiva, who is the equivalent of Asar, also lost his phallus in one story. In Egyptian and Hindu-Tantra mythology, this loss represents seminal retention in order to channel the sexual energy to the higher spiritual centers, thereby transforming it into spiritual energy. Aset, Anubis, and Nebethet "re-membered" the pieces, all except the phallus which was eaten by a fish. Asar thus regained life in the realm of the dead and engendered the life of Horus while conserving the Life Force energy and using it to impregnate Aset, symbolizing his own resurrection.

According to the Ausarian Resurrection story, the principles represented by the God Set include physical strength, sexual promiscuity, passion and brute force. Set has one more important meaning with regard to sexuality. The derivative word ***SETI*** which comes from Set also means "to shoot," as in shooting an arrow or as in ejaculation. From several mythological stories, it is clear that Set cannot control his sexual desires nor does he have the ability to contain his semen. In one episode of the battle between Horus and Set, Set tried to catch Aset in order to have intercourse with her. Unable to do so, he ejaculated on the ground, frustrated. Thus, Set represents the animal tendency to direct energy out of the body without control and to think passionately, reacting to life events without thinking. Min is the aspect of Horus who restores justice after the brutal murder of Asar. As *"The victorious one over the enemies of his father"*, Min, as a form of Horus, is victorious over the primal animal tendencies to passionate behavior and ejaculation (Set). Min's victory is not one of destruction over the primal forces, but one of mastery, control and sublimation.

Sexuality in The Ausarian Iconography

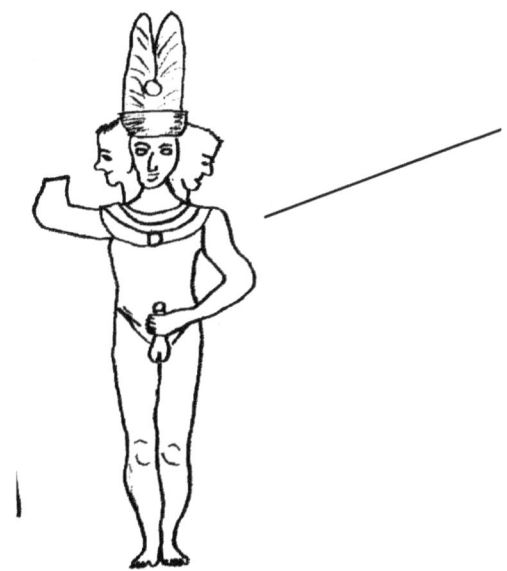

At left: The god Osiris in the Min aspect including the triune heads symbolizing the Lord of the Trinity.

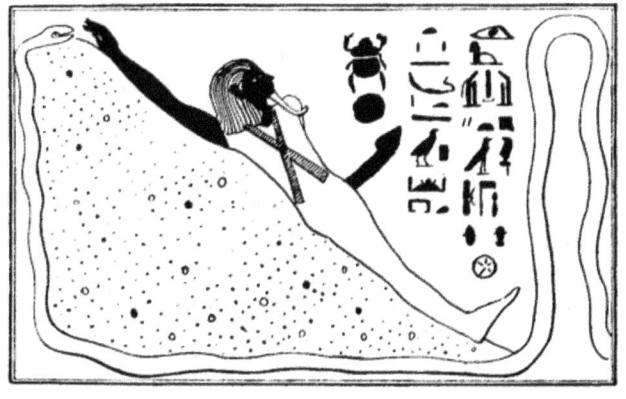

Left: Osiris as the creator who engenders Life Force energy into creation through the Mehen Serpent (Power) of the Primeval Waters.

Mystical Philosophy of Universal Consciousness

Sexuality in The Ausarian Resurrection Myth

125 "Souls, Horus, son, are of the self same nature in themselves, in that they are from one and the same place where the Creator modeled them; nor male nor female are they. Sex is a thing of bodies, not of souls."

The quotation above comes from the Ausarian Resurrection epic. It embodies the highest teaching related to the nature of the soul and its relationship to the physical body. As stated earlier, the relationships of certain gods and goddesses in the epic, give important insights into the source and purpose of sexual energy. The same teaching may be found in the Egyptian Book of Coming Forth By Day Chapter 175:

The Asar, the scribe Ani, whose word is truth, saith:- Hail, Temu! What manner of land is this unto which I have come? It hath not water, it hath not air; it is depth unfathomable, it is black as the blackest night, and men wander helplessly therein. In it a man cannot live in quietness of heart; nor may the desire for love-making be satisfied therein.

Temu: The state of the Spirit-souls has been given unto instead of water and air, and the satisfying of the longings of love, and quietness of heart has been given instead of cakes and ale.

Sexuality and the pleasures which human beings seek are in reality only activities which can be performed in the physical realm and only when there is a physical body, mind and senses to experience with. The Sahu or spirit-soul (Living-soul) state is beyond physicality and beyond time and space. Thus, in order to achieve this level of consciousness it is necessary to renounce and leave behind the ignorant and egoistic notions of the lower desires and the needs of the body. This process is outlined in the *Ausarian Resurrection Myth* as well as in the *Book of Coming Forth By Day*.

The main characters in the Ausarian Resurrection Myth may be seen as stages which every human being must pass through in the journey toward spiritual enlightenment. Beginning with Set at the lowest level, the psycho-spiritual awareness develops through Anubis-Maat, Horus-Hathor and Min until it discovers and unites with the absolute, transcendental reality Asar-Aset.

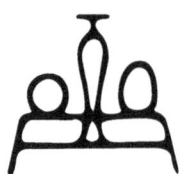

EGYPTIAN TANTRIC YOGA

Asar-Aset
(Pure Spirit - Absolute -
Transcendental - Supreme Self)

"The soul belongs to heaven-body to earth."

Ancient Egyptian Proverb

Asar represents the human soul which assumes physical existence. Ancient Egyptian mysticism expresses the true nature of every human being as composed of a soul, an astral or subtle body and a physical body. The Soul or the Self is singular and pure. Therefore, it is likened to a dot. The soul develops a mental process through association with its subtle nature and with desires. Through this process, a form of ignorance of its true nature develops. The soul becomes submerged, as it were, in the sea of thoughts and impulses from the mind and senses. It remains as a latent witness in the deep unconscious level of the mind, caught in the powerlessness produced by the web of ignorance it has spun for itself. Through the mind and senses of the individual human body, it experiences the universe, life, death, happiness, sadness etc. However, in reality the soul is never touched or affected by the occurrences of life but nevertheless experiences them as being real and compelling. The belief in mortal existence as being real prevents it (the soul) from discovering the deeper, transcendental reality, therefore, the Soul travels on a journey which involves many experiences of birth and death into a physical existence as well as the myriad experiences which occur in dreams along with those of the after death state.

```
                    Asar
              (The Immortal Self)
                  ↙ ⇧ ⇧ ↘
                ↙   ⇧ ⇧   ↘
              ↙     ⇧ ⇧     ↘
Aset    ⇨ ⇨ ⇨  ⇨ ⇦ ⇦ ⇦ ⇦    Nebethet
(Life)                          (Death)
```

The mystical teaching outlined above is the reason why every human being is referred to as Asar. Every human being is endowed with three important principals embodied in the character of Asar. He experiences immortality as a human being, he experiences life as a human being and he experiences death as a human being. The innermost Self of every human being is none other that the Supreme Self, who has assumed the form of all living things. The highest task of every life form is to throw off the veil of ignorance and to discover the Higher (immortal) Self within. The picture of Asar, Aset and Nebethet in the inner shrine (see cover) is a mystical representation of human existence. Asar is accompanied by Aset and Nebethet, who represent life and death. However, Asar in reality transcends them and also encompasses them. In other worlds, they are emanations of himself but in reality this expression of duality in the forms of Aset and Nebethet is only a projection of himself which is essentially one and whole. Therefore, while there appear to be three principles (Asar-Aset-Nebethet), in reality there is only one being, one consciousness in existence, which has caused an image to appear in the vast ocean of

Mystical Philosophy of Universal Consciousness

consciousness (the Creation) just as a movie projector causes an image to project upon the surface of a screen. In the same way, the experiences of birth, life, death, success, failure, etc. are produced by every individual just as dreams are projected in the lake of the mind during sleep and these experiences do not hurt or destroy the innermost Self of an individual. However, just as a person becomes lost in the action of a movie and feels identified with a character who is experiencing happiness or sorrow in the movie performance, the human soul sees itself as an individual entity cut off from the rest of the universe and has become lost in the experiences of human life and has forgotten its true nature as being one with the Supreme which encompasses all that exists. However, regardless of the depths of ignorance which the soul may reach it is possible for every individual to undo the web of confusion in the human heart through the process of yoga.

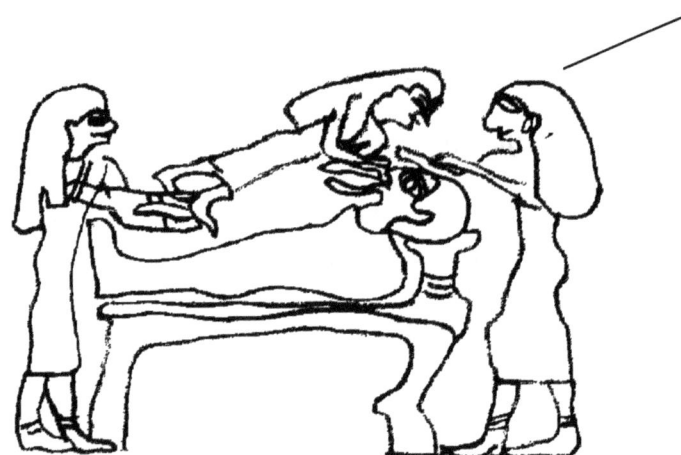

Isis (representing the subtle-lucid aspect of nature-creation) and the dead body of Osiris (representing the spirit, that essence which vivifies matter) are shown in symbolic immaculate union begetting Horus, symbolizing to the new birth of the spirit which takes place at the birth of the spiritual life in every human: the birth of the soul (Ba) in a human is the birth of Horus.

From a Stele at the British Museum 1372. 13th Dyn.

Asar and Aset in reality are one entity. The Self (Asar) and the wisdom of its own self (Aset) are in reality one and the same. When the soul transcends the state of Horus (having lived life based on Maat, having acquired wisdom (Aset) become enlightened to the Divine Self within, and having vindicated Asar, having vanquished ignorance, anger, hatred and greed (Set). In the scenes below from the Temple of Hetheru at Denderah the union of Asar and Aset and the dramatic resurrection are outlined.

EGYPTIAN TANTRIC YOGA
Scenes of the resurrection of Osiris from the Temple of Denderah

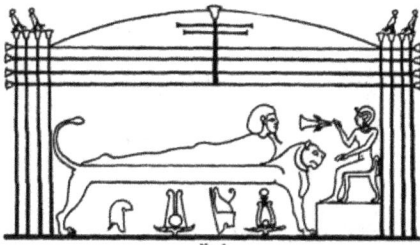

Horus presenting a Lotus Flower To Asar

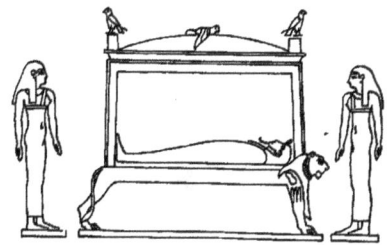

Asar lying on a funeral bier as Aset and Nebthet look on.

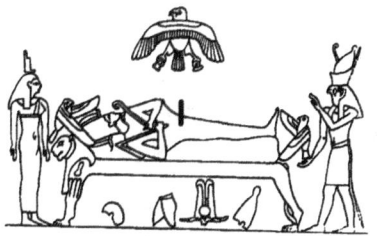

Asar, ithyphallic, wearing the Atef crown, with Aset and Heru.

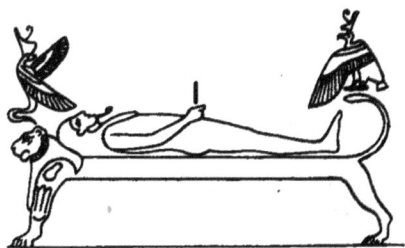

Asar, ithyphallic, with the vulture goddess Nekhebet at the foot and the Uraeus goddess Uatchet at the head.

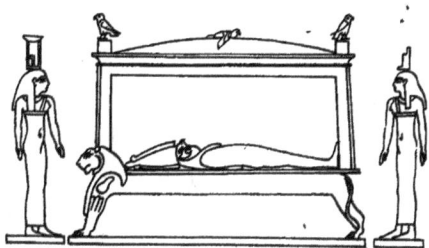

Asar lying on a funeral bier as Aset, at the foot, and Nebthet, at the head, look on.

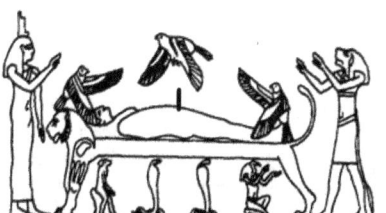

Asar, ithyphallic, being watched over by three hawks, a frog headed Heru, Aset, two apes and two snake goddesses.

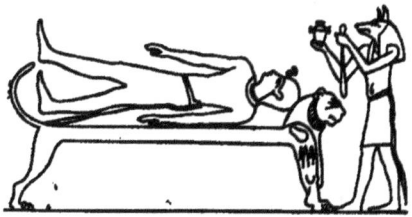

Asar lying on a funeral bier as Anpu embalms him.

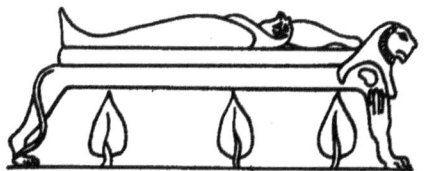

Asar as a hawk headed mummy with three trees below his bier.

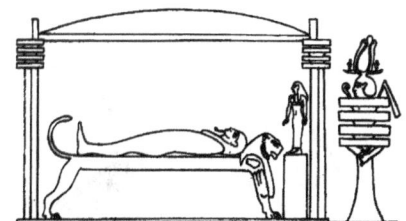

Asar lying in his chest with Isis at his head, and Asar in the form of the Djed Pillar looks on holding crook and flail.

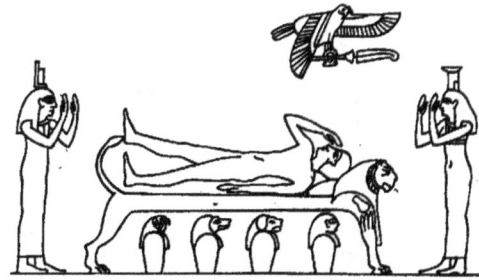

Asar lying on a funeral bier as Aset, at the foot, and Nebthet, at the head, look on. Below are the canopic jars in the form of the four sons of Horus.

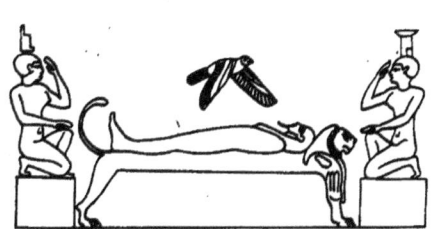

Asar lying on a funeral bier as Aset, at the foot, and Nebthet, at the head, look on. Above is a hawk.

Mystical Philosophy of Universal Consciousness
Scenes of the resurrection of Osiris from the Temple of Denderah

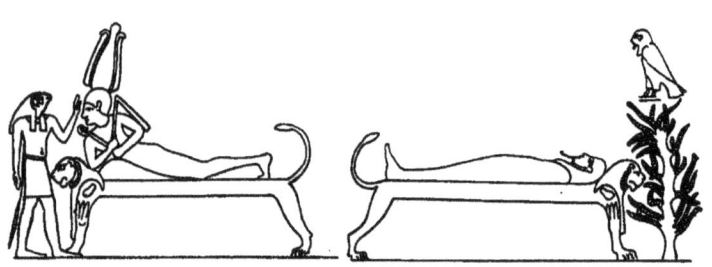

Left: Asar rising up at the command of Heru.
Right: Asar lying in his bier, at the head of which is a *persea* tree. Above the tree is his soul.

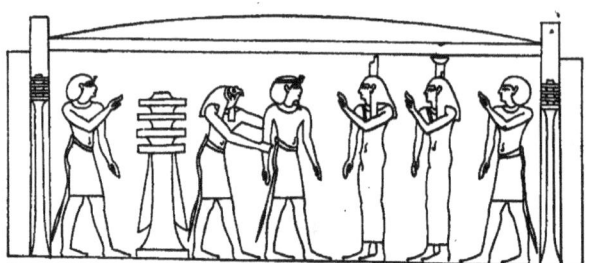

Heru, Aset and Nebthet raise up the pillar of Asar, and raise Asar himself.

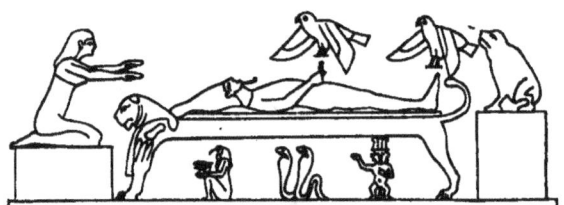

Hathor kneels before Asar, who is conceiving Horus with Aset (swallow-hawk), as the frog-god at the foot looks on. Below are Djehuti who is holding the Utchat (Eye of Heru), the two serpent goddesses and Bes.

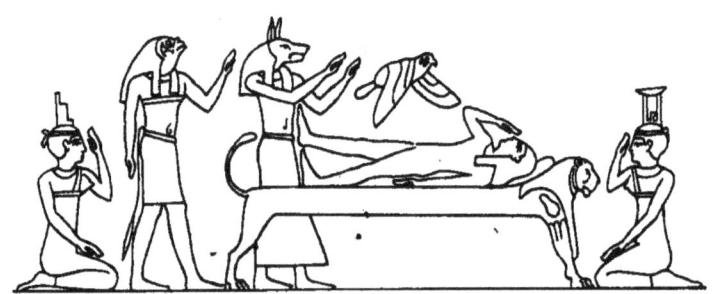

Anpu addressing Asar lying on a funeral bier as Aset and Heru, at the foot, and Nebthet, at the head, look on. The swallow-hawk hovers above.

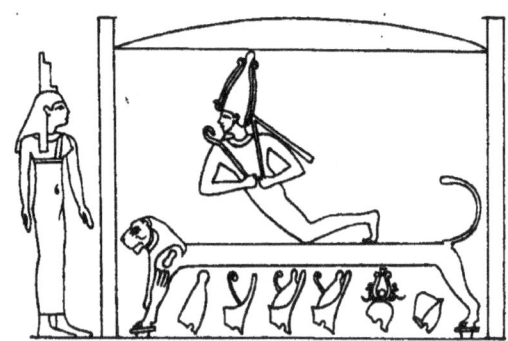

Asar rising as Isis looks on at the head of the bier. Below are his crowns.

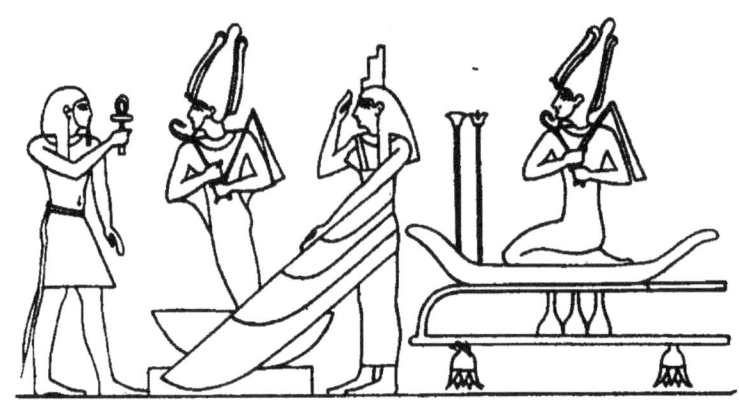

At left, Asar is rising as Isis looks on.
At right, Asar kneels on a boat at the head of which are a Lotus plant and a Papyrus plant (Upper and Lower Egypt). The boat sits on a sledge which is supported by two inverted Lotuses - symbols of the morning, the dawn, which brings new life.

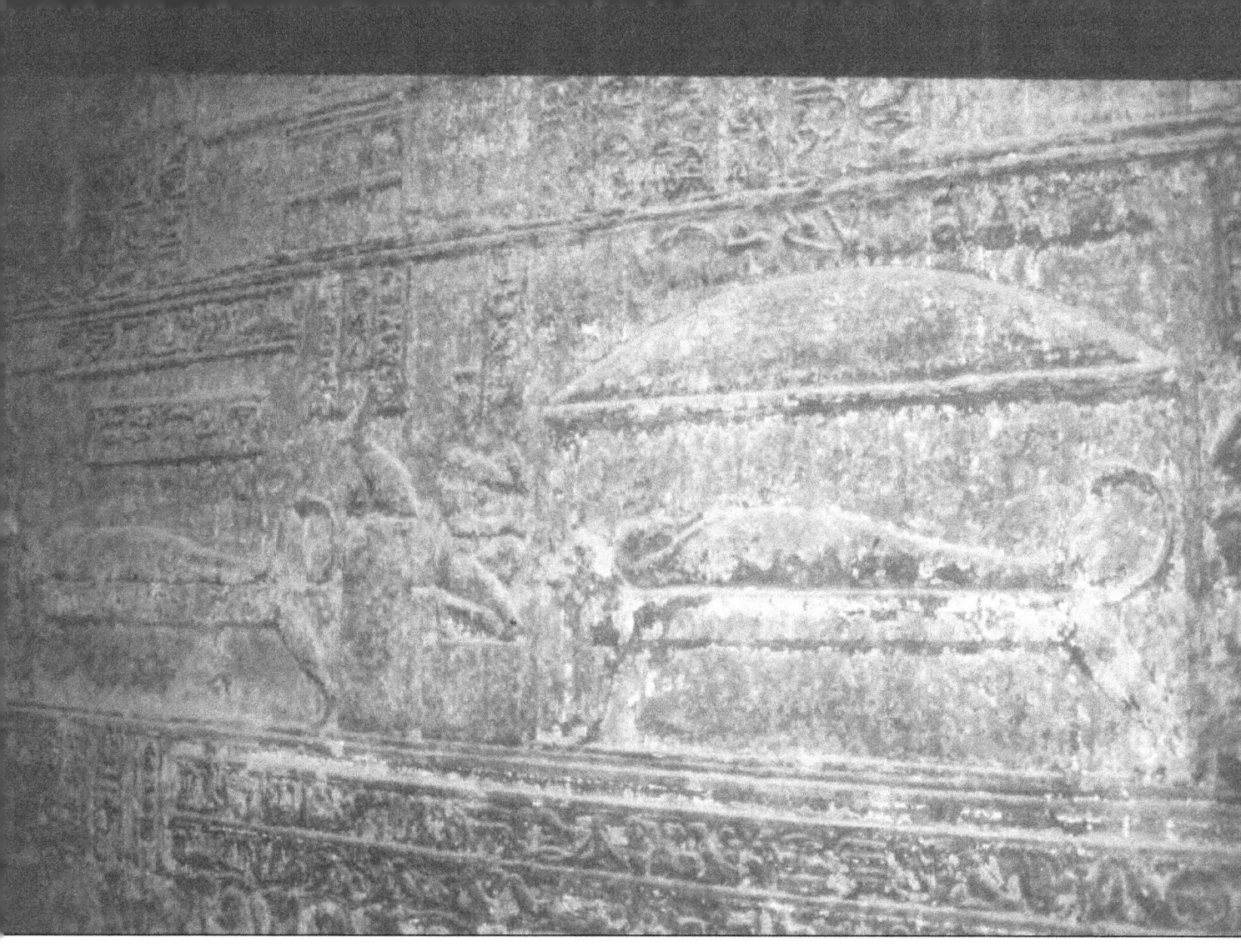

Above: one of the scenes presented in the series of line drawings in the previous pages of the resurrection of Asar.

Mystical Philosophy of Universal Consciousness

The Body: Magnetic (Female) and Electric (Male)

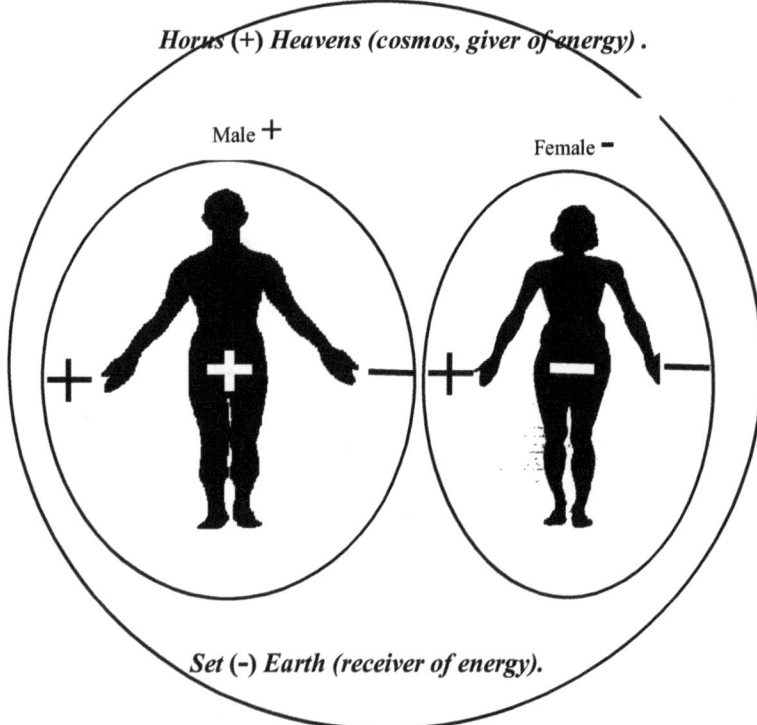

At left: diagram showing the poles of cosmic energy in nature and the human body.

It is important to understand that cosmic (sexual) energy is one energy but with different poles. The different poles give rise to an interplay of molecules which then appear to give rise to separate objects. Indeed, all objects in nature and the human body are composed of the same material: energy, which is controlled by mental vibrations. This is the interplay of Horus and Set.

The Androgynous quality of the Human Body.

EGYPTIAN TANTRIC YOGA

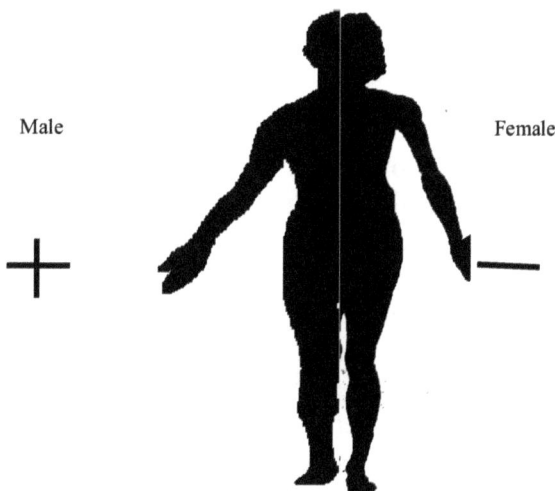

It is important to understand that each human being contains a male and female half. As we move toward universal understanding (Horushood), we become "more androgynous" as we gradually allow the androgynous spirit within us, Asar, to have control of our being. It is only due to the identification with the ego-personality and its desires and fanciful notions that we believe we are members of a certain sex, race, country or planet.

Nebethet-Set
(Slave to the Lower Self)

The relationship between Nebethet and Asar gives deep insight into the innermost desires of the human heart. Nebethet is the very embodiment of nature, as such she is devoted to Asar because Asar (Supreme Being) is the source and master of all that exists. Thus the desire of Nebethet to unite with Asar in reality represents the innermost desire of the soul in every human being to unite with God. Asar is the embodiment of the Self (the Spirit), and it is the innate nature of the Spirit to unite with Nature. Thus nature and the Spirit are in love with each other and nowhere is this better expressed in ancient Egyptian iconography than in the images of Geb and Nut through the mythology surrounding their union and separation. This relationship between Nature and the Spirit is also paramount in the Tantric symbolism of Hindu mythology in the form of Shiva (God, the Spirit) and Shakti (Nature). This union is the cause of the proliferation of the myriad forms of life on earth and throughout the universe. In this respect, the union between Asar and Nebethet cannot be seen as an illicit or adulterous relationship. It is to be understood as the symbol of the soul (Asar) in every human being which has become intoxicated as it were by the promise of human experience. It is a union which occurs based on the innermost urges of the heart, however it is a movement based on ignorance of the truth about one's true identity. When the soul's intellectual capacity for reason in a human being is clouded by ignorance the desires of the ego hold sway over the feelings, thoughts and actions of the soul. Thus the desire to unite with the self, instead of being understood as a need to discover the higher Self, becomes degraded into a movement toward overindulgence in sexuality, material possessions, vanity, and many other detrimental desires. Based on the erroneous idea, propagated by society, that life is to be lived for the purpose of indulging in sexual desire, amassing wealth and possessions, and gaining fame in society, people constantly seek to engender situations

Mystical Philosophy of Universal Consciousness

which are considered prosperous in the form of sensual pleasures and egoistic indulgences which only lead to more psychological pain and disappointment as well as physical and mental depletion.

Set represents the human condition wherein a person is under the control of their mind, senses and ego. This is the most degraded state of human existence. The lower self and its qualities hold sway over the mind and every aspect of the person's life. When this occurs the consequences are invariably disastrous. The qualities of Set develop in a person when there is dedication of one's thoughts to worldly or material goals and there is intensification of the negative qualities such as anger, hatred, greed, etc. in the mind. This principle of desiring what is gross is symbolized by his marriage to Nebethet (earth, death, decay, etc.). While Aset symbolizes subtle nature, Nebethet symbolizes gross physicality, concrete nature. Throughout the story, Set's sexual desire for Aset is also expressed. Like Nebethet, Set is desirous of Aset but this desire is of an impure nature. Set does not want Aset for who she is but as a possession to be held and experienced in the gross way as one might possess property or chattel for the purpose of pleasure alone. Set's intellect, being clouded by the pressure of desire, renders him powerless against the strategies of Aset and he ultimately fails in all his desires to possess her. Achieving union with the Self (Asar-Aset) can only be achieved by putting the desires of the lower nature in a subordinate position and developing an increasing understanding of the higher reality beyond the egoistic desires, feelings and thoughts of the lower self.

Set's attempted sexual assault on Horus is also an expression of the same movement of the distorted desire to unite with the Spirit (Horus). As an expression of his uncontrolled pride, vanity, conceit, and ignorance, Set is compelled to do whatever is necessary to achieve his object of desire no matter how unrighteous the means. The movement in ignorance (Set) is a metaphor for the Soul which is beset and overpowered by egotism and desires of the lower nature. Negative thoughts deplete will power and the ability to reason clearly. The negative thoughts, those based on ignorance, desire, greed, hatred, lust, etc., constantly seek to impregnate, as it were, the unconscious mind. If the ignorance is strong enough and the mind is weakened by the negative desires it will be susceptible to the negative thoughts and therefore demoniac qualities develop. However, if the mind is nurtured by Self-knowledge and righteousness it can capture the seeds of negativity and easily destroy them and at the same time establish its own seeds of understanding, love, and spiritual energy. This is the deeper significance of the sexual struggle between Set and Horus. Self-knowledge and wisdom (Aset) cannot be achieved by brute force or egoistic schemes. Likewise, uniting with the Spirit (Horus) cannot be achieved on the gross plane of nature.

The desire for objects and situations of happiness from the world of human experience is the source of all negative qualities in a human being. The inability to satisfy the desires leads to anger and hatred toward the person or situation which is perceived to be the obstacle preventing the achievement of the object of desire. This flaw in the character of Set is evinced in his attitude toward Horus, Aset and Asar as well as anyone who comes between him and the throne of Egypt. When the desire for self-discovery and creativity becomes degraded it expresses as an abnormal desire for sexuality and sensual pleasures as well as an unnatural desire for possessions and social acclamation. When the desire of self-discovery is understood and promoted, the desires for sexuality and for material possessions naturally assumes its proper place in life. Life can become more harmonious, peaceful and productive when virtuous principles are upheld. The righteous person engenders a movement toward expansion and creativity in consciousness rather than a desire for procreation and the pleasures of the senses. Expansion in consciousness implies the discovery, in greater and greater degrees, that the higher reality, the spiritual essence within, is greater, abiding and more fulfilling than the transient pleasures of the mind and senses. This is the mystical process of sex sublimation. When society is governed by the desires of the lower nature, disharmony and criminality are engendered. When society is based on the principles of spiritual truth, the lower nature is sublimated and it evolves into a great tool for spiritual and material achievement in the form of art which stirs and inspires as well as great accomplishments in science which benefit all life and leadership (both secular and non-secular) which brings out the best in humanity.

Consider the following, when you desire some object or situation and you develop attachment toward that thing you are actually allowing that thing to control you. Many people learn that they can only feel happy if they get something they desire. Therefore, if they can't get it there is anger and frustration. If per chance they do succeed they develop greed and want more. so there is never satisfaction and contentment, only more tension and unrest. Both succeeding or failing leave the mind in a state of agitation and when there is mental agitation there cannot be clarity of vision or spiritual awareness, but only egoism and the struggle to fulfill one desire after the next. Thus when there is no mental peace there is no real peace. Therefore, what most people consider to be rest, pleasure and relaxation when they acquire some object or situation they desire, is in reality, a modified form of mental agitation which temporarily creates the feeling of satisfaction or contentment but which soon after leads the person on a new quest to satisfy a new desire for satisfaction often through the same activities. From a mythological standpoint, sin is to be understood as the absence of wisdom which leads to righteousness and peace and the existence of ignorance which leads to mental unrest and the endless desires of the mind. Sin operates in human life as any movement which works against self-discovery and virtue is any movement toward discovering the essential truth of the innermost heart. This state of ignorance will end only when the mind develops a higher vision, it must look beyond the illusions of human desire and begin to seek something more substantial, more substantial and abiding. This is when the aspirant develops an interest in spirituality and the practice of order, correctness, self-improvement and intellectual development. These qualities are symbolized by MAAT and Anubis is the symbol of the discerning intellect which can see right from wrong, good from evil, etc.

Horus-Hathor
(Righteous Action -
(Virtue - Spiritual Power and Sexual Energy)

Horus embodies the following principles of initiation. **"Have faith in your master's ability to lead you along the path of truth," "Have faith in your own ability to accept the truth," "Have faith in your ability to act with wisdom," "Be free from resentment under the experience of persecution" (Bear insult), "Be free from resentment under experience of wrong," (Bear injury).** In the Ausarian resurrection story, it is described how Horus developed faith in his master, Aset. Even after being slighted by the Ennead and after being insulted by Set,

Mystical Philosophy of Universal Consciousness

Horus was able to go beyond egoistic feelings of being insulted and of feeling resentment. He steadfastly pursued Maat, righteousness, and thus was able to succeed in the end.

Horus represents the state of consciousness wherein there is awareness of the underlying unity of spirit and matter. Having been nurtured by Aset (study of wisdom teachings) and encouraged by Asar (communion with the Divine), the soul's latent divine qualities and boundless power emerge. This stage implies an attenuation of the negative qualities and an unfoldment of Divine glory in the human heart. At this stage the soul becomes associated with Hathor, the power of the Divine, and is able to act heroically in all areas of life in order to succeed against evil in the form of inimical personalities but more importantly, in the face of negative thoughts, feelings and inner fetters (anger, hatred, greed, etc.).

Hathor represents the power of the Sun (God), therefore, associating with her implies coming into contact with the boundless source of energy which sustains the universe (God). This movement implies performing actions which are in accord with Maat. When action is in line with the Divine Will (Maat) there are boundless positive resources and energies which move toward that action. When there is unrighteousness, obstacles arise and depletion of energy occurs. Therefore, making contact with Hathor implies the development of inner harmony which engenders clarity of vision that will lead to the discovery of what is righteous and what is unrighteous. A mind which is constantly distracted and beset with fetters cannot discern the optimal course in life and unrighteous actions develop.

The principle of sexuality is another important element in the symbolism of Hathor. She does not represent promiscuity or vicarious sexual pleasure, but the very purest form of sexual energy. Sexual energy is the source of all forms of action. It impels all life to move, grow and develop. The question is will this movement be toward progress and positive development or toward degradation and de-evolution? Sexual energy is the most basic instinct in human nature and it is engendered from the primordial need of the soul to unite and make itself whole. When the energy is led by ignorance, such as in the case of one who is not aware of the deeper essence of the Self within, the energy externalizes, as a person searches for fulfillment in the environment. The energy becomes refracted or distorted, as it were, and the person seeks to unite sexually with others or with objects by possessing these and thereby drawing some satisfaction. However, this form of activity cannot bring true satisfaction because it is fleeting and limited. Therefore, when the sexual energy is sublimated it can be directed toward a process of spiritual discovery wherein the lower nature composed of primitive sexual desires is led to unite with its own true source, the Self. This process involves the control of sexual energy and its direction toward an integrated development of mind, body and spirit wherein the emotional and intellectual faculties of the mind are gradually expanded to encompass all creation. This is why Hathor represents the principle of sexual energy (creation and sustenance) and the principle of destruction at the same time. Used in the proper way, sexual energy destroys evil and ignorance. When used in an improper way sexual energy destroys the physical constitution by depleting its vitality, will power, reasoning ability and the ability to experience true mental peace. Overindulgence in sexuality leaves the mind longing for more pleasure and the pursuit of pleasure clouds the intellect and agitates the unconscious, engendering more thoughts and desires endlessly.

EGYPTIAN TANTRIC YOGA

As old age comes along, the mind which has not discovered a deeper reality beyond the values of the masses, which stress of sexual prowess, financial wealth and social popularity is left in a position of frustration and despair because none of these (sex, wealth, popularity, etc.) can be maintained. Therefore, it is wise to develop a movement in life which leads to the discovery of a deeper, more stable essence in life, an essence which is not dependent upon the transient nature of life in the phenomenal universe or on youth and its deceptive qualities, but which transcends these. This is the purpose of yoga and mystical spirituality and it is the ideal in a society which is based on the principles of MAAT. In short, a person should develop independence from the lower nature as they grow older. Most people grow mentally feeble, weak, dependent and frustrated instead.

The Illusoriness of Sexuality

The illusoriness of sexuality and of relationships is underscored by the process of nature itself. It is only due to a lack of reasoning and will power that the truth is not realized and accepted by people. When the body grows and sexual maturity arises in adolescence the sexual drive, the need to discover and unite, arises. This drive is the basic force of nature and it must be fulfilled one way or another. When this drive is mixed with ignorance, base emotions and feelings it is directed toward physical sex when a certain form is perceived as a stimulus to the senses or when the mind formulates sexual thoughts. But what are these forms and thoughts? In reality, thoughts and forms are an expression of nature which in themselves have no reality. Think about it, when you decide that you like something it is because you have associated a positive or pleasurable feeling with it, however other people may feel that the very same object is not desirable. So what does this mean? Beauty and desirability are conditioned responses of the mind, based on its past associations or learned responses. So you have learned to feel desire for certain objects, relationships and situations as well as disgust towards others. In and of themselves, the objects, relationships and situations of life have no value except that which you have placed upon them.

A scientific examination of the human body reveals that it is composed of elements which are composed of atoms, molecules, etc. If you were to place a lump of matter containing the elements of an average human body, equal to the volume of a human body, on a table would you feel desire for it? Of course not. Desire is based on the conditioned response to forms as well as the mental association of that form with an idea of pleasure which that form will bring. The inability to control one's desires and to see the world objectively (as being composed of a homogenous essence) is a factor of one's dependency upon forms of nature (attractive people, objects and situations) as sources of pleasure. The best way to control desire is through the discipline, restraint and control of the sexual urge while at the same time gaining insight into the nature of sexuality and the nature of your true identity. Along with this a person should ask why it is that a mother or sister, father or son is not seen with sexual arousal even if they are attractive. Sexuality is a mental concept and it can be unlearned or sublimated according to your will.

Stark examples of the illusion of human life are to be found in the discoveries of modern physics and in the discipline of genetics. Most people look at each other as individual and

Mystical Philosophy of Universal Consciousness

separate entities, not realizing that they are all parts of a whole organism. Even as you breath air you are communing with the atmosphere. As you breath, minute particles of your lungs leave your body through the breath and go into the atmosphere. This happens to all beings on earth. Thus as you breath you are ingesting the particles of the bodies of other people from your community and from around the world since the world atmosphere carries particles across the world in a short time. Further, you are communing with the cosmic particles of dust which have traveled across the universe into the earth's atmosphere .

Modern medical science and genetics reveal that while human beings appear to be different on the surface (sex, race, etc.) in reality all human beings are remarkably alike. They make use of the same food and their bodies are made up of the same substances although these are arranged in slightly different ways. Skin coloration is mostly a difference based on the arrangement of pigmentation in the skin. Some people have more and some less but all have it in varying quantities, therefore all are in reality the same.

Sexuality is another example. Upon close examination, men and women are found to possess the same organs although arranged slightly differently and exhibiting different emphasis on certain levels of development. For example, the male penis has its counterpart in the female clitoris, the male testicles in the female ovaries and the male prostate with the female uterus. It is this understanding of the oneness of the androgynous nature which underlies male and female human bodies which is at the heart of Tantric philosophy. When this understanding is reached and integrated in the human heart it constitutes an extension (Tantra) from limited consciousness based on a sexual (dualistic) understanding to an awareness of the non-duality which is the ultimate reality. Thus while sexuality exists as a practical reality of life the practitioner of Tantra discovers the a-sexuality of existence as well, thereby expanding in consciousness to encompass all (sexuality and androgyny, duality and non-duality, etc.)

Many more examples could be given. The point is that the true identity of a human being is not sexual, not the body, mind, senses or anything which is in the realm of time and space because the realm of time and space is the realm of duality and illusion. Sexuality is only an expression of the personality based on an emphasis of the spirit which has tended toward a pole within the range of human consciousness (male-polarity, female polarity). Human existence is based on the karmic desires of an individual soul which is expressed within the limits allowed by the genetic basis of the organism. This means that the spirit can express as the DNA of the particular life form allows it to. These limits are divinely ordained and this is why they follow set rules (cosmic law-MAAT). Thus the spirit can manifest (incarnate) as a male or female within the given species. This is the range of expression which is allowed by the Divine Will which created and supports all life in the universe.

Simply stated, the spirit operates through the genes and is limited to the modes of expression which are dictated by the genes which fall within the range of either male at one extreme or female at the other. However, human beings are in reality the same essential being. In other words, all human beings are of the self-same nature. This factor becomes most evident when the egoistic feelings and sentiments of desire are cleansed from the heart. When this occurs the underlying unity which supports the appearance of duality, which expresses as sexuality, becomes most evident. These are only a few examples out of hundreds which can be presented to show that in reality human life is not separate and individual. Sexuality is a factor of nature and not of consciousness and consciousness is the essential innermost essence of every human being. Therefore any notions to the contrary are based on illusion and ignorance. Further, when the mind and its dualistic notions are transcended (through yoga practices) a person can discover that they are not the body, neither male nor female, but spirit. (For more on the findings of modern science which corroborate the ancient mystical teachings of Yoga and Tantric Philosophy see the book, *The Hidden Properties of Matter* by Muata Ashby).

Thus it is the creative energy which flows from the spirit which manifests as sexual desire in human beings. Nature has implanted an innate need to unite, to procreate. All things seek their mates in nature. Therefore it is in the polarity of males and females that the attractive force can be seen most prominently. For a person who has not understood this teaching there is no escaping the force of nature. That person is compelled by nature to enter into sexual relationships which lead to family relations and responsibilities or other forms of entanglement (karma). For one who has transcended these impulses the energy is redirected towards creativity of a different order, the expansion in consciousness which is the source of great achievements in spirituality as well as in art and social advancement of humanity.

Thus, upon closer reflection you must understand that sexual attraction is based on mental delusion due to the mind's being overpowered by the desires of the body (nature) and ignorance of the greater truth. Attraction and repulsion in the human mind are based on passion, restlessness and distraction. The force of passion compels one to search for ways to fulfill desires and the weakened mind which arises from living a life of distractions, due to giving way to emotions and feelings, renders a human being incapable of resisting the urges of the lower nature. the lower self then controls a human being. If the urges are resisted without a higher order of spiritual integration the force can lead to all manner of anxieties, perturbations, feelings of emptiness, frustration and even insanity and sexual violence. So passion may be understood as a form of intensified infatuation with certain forms in nature as well as the belief in the illusion of pleasure which is thought to be derived from them.

Many people believe that if God (nature) gave them the ability to do something that they should go ahead and do it. Therefore, they think "If I have sexual desires I should try to fulfill them, otherwise I cannot enjoy the pleasure of life." People do not reason out that they have many possibilities in life and why do they not follow those possibilities as well? For example, a person could easily commit suicide in various ways so why not do it? Just because there is a possibility to do something does not necessarily mean that it should be done. God has provided human beings with free will and the means to act out that will within certain limits. Through those actions experiences are generated and these experiences lead the soul to self-discovery. However, if you live life according to the dictates of nature (lower instincts and desires) you will be led to some fleeting experiences of elation but these will inevitably lead new desires and urges along with pain and sorrow at some future time.

The world is purposely designed in such a manner that there is more pain and sorrow than happiness and bliss to be found in human situations. Therefore it is up to the individual to act righteously or un-righteously and to reap the rewards for those actions (karma). Righteousness and self-control lead to peace and prosperity. While unrighteousness and unruliness leads to

Mystical Philosophy of Universal Consciousness

adverse situations. The weak willed person has no choice but to follow the dictates of the imagination, longings and the hormones as they flow through the body and engender feelings of sexual desire. Thus, a weak willed person is controlled by their ego-self (desires, feelings, emotions) rather than being in control of it.

Upon closer reflection, sexual desire cannot be understood as something which is stimulated by something that is outside of oneself. If this were so then it would only be possible to cause sexual arousal by means of contact with a "real" person. However, sexual stimulation can arise simply by looking at some suggestive printed matter or even through imagination. Therefore, sexuality is not an external development but an internal one, based on the feelings and desires which have developed in and which make up the content of the mind. As such it can be controlled in and through the mind itself when the distractions of the mind in the form of strong emotions such as lust, anger, hatred, greed, desires, etc. are reduced and when the inner Self is discovered. This is not only true of sexuality but of everything that involves the mind and its endless desires. Thus, the thinking process itself must be well understood and purified if there is to be any hope of controlling the feelings and actions of the body.

When a soul's consciousness tends toward femaleness or maleness there is never peace because the soul is innately androgynous and so the internal force is engendering a desire for wholeness. This innate desire is translated by the ego as a desire for another human being. No matter how much two people may profess undying love, some day they will part as mysteriously as they came together. Is this not sufficient motive to question the nature of human existence? Is this all there is? A fleeting interlude in the vastness of creation. Is there nothing more? Most people do not even want to consider these questions. They simply try to grab at whatever pleasure they can as they shut the voice of their intellect. However, as old age sets in and the important questions of life are not answered they develop sorrow, regrets, irritability and frustration along with fear of death and the frantic search for a means to prolong life, no matter how degraded it may have become since they know of no other reality besides this one and they ignorantly believe that after this life this is nothing more.

When the desire for personal satisfaction is foremost in a relationship the movement towards understanding is negative since there is only interest in one's own gratification. When there is selflessness in a relationship there can be true caring, peace and freedom. Thus understanding the opposite sex and the relations between male and female comes from expanding one's consciousness beyond the limited thought patterns and desires of one's own gender and one's own personal desires. This means that true harmony is to be found by discovering the inner androgynous essence of one's own being whether in a relationship or not. When real understanding and selflessness is present in a relationship it will blossom into an expanded experience which transcends physical sex. However when partners are interested in satisfying their personal (egoistic) desires the relationship will suffer from all kinds of conflict, infidelity, misunderstanding, frustration, anxiety and hatred. Therefore, sex is in reality a deeper means toward love and understanding when used in accordance with reason and control but it can be a means to deeply negative experiences in life.

EGYPTIAN TANTRIC YOGA

Discipline, Restraint and Control

Discipline, restraint and control of the sexual urge are strongly related. All are necessary for a viable spiritual discipline and they are the foundations of continued success because they allow you to practice (meditation, study and reflection on the teachings. Self-control etc.) for a long enough period of time to see some results of your efforts. What good would it do you to set out on a search for a treasure if you cannot discipline yourself to do what is required to perform the search (read the map, follow the instructions, travel to the location and dig until you find what you know is there? Similarly, what good would you derive from your spiritual search if you could not maintain the required amount of concentration because you are continuously distracted by other objects which also appear to be treasures but as soon as you grasp them, they fade into thin air, in a short time? In this example, the treasure is Spiritual Enlightenment and the objects which appear to be treasures, are in reality, objects which you sought to acquire because you thought they would bring you happiness (desires) but after a short time lost your fascination and ceased to elate you. Enlightenment is a treasure of boundless proportions. It does not fade and is ever full of eternal expansion. Which is the real and which is the illusion?

Whenever an uncontrolled feeling of lust arises, use the prescribed yogic process to control it. Sexual desire is a normal part of the animal aspect of the body and it is a tremendous source of energy which may be used to accomplish great deeds. However, if these feelings are unrestricted, the sheer force of the energy behind them is irresistible to the mind. One who is dominated by passion and sexual desire cannot aspire to great accomplishments in the relative world or in the spiritual because they are ever caught in the mire of nature's temptations and the pursuit of worldly pleasures. This is why the Sages and Saint of all faiths have enjoined the practice of celibacy in order to control the sexual urge. Even yoga practices, which include the cultivation of sexual energy such as the Left Hand Path of Tantrism, also require the practice of celibacy and control of the sex urge. Celibacy must be practiced along with exercises for sexual sublimation, otherwise, the un-channelized sexual energy will cause tremendous pressure on the mind and body.

The failure in the practice of celibacy comes from the ignorance and immaturity of the practitioner. Many people do not even want to think about stopping or controlling their sexual urges. After all this is the source of all pleasure in life isn't it?

The view described above is of immaturity and weakness. Also it is self defeating and the source of all obstacles which prevent a human being from discovering true pleasure and sexual fulfillment. The mind is strong in its own way. Also it has the ability to tenaciously go after and hold onto whatever it perceives will bring the most pleasure and satisfaction. This is why people cannot give up their vices and whatever it is that they perceive will bring happiness, be it partying, spending money, seeking thrills, fame or even sexuality. There is a very important secret which every spiritual aspirant must understand, especially those who have not yet attained control over the sexual urge. When the human mind discovers a higher form of satisfaction or happiness it begins to leave the lower one behind in favor of the higher in much the same way as an adolescent leaves behind the toys once used in the preteen years. Likewise, a mature adults leaves behind the urges of the adolescent in favor of the higher satisfaction of adult life. A spiritual aspirant should leave behind the accepted or prescribed practices and customs of society which lay down the norms of adult behavior. In deed from the yogic point of view, what modern society considers normal is abnormal.

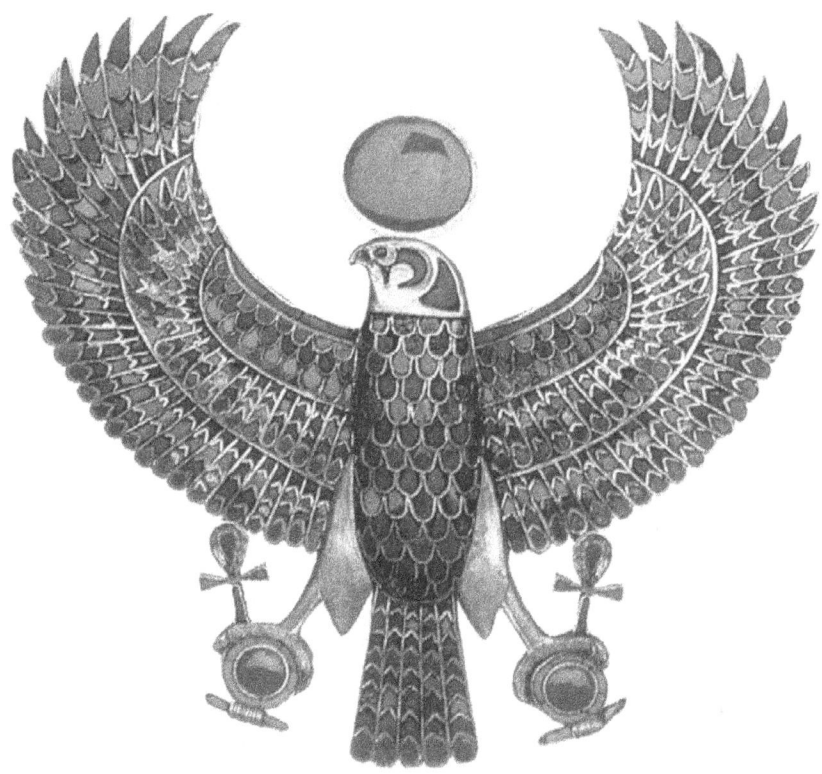

EGYPTIAN TANTRIC YOGA

The Tantra of the Soul and the Body

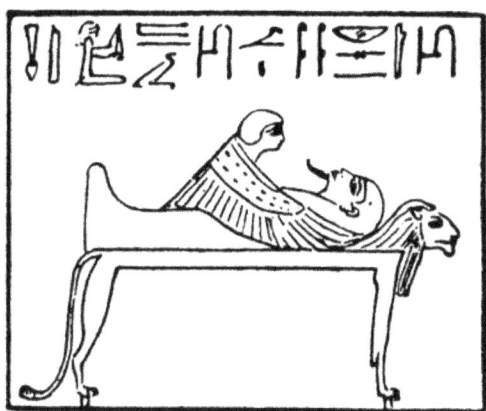

The soul of the scribe Nebseni visiting its mummified body in the tomb.

Above, from the papyrus of Nebseni, nebseni's soul visits the mummy (physical body of Nebseni) in Nebseni;s tomb. The Ba assumes the "Aset Position" a tantric sexual posture wherein she revives the body of Asar long enough to receive his seed and produce offspring, Heru-sa Asar sa Aset (Heru the son of Asar and Aset). This signifies the transference of the life essence to soul form. The soul is the intermediary aspect of the personality between the physical and the spiritual.

The Highest Tantra: Supreme Love

True love is unconditional. This does not mean that people should not be told when they are acting improperly. It means that love should not be affected by externalities. What someone does, says or feels is an externality. If these affect the feeling of love then it is in reality not love at all. It is an attachment to an externality in that individual which is no longer pleasing to you and is now causing strife and anger. Therefore, a true relationship is one which is growing beyond the externality and is discovering the deeper essence of the soul within the other person, the soul which is a reflection of the Divine.

The soul within one's partner or loved ones should be the true object of love because it is the true essence of that person. It is beyond any capacity for greed or lust and it is eternal and immutable. It does not demand or expect anything from you but it is ready to open up to all. The external personality of a person is like an illusion, a reflection or shadow of the soul, much like a world which is seen through colored glasses. Every part of the world is tinged with the color of the glasses so the reality cannot be seen the way it really is. Further, the external personality is ephemeral and flawed. The outer expression of the soul in the human personality is based on the level of spiritual ignorance and immaturity of the individual. Through this ignorance the selflessness and radiance of the soul becomes refracted into lust, greed and desire which reflect in the egoistic human personality. Therefore, the cure for the human condition of ignorance is spiritual knowledge and spiritual practice (selfless service to humanity. Having discovered the true essence of the soul within, the personality of a Sage or Saint reflects the light of reason, selflessness, peacefulness, contentment and universal love. To the extent that these are reflected, the level of spiritual maturity in an individual is also reflected. Further, to the extent that one is

Mystical Philosophy of Universal Consciousness

established in one's spiritual knowledge of the truth, the universal Self, to that extent perfection in the plane of the ego-personality is manifested. So one who has discovered the essence within (Sage, Saint) is perfect in consciousness. Therefore, spiritual maturity implies an increasing understanding, tolerance and forgiveness of others mistakes, wrongdoing, and sinful behavior. It allows true love to develop within the human heart. True love means joining with the soul of all that exists, its true essence, to become one with the Self which is at the heart of all. This is the highest expression of sexuality.

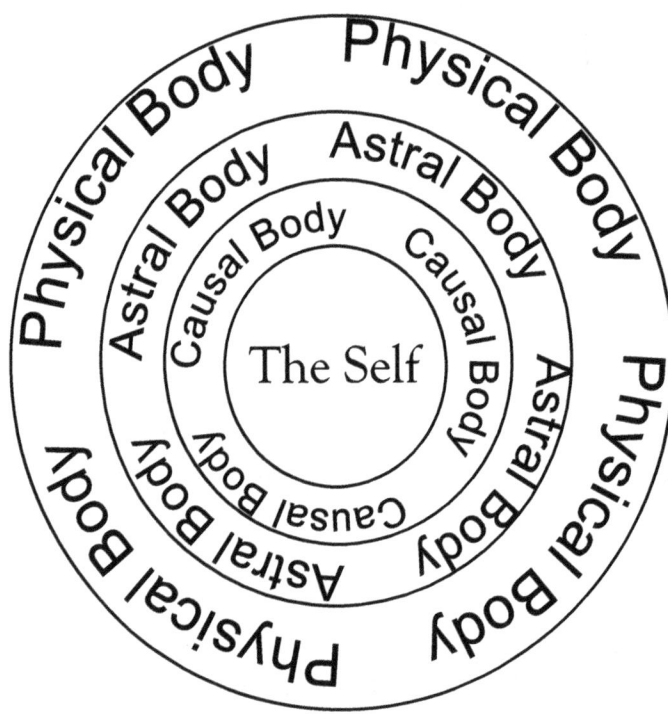

Above: a two dimensional schematic drawing of the subtle human constitution and its relationship to the Self or Soul.

The Self, in every individual, emanates the Life Force energy which creates and sustains the three bodies: Causal, Astral and Physical.

The Causal Body consists of the unconscious mind with the sum total of karmic impressions which impel an individual to have desires and aspirations. The Astral Body is composed of the mind and senses.

The Physical Body is the gross, visible manifestation of the Life Force energy through increasingly more dense (condensed) subtle matter.

People who grow up in a family with erroneous values, where sex and sense pleasures are seen as the greatest purpose and goal of life, develop in an atmosphere of mistrust, frustration and greed, born from the endless desires and their egoistic search to fulfill themselves. This search drives people to repeated negative relationships with others as well as a failed search to acquire material wealth in order to "feel happy". Thus, those who advocate the idea that life is meaningless without sexuality, fame, or wealth as well as those who write books which promote ways of intensifying and pursuing the egoistic pleasures are in reality expressing their ignorance about inner life as well as intensifying their own egoism and that of others. Further, they are working toward the degradation of society by inducing others to indulge their egoism. This has been the result of much of the work which writers and researchers in the area of sexuality in modern culture have produced. The teachings of tantrism have been confused with sexuality and sensual pleasure. The erroneous understanding promotes the idea that personal fulfillment is to be equated with sexuality and material fulfillment. The resulting philosophy is one of permissiveness, indulgence in the pursuit of pleasure and lack of restraint and reason. This kind of life leads to an endless and fruitless search for fulfillment through satisfying the selfish desires of the mind and body. In reality it is a living hell in comparison to the peace and inner contentment which can be discovered through self-discovery as promoted in yoga science.

Through increasing spiritual understanding and sacrifice of the personal desires in order to serve others, an understanding that true love is universal arises. In reality the lower forms of relationships such as physical contact, sexuality and sentimental attachments become obstructions to the experience of higher feelings. As people get older the inability to perform acts which society deems as "good" causes feelings of worthlessness and anguish in their minds. They view themselves as passé and worn out, with no purpose. Having indulged in the frivolities of modern culture, they have developed minds which cannot experience peace or understanding for others. Having lived with the ideal of youth and the disgust for old age they begin to resent and revile themselves. Thus there is bitterness and frustration. Old age should be a culminating point in the development of a human being. Other cultures in the past have recognized the wisdom and worth of the older members to the extent of according them elevated status in society. The modern tendency toward denigrating old age is an extreme example of ignorance and self-deprecation which fuel the feelings of hatred and self-destruction since younger people know, deep down, that they too will grow old, be unable to perform the activities of their youth and die some day.

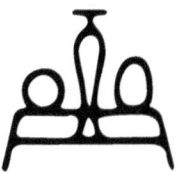

Mystical Philosophy of Universal Consciousness

Tantric evolution through Kemetic Ritual

Tantric evolution is promoted in Kemetic Spirituality through the certain secret rituals which will be described here but will not be explained in detail, due to their sacred and secret nature.

Ritual of the Journey of The Divine Boat

The first important ritual is the journey of the Divine Boat. Several temples had this ritual. The ritual entails the transportation of a divine image from one temple to another. The image is placed on a boat, which symbolizes the movement of the first boat that first stirred up the primeval waters and thus created the forms that became the objects of Creation. The ritual is to be carried out each year so that the act of creation may be renewed for another period of time. It constitutes a metaphysical reenactment but also an actual participation in upholding the laws upon which the universe and the religion itself is based.

In Ancient Kamit the annual ritual of carrying the Divine Boat (vehicle of the god or goddess) from one Temple to another was a means to maintain the order of the cosmos, as the movement of the boat engenders and sustains Creation itself. This same act of Creation was re-enacted by the Priests and Priestesses of Ancient Egypt. In Kamit, pallbearers would carry the boat while a Priest opened the way by burning incense on the path. A long procession would follow behind, some playing music and others dancing and others uttering chants. .

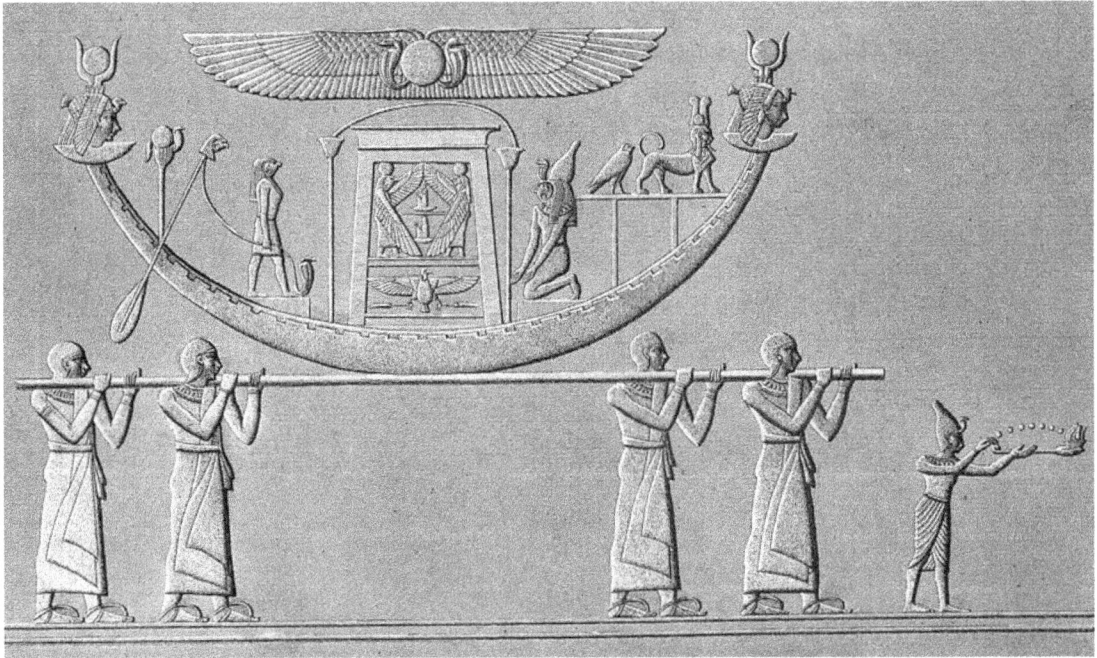

What is less understood by most people is that the ritual is often dedicated to bringing two divinities closer together so that the may copulate and thereby give birth to the force that sustains Creation. The divinities are male and female. The female travels to her beloved and unites with him. This was the case with Amun and Mut (Procession from Karnak to Luxor) and Hetheru and

Heru (Procession from Denderah to Edfu). Below is a drawing of the actual Divine Boat of Sokkar and the boat of Tem.

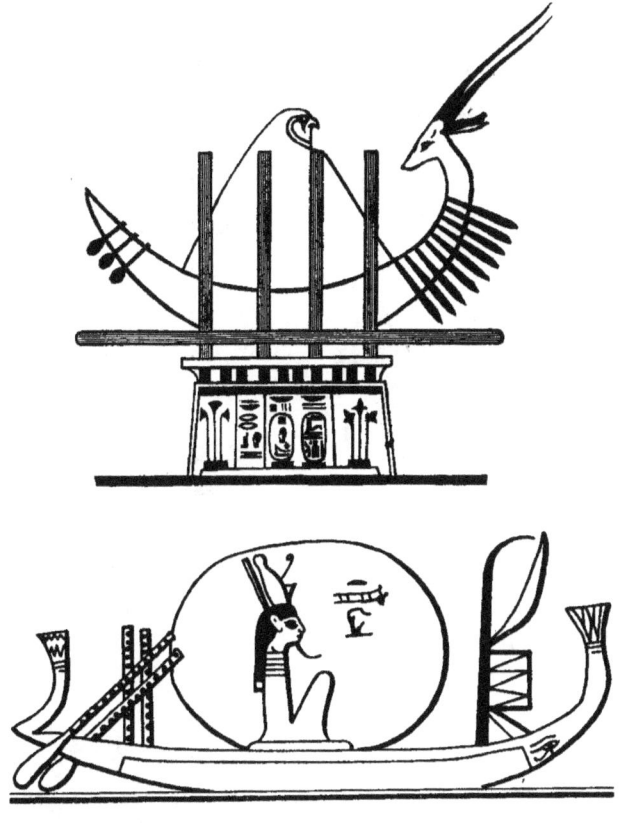

On the following page:
Above: actual ritual boat of Heru (Temple of Heru, Edfu, Egypt)

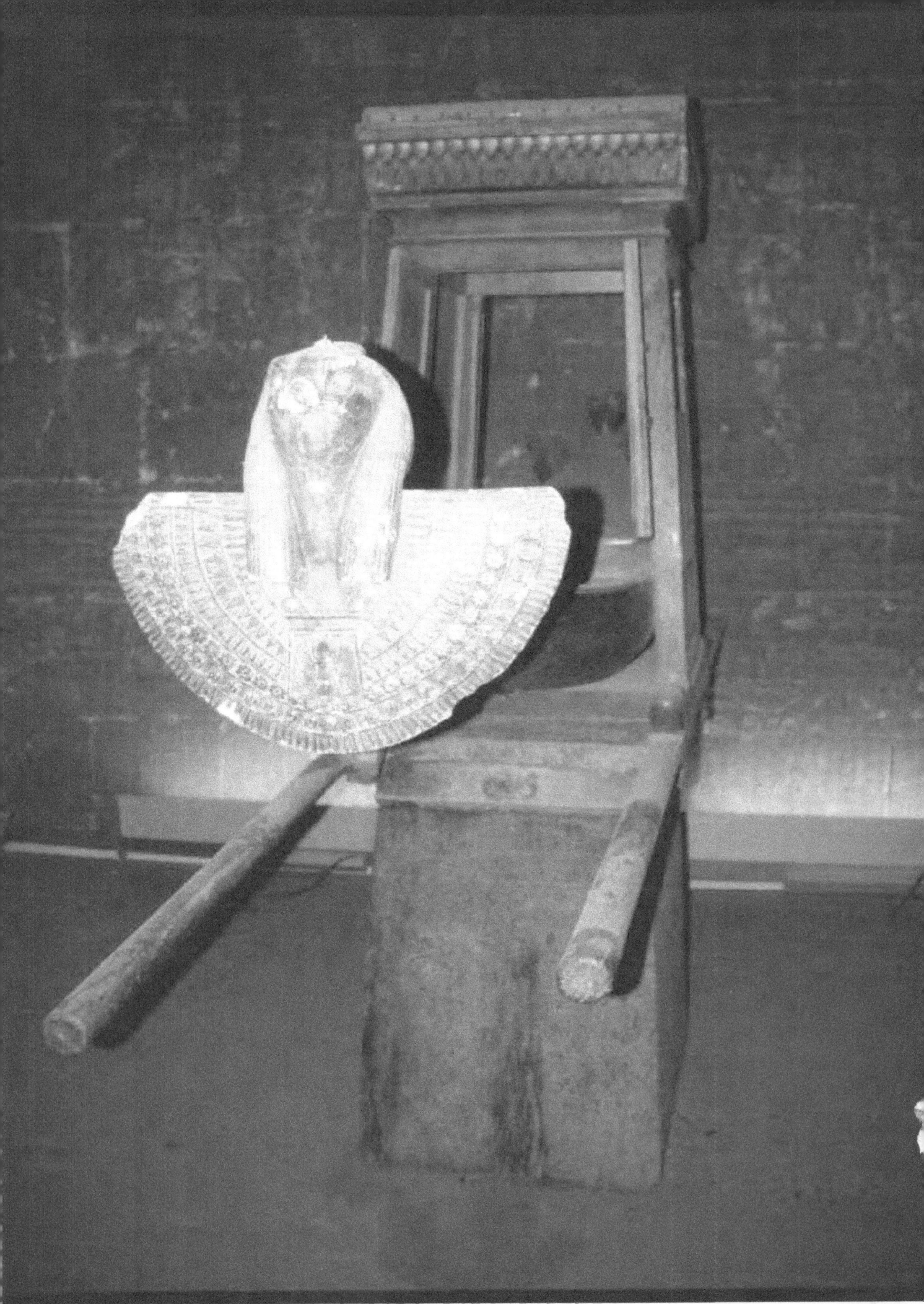

EGYPTIAN TANTRIC YOGA

Mystical Philosophy of Universal Consciousness

Ritual of the Dawn at Denderah Temple

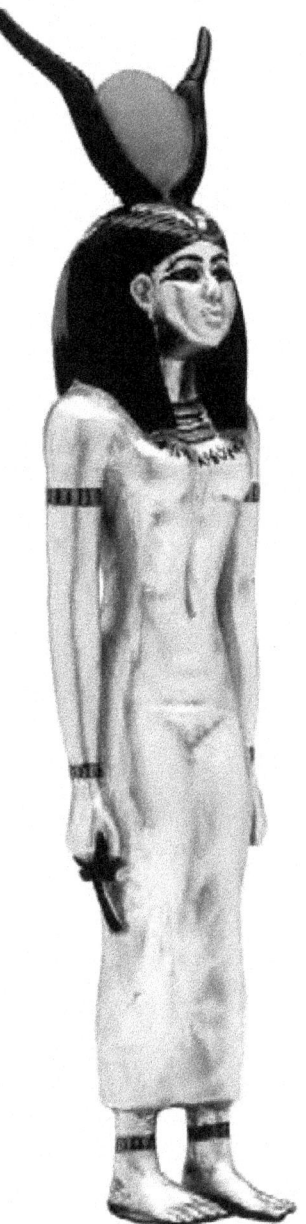

Statue of Goddess Hetheru

At the Denderah temple there was another kind of tantric ritual. Each year the image of the goddess Hetheru was brought out before dawn, following a procession of priests and priestesses, uttering chants and bringing offerings to the roof of the temple. There they waited for the dawns first light, which would touch the naked goddesses body and thereby be impregnated with the life force of the sun (Heru) and thereby the cycle life and prosperity continues on for the next year.

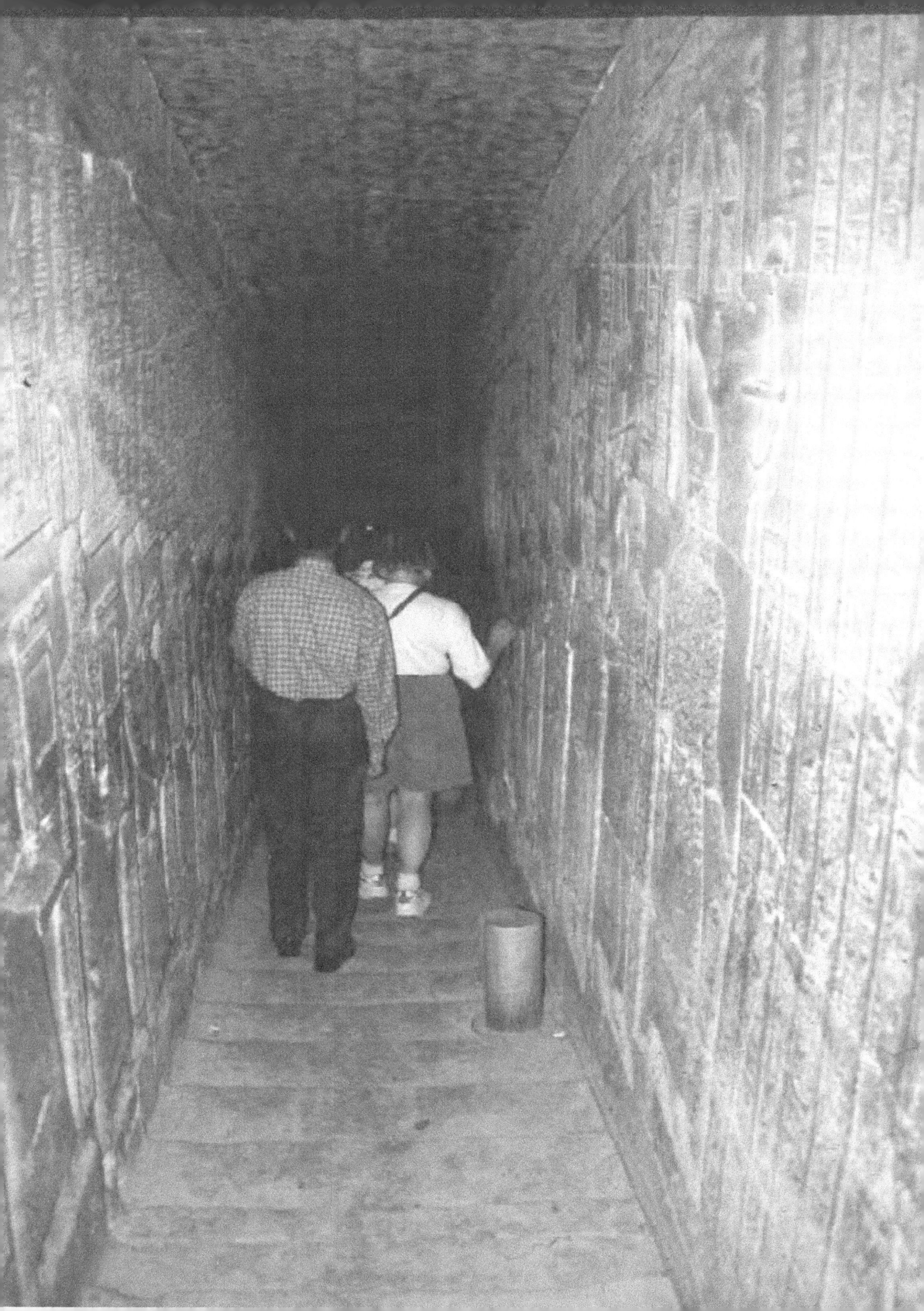

Mystical Philosophy of Universal Consciousness

Above: a stairway from the inner portions of the temple of Hetheru leads up to the roof. The images of priests and priestesses carrying offerings and artifacts are inscribed in the wall itself. (Denderah, Egypt)

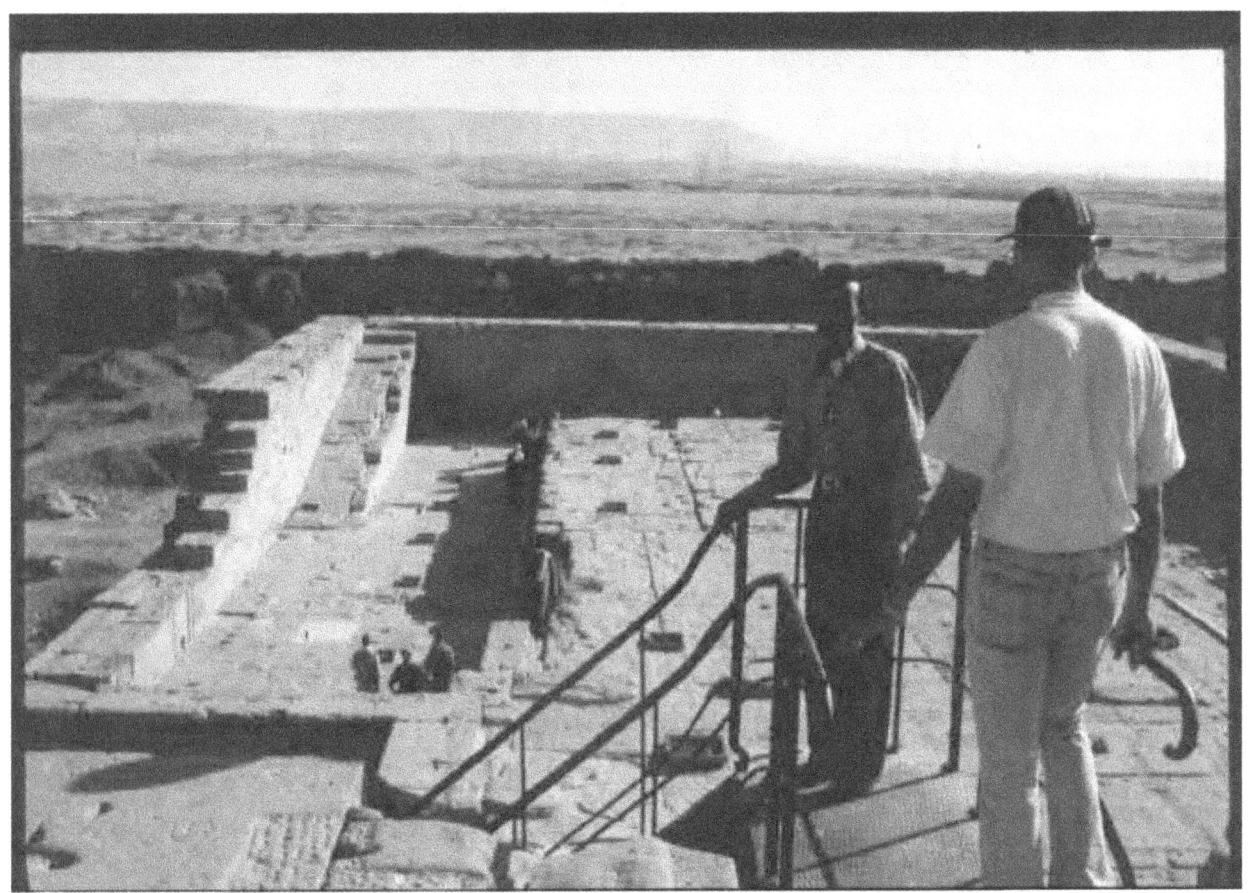

Above: roof of the temple of Hetheru. (Denderah, Egypt)

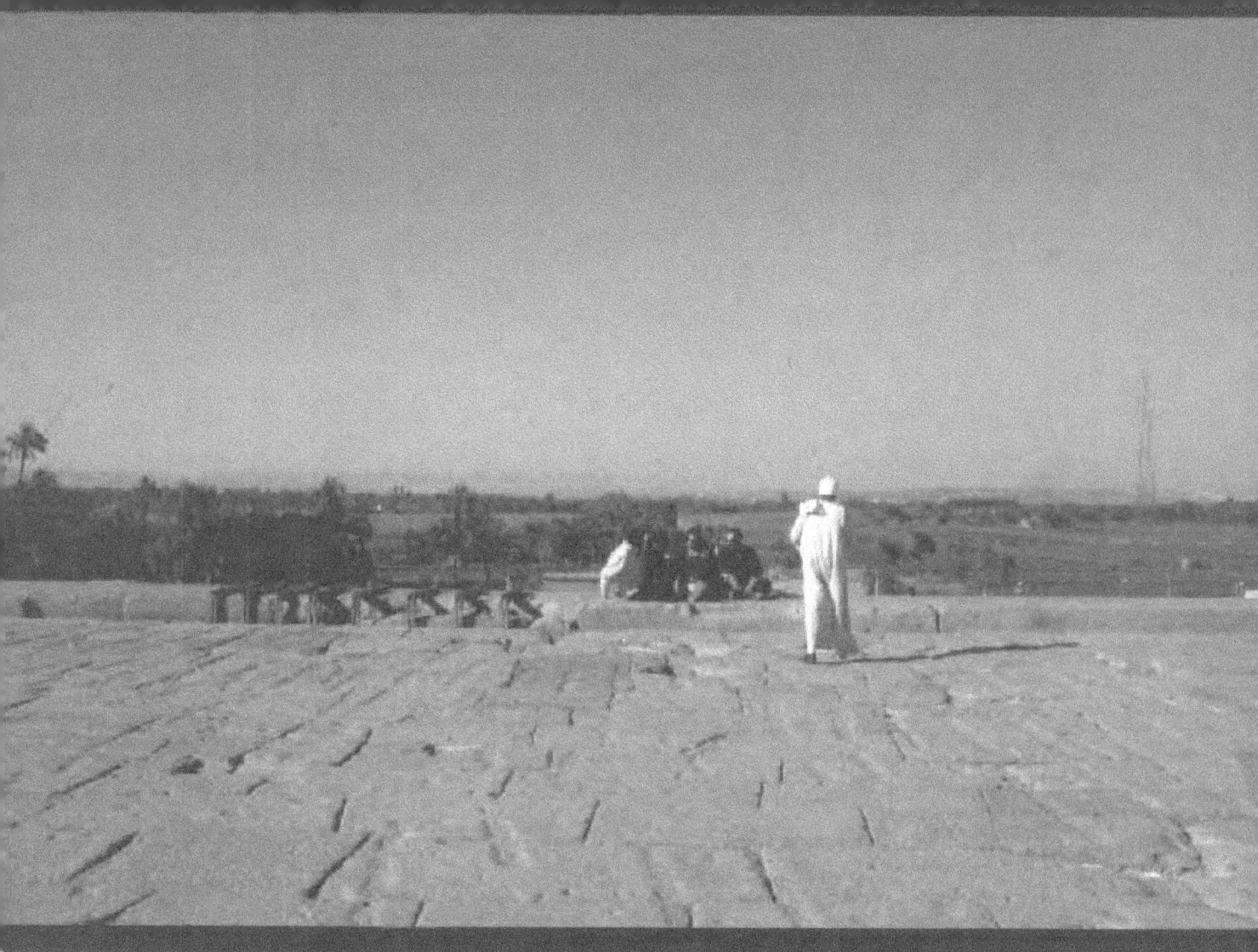

Above: roof of the temple of Hetheru. **(Denderah, Egypt)**

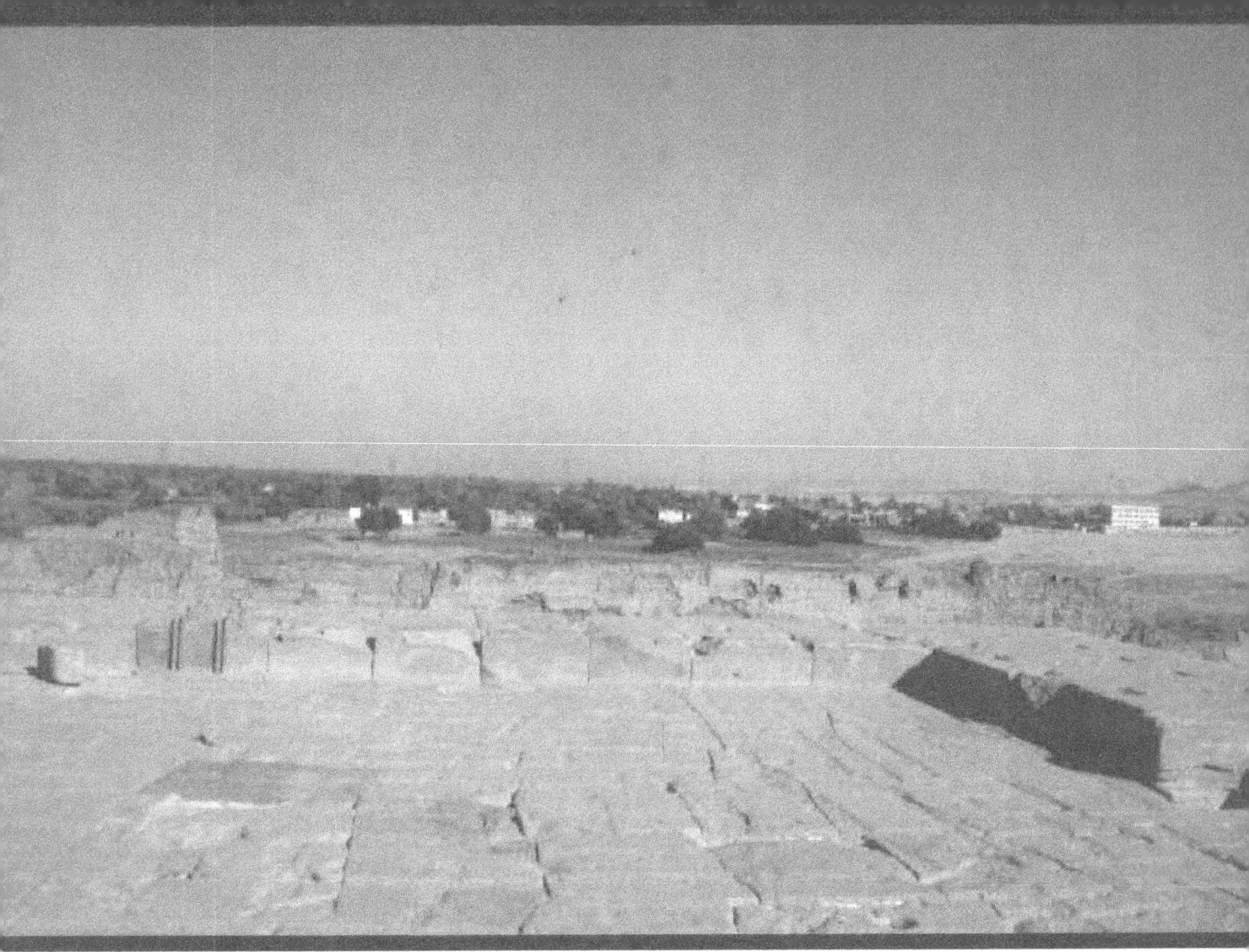

Above: roof of the temple of Hetheru showing the boundary between the green Nile irrigated lands and the desert. (Denderah, Egypt)

EGYPTIAN TANTRIC YOGA

Ritual of the Divine Embrace

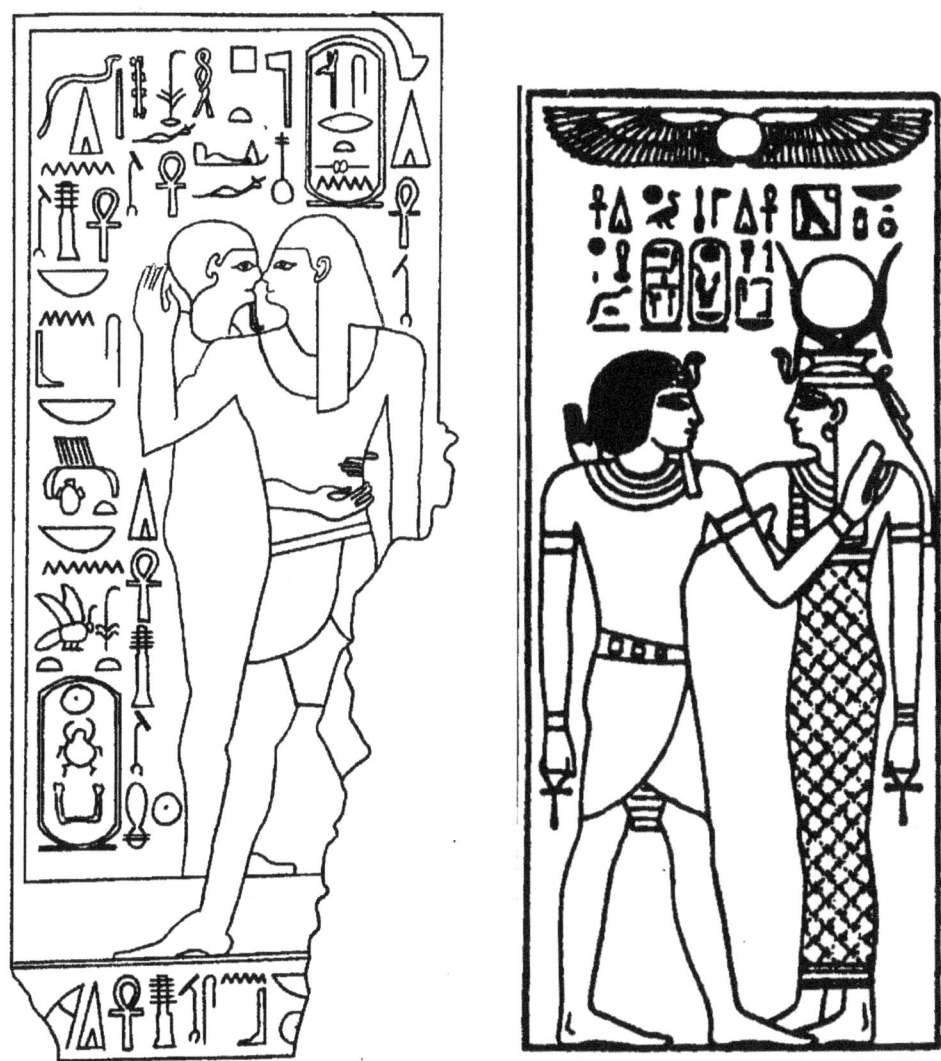

Above left: King Senusert and the God Ptah (Pillar from Temple of Senusert at Karnak
Above right: Goddess Hetheru embracing the king.

The Waset Temple (Karnak) is a prime example of one of the most important tantric rituals, the Divine Embrace. This ritual is to be performed by the most elevated initiates as it symbolizes the sexual union with the Divinity him/her self. No more will be said on this ritual as it is reserved for advanced practice.

The visualization is one of unity with the Divine through a loving embrace which encompasses parental, and spousal relationships. Men can see themselves with the goddess or with the god because "he" is understood to be androgynous. Women can visualize the tantric unity in the same way.

Mystical Philosophy of Universal Consciousness

Tantric Symbolism of Gods Hand

Especially in the New Kingdom Era and in the tradition of Amun, the High Priestess of Amun took on the title of God's Hand. This tradition followed the ancient history about how God (Amun) brought Creation into existence by masturbating. His seed fell on his own hand and thus his own hand became pregnant and Creation came forth from his own hand. So the priestess performs certain secret and sacred rituals to keep the seed flowing so that Creation may be continually (daily) extended. In so doing she is reenacting the first act of creation and engendering more creation while become one with the Divinity.

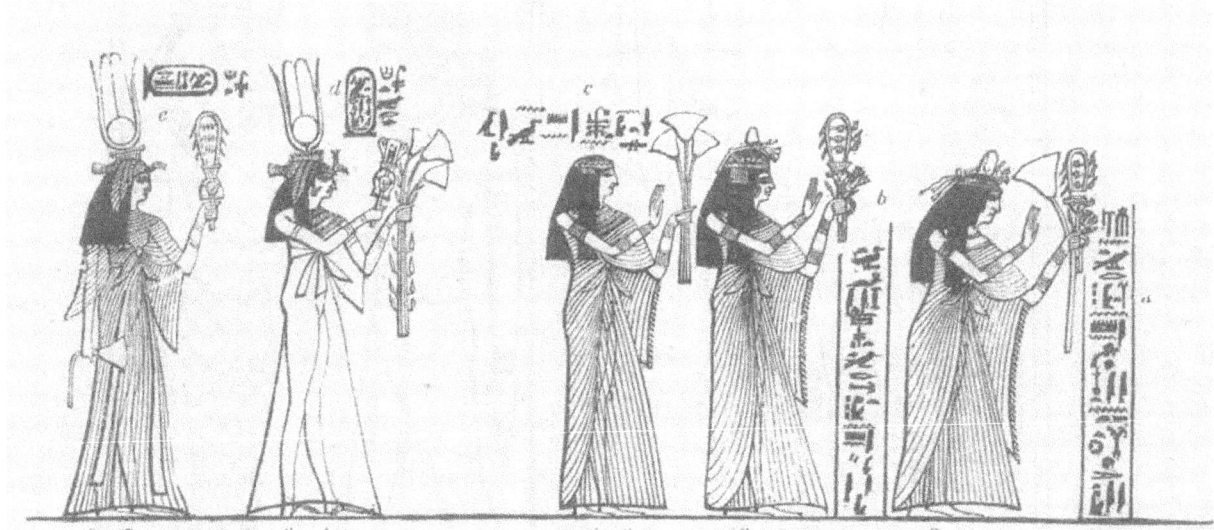

sacred women priestesses making offerings

EGYPTIAN TANTRIC YOGA

The Sublime Vision of Egyptian Tantra Yoga Part I

Tantrism is the recognition that there is no separateness in the universe. It is an understanding that all parts are inseparably related to the whole of creation. The love which most people experience for loved ones exclusively, is a contradiction to the tantric movement. True love is universal and unrestricted. Even though certain things can be loved by you, true love cannot be reserved for a certain person, family, country or planet alone. It is an understanding that the entire universe is an expression of the Divine and as such, worthy of love. Thus, the true expression of love is through service to others in order to promote peace, understanding, harmony. True love requires the sacrifice of the lesser expressions of love (physical contact, sexuality, egoistic desires and sentimental attachments) in order to experience the boundless source of love which is the very nature of the Divine, just as the sun shines on all alike. True love is to be expressed towards all creatures and all existence. This is the epitome of the tantric movement. Love which is reserved for close family members or friends or for a certain country or group, is very limited and constricting to the soul. The soul must evolve to discover an all-encompassing love for the entire universe. When this movement is underway, the drive toward the lower, constricting, forms of love and sexuality are transcended and the sex-energy (Life Force) is sublimated to the fullest degree. This is the kind of love which God has for all creation. When this state of awareness is reached by a human being, there is a transformation which occurs in the human heart. The individual becomes one with all and this transcendental movement is the goal of Tantrism.

As you develop the vision of tantrism through the practice of the teachings outlines here you will begin to realize that all creation is part of a whole and in reality there are no opposites, no separations and no differences. Everything is connected and the outward appearances are only illusions of the senses. Modern science has shown that all matter is composed of the same material. This confirms the Tantric wisdom of ages long past. In reality there is no separation or difference between the Self, the Causal plane, Astral plane and the Physical plane. All creation is in reality one unit which expresses in ways which appear different, through the magic of the opposites. This illusion, known as the *Veil of Aset* in Ancient Egyptian mythology and as *Maya*, the veil of ignorance, in Indian mystical philosophy, when understood, opens the door to discovering the innermost reality of the universe and of the human heart.

With this understanding you should not be deluded by the outward appearances. You should be able to discover inner peace and contentment wherever you are and under any conditions. You should be developing a sense of independence from the externalities of the world. This includes situations of prosperity or adversity, the presence or absence of objects you desire, the presence or absence of loved ones and your own body. As you discover deeper and deeper levels of your own existence the outward manifestation you have up to now considered to be yourself and held so dear will transform into a recognition of your own immortality, infinity and boundless reservoir of universal love.

Mystical Philosophy of Universal Consciousness

Part 5: Icons and Symbols of Kemetic Tantra Mysticism

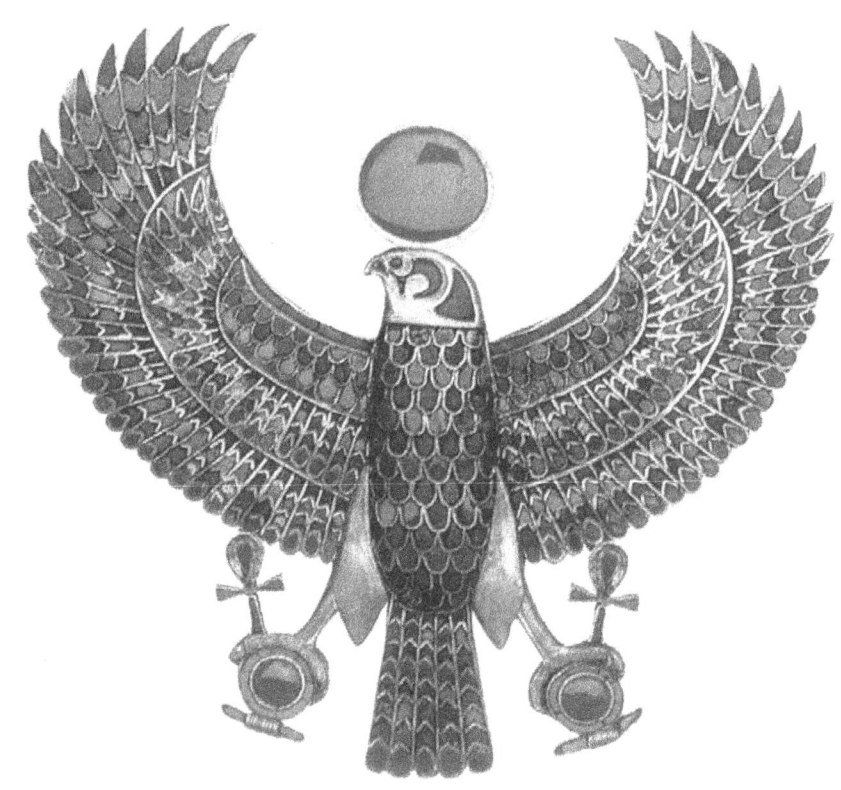

EGYPTIAN TANTRIC YOGA

The Tantric Menat Symbol of Ancient Egypt

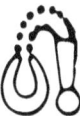

The Menit (menat) necklace is a distinctive ornament of the goddess. The Ancient Egyptian word "Menit" is synonymous with "Hathor" and its root is the Ancient Egyptian word for "nurse". It is held to be the combination of the male and female generative energies combined and so it is the goddess who lifts up the necklace in order to transmit the Life Force energy to the initiate. The energy arouses a movement toward spiritual aspiration and self-discovery leading to Enlightenment.

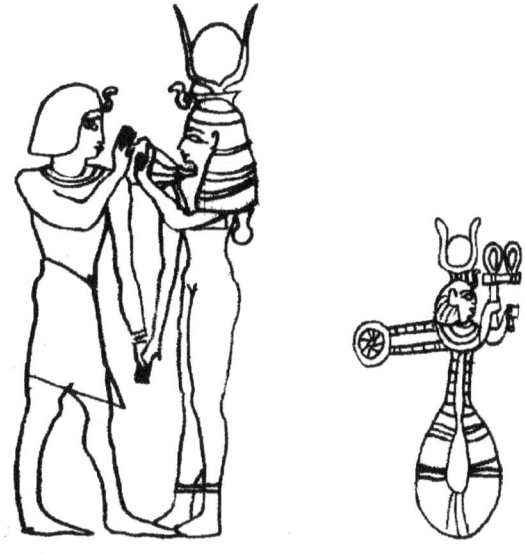

Above: Hathor offers the Menat necklace to a King.

The *Menat* Necklace

Mystical Philosophy of Universal Consciousness

Goddess Hetheru extends the Menat to the King

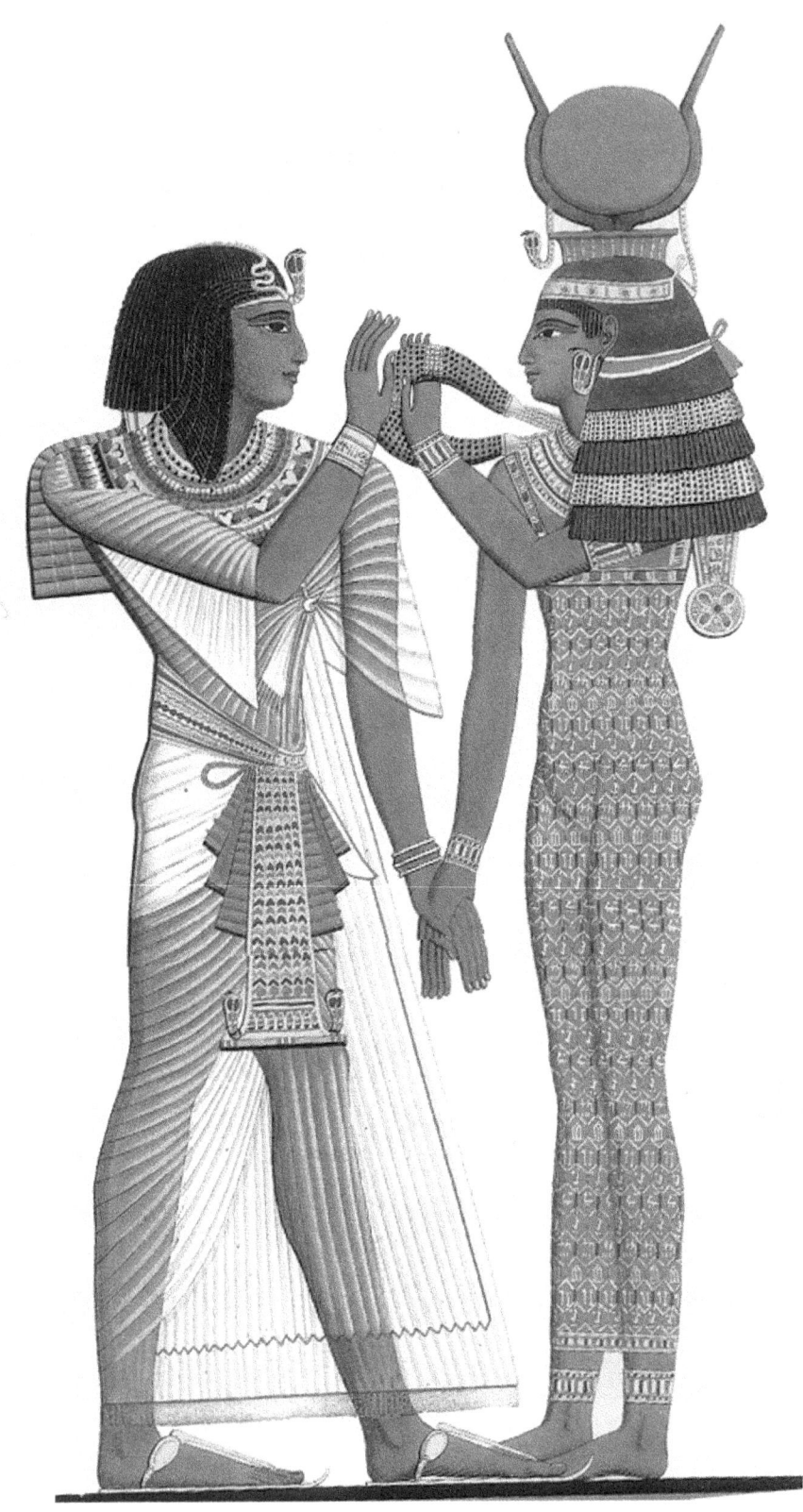

EGYPTIAN TANTRIC YOGA

Tantric Symbolism of The Mystical Ankh

The Ankh, ☥ , is the symbol of the imperishable vital force of life. Related to the life giving properties of air and water, the Ankh depicts three symbolic principles found in creation: 1. the circle (female member) 2. the cross (male member) and 3. unity (the male member united with that of the female). Life literally occurs as a result of the union of spirit and matter, the circle representing the immortal and eternal part (absolute reality) and the cross representing that which is mortal and transient (illusion-matter).

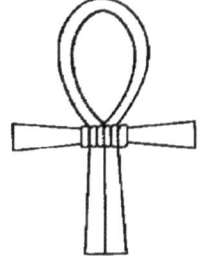

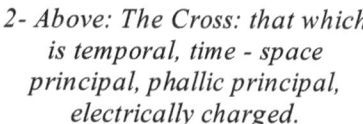
The parts of the Ankh

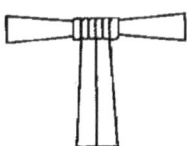

Thus the Ankh refers to life in the form of a human being.

2- Above: The Cross: that which is temporal, time - space principal, phallic principal, electrically charged.

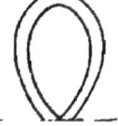

1- Above: The Shen ring: eternity, feminine principal, womb, magnetically charged.

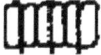

3- Above: The Ankh Knot: That which holds the two principals together, (eternity-temporal, immortal-mortal, spirit-body) creating the human being.

FEMALE

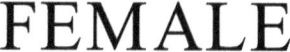
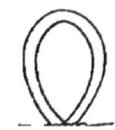
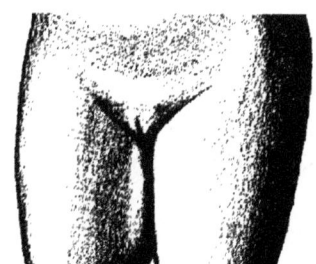

MALE

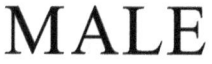
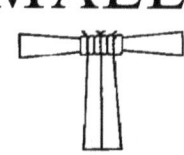
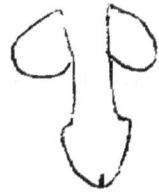

Mystical Philosophy of Universal Consciousness

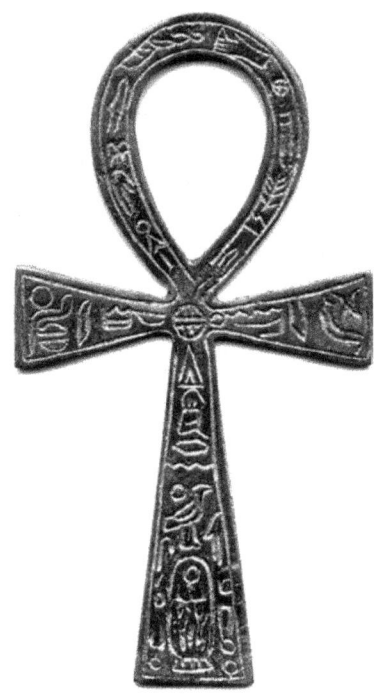

Above: the ancient Egyptian Ankh.

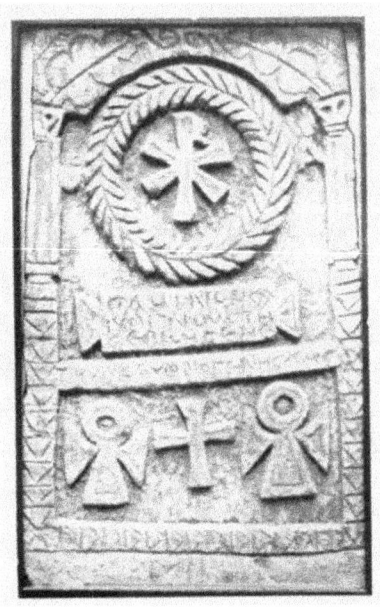

Left: the Christian Ankh Cross as used by the Christians in Egypt (c. first century A.C.E.

At far right: the Christian Ankh.

The Ankh, ☥ , was one of the most common and important symbols of the ancient Egyptian deities. It symbolized life. It was later adopted by early Christianity and also by Hinduism.

EGYPTIAN TANTRIC YOGA

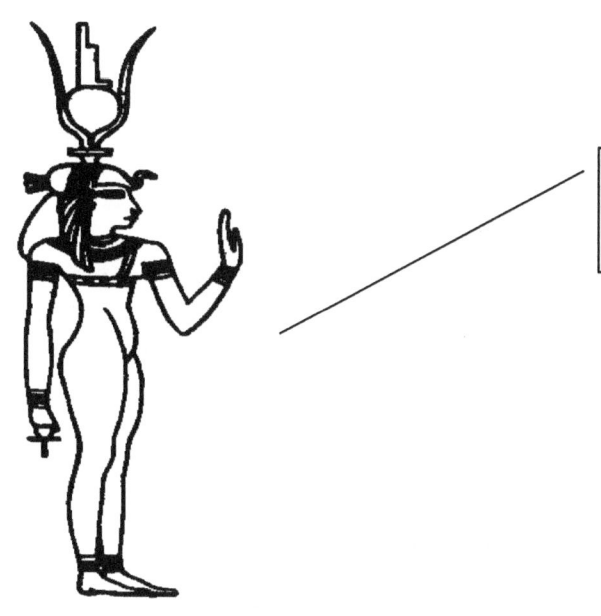

the ancient Egyptian Goddess Isis holding the Ankh.

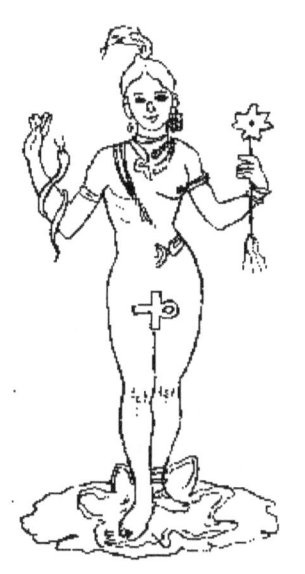

Below right: the Indian-Hindu God/Goddess Ardhanari-Ishwara, displaying the Ankh at the level of the genitalia.

Mystical Philosophy of Universal Consciousness

Thus, as with the Ying and Yang symbol of the Chinese Tao philosophy, the Ankh also symbolizes the balance between the two forces of life, which translates into pairs of opposites, positive-negative, light-dark, long-short, female-male, etc. If properly balanced and cultivated, the power of harmony (union of opposites) is formidable. The top of the Ankh, the circle, represents the Shen, the Egyptian symbol of eternity. In Indian - Hindu Mythology, the Ankh is depicted in the pictures of the androgynous God-Goddess **Ardhanari.** The left side of Ardhanari is female and the right side is male. In Chinese philosophy, the word Shen represents the life force in the cosmos; it is the wisdom-consciousness, the spirit.

The Ankh is also known as the *"key of life."* To give an Ankh to someone in thought or deed is to wish that person life and health. A most important feature of the Ankh symbol is that it is composed of two separable parts. That is to say, the loop at the top (female) and the cross at the bottom (male) are only "tied" together as it were. Therefore, it is possible to loosen the bonds (knots) that tie the spirit to the body and thus make it possible for the soul to attain enlightenment. Ankh may be uttered chanting repeatedly (aloud or mentally) while concentrating on the meaning behind the symbolism. Staring at the symbols either alone or in conjunction with the hekau or simply concentrating on it (alone) mentally will help steady the mind during concentration and meditation.

Tantric Mysticism of the Hetep Offering Table

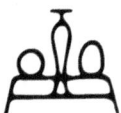

The "Hetep Slab" or Offering Table is another most important tantric symbol from Ancient Egypt. It is composed of a stone slab with male ⟿, thigh, and female ⟿, duck, symbols carved into the top, along with the symbol of Supreme Peace, ⟿, or Hetep, which consists of a loaf of bread, ⊙, and an offering mat, ⟿, which was composed of woven reeds (in predynastic times) and two libation vessels ⫯⫯. In ancient times the actual offering mat consisted of the articles themselves (loaf, thigh, duck and libation fluids (water, wine or milk) but in dynastic times (5,500 B.C.E-400 A.C.E) the table top or slab contained the articles as engraved glyphs. The top of the table has grooves which channel the libations around the offering toward the front and center of the table and then out through the outermost point of the protruding section. The hetep symbol, ⟿, means "rest", "peace" and "satisfaction" and when it is used in the hetep offering ritual it refers to the satisfaction of the neters (gods and goddesses) which comes from uniting the male and female principles into one transcendental being. More specifically it refers to the union of the male and female principle within the human heart, the opposites, and discovering the androgynous Supreme Spirit within. The Hetep Offering Table can be seen in the innermost shrine of the Papyrus of Ani (Book of Coming Forth By Day of Ani) where he is making two offerings, one female and the other male.

EGYPTIAN TANTRIC YOGA

HETEP OFFERING TABLE TOP

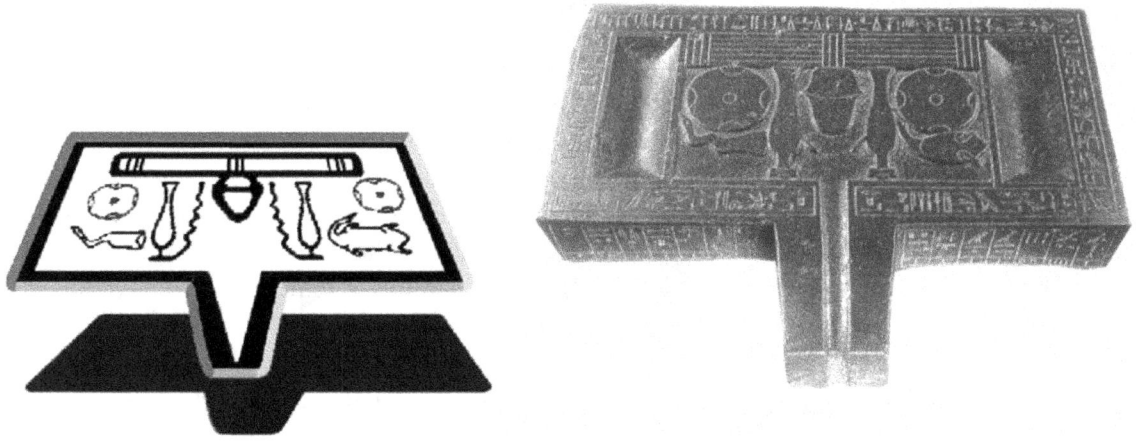

The Hetep Ritual Slab of Africa and the Lingam-Yoni of India

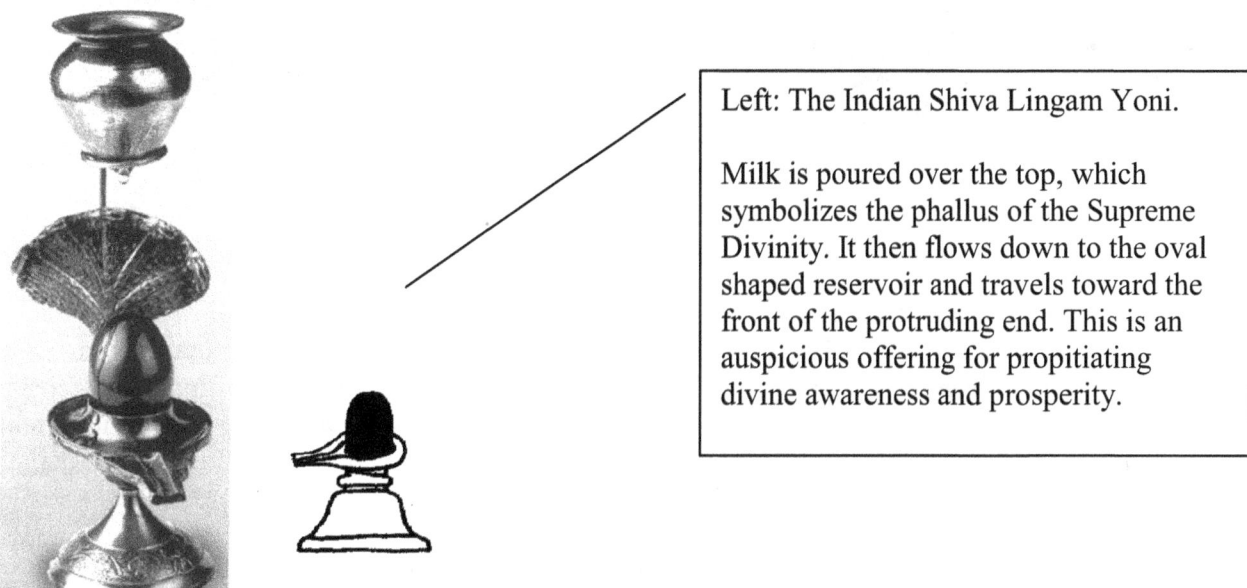

Left: The Indian Shiva Lingam Yoni.

Milk is poured over the top, which symbolizes the phallus of the Supreme Divinity. It then flows down to the oval shaped reservoir and travels toward the front of the protruding end. This is an auspicious offering for propitiating divine awareness and prosperity.

The *Lingam-Yoni* from India is used in the same way as the Hetep Slab of Ancient Egypt. The protruding section symbolizes the male phallus of God (Shiva) and the oval base represents the female vulva (Creation). It symbolizes the union of the male and female sex organs. The libation is poured over the Lingam and it runs down to the Yoni and then it is channeled toward the front and center of the structure and then out through the outermost point of the protruding section. The libation is poured continuously and symbolizes a continuous flow of thought and feeling towards the Divine. Milk is often used in the ritual involving the Lingam-Yoni.

Mystical Philosophy of Universal Consciousness

The Ithyphallic Symbol

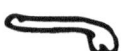

There are many examples of the Ithyphallic (erect penis) motif within Ancient Egyptian symbolism. It implies burgeoning sexual power which impregnates matter and causes life to be. The male god with the erect penis is often seen unmoving, static, while the serpent (the goddess) is coiled around him, in motion. This symbolism may be found with most emphasis in Ancient Egyptian and modern Indian Tantric-mystical iconography. Thus, the iconography of the god and goddess with sexual determinative (erect penis) again points to the union of the opposites. The power which engenders the universe is male and the manifestation is female.

Some of the most important Ancient Egyptian ithyphallic symbols include Asar, Min, Geb, Nebertcher (The All-encompassing Divinity), and **Sekhmet-Bast-Ra, The All-Goddess.**

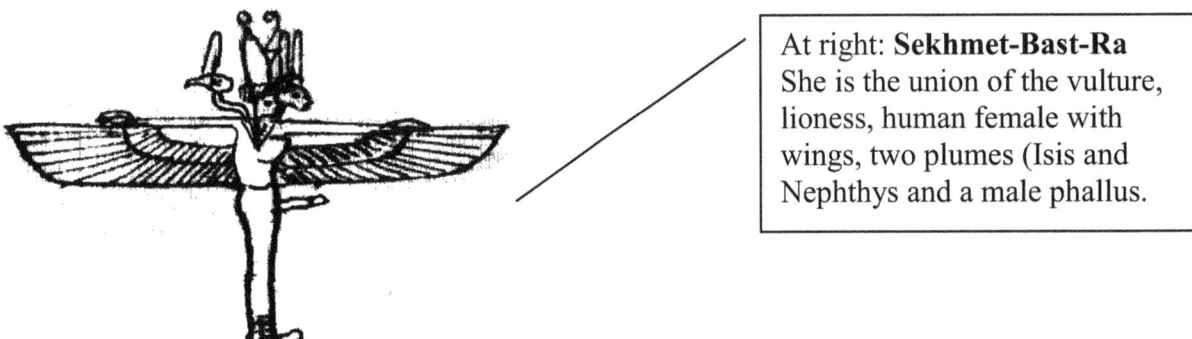

At right: **Sekhmet-Bast-Ra** She is the union of the vulture, lioness, human female with wings, two plumes (Isis and Nephthys and a male phallus.

Sekhmet-Bast-Ra is a composite depiction of the goddess encompassing all of the attributes of the goddesses as well as the attributes of the gods. This is a recognition that all things in creation are not absolutely female or male. All of creation is a combination of male and female elements in varying proportions. Therefore, since creation is androgynous, so too Divinity and the human soul are also androgynous. This understanding is reflected in the following instruction from Aset to Horus from the Ausarian Resurrection.

"Sex is a thing of bodies, not of souls"

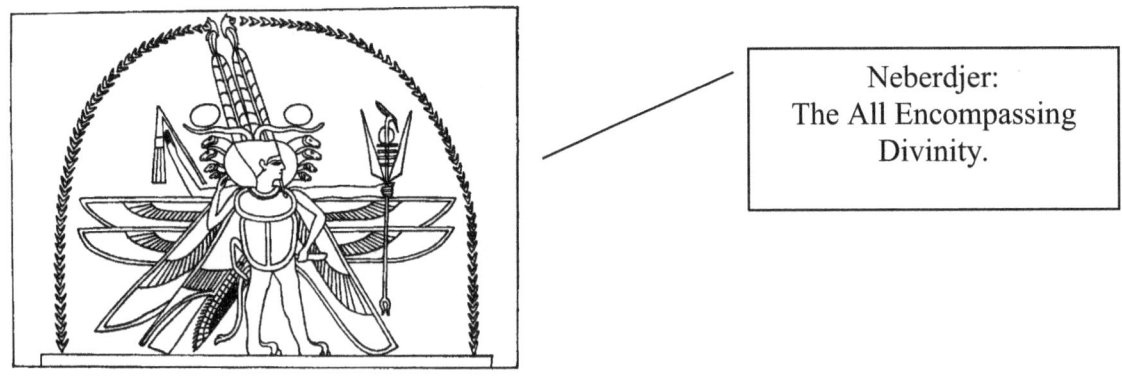

Neberdjer: The All Encompassing Divinity.

EGYPTIAN TANTRIC YOGA

The Lotus Symbol of Ancient Egypt

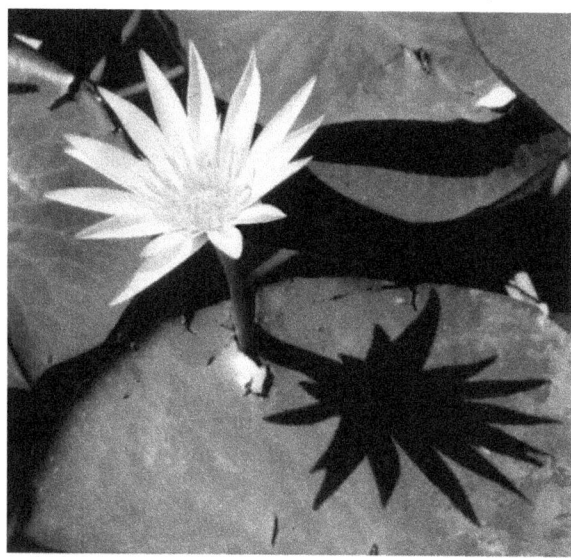

Plate: Above: Sushen -Lotus from Egypt

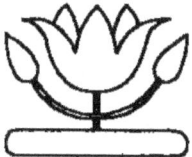

The lotus is the quintessential tantric symbol because it signifies the essence of nature, the Creation, as well as the essence of the Divine Self. The horizontal line at the base of the symbol signifies the primeval ocean. The lotus comes out of the primeval ocean and it itself constitutes Creation itself. That is, the lotus is an extension of the primeval waters, which is itself the body of the Divine Self, God in the form of Ra-Atum. Therefore, the lotus metaphorically relates to the tantric idea that Creation is itself a part of the Divine and that God manifests as Creation. Thus, the underlying non-duality is expressed in one simple and concise image. The philosophy extends our awareness from believing that the Creation and Creator are separate entities to making the connection, bridging the gap to understand the underlying unity of all.

Figure: Below- The God Heru (left) sitting on the lotus.

The symbolic usage of the lotus we just saw in the previous item for comparison is taken to another level when the correlations between the lotuses of Egypt and India are examined more closely. First, in both mythologies the lotus symbolizes the number 1,000 (manifold). Since the lotus opens and turns towards the light of the sun, it is a natural symbol in both Neterianism and Hinduism of turning towards the light of the Divine Spirit. Further, the lotus symbolizes dispassion in both mythologies as it grows in the muddy waters but remains untouched by the waters due to a special coating. So too a spiritual aspirant must remain detached from the world even while continuing to live and work in it, while at the same time turning away from the world and towards the Divine. In both mythologies the symbol is used to represent the creation itself, which emerges out of the murky, disordered waters of primeval potential in order to establish

Mystical Philosophy of Universal Consciousness

order and truth and make a way for life. The lotus also symbolizes the glorious fragrance of the Divine Self as well as the state of spiritual enlightenment. Thus, the symbol that was first used in Ancient Egypt was adopted in India, and though the name changes from Sushen (Kamitan - a source for the English name "Susan") to Padma (Hindu) its symbolism, number, myth and usage remained the same.

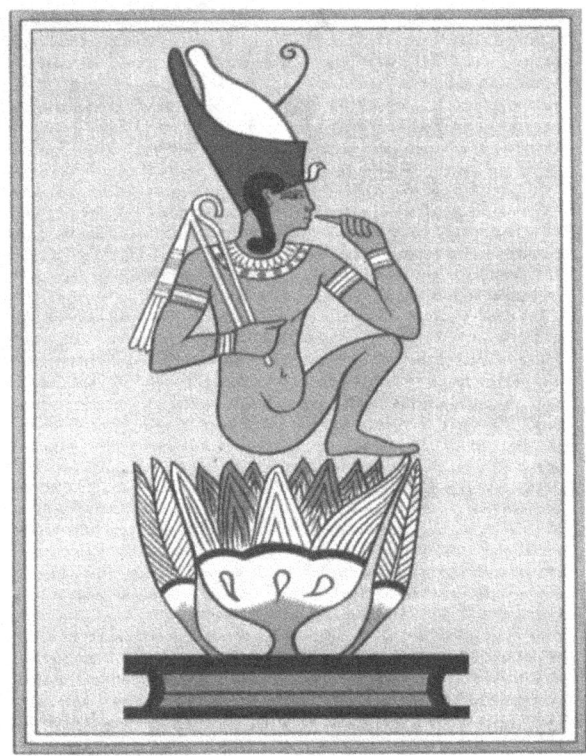

The God Heru-Nefertem symbolizes the archetypal ideal of spiritual mastery and absolute consciousness. He sits on the lotus as its master, pointing to the mouth as the controller through word-sound. Nefertem means "beautiful-completion" signifying absolute wholeness, fullness and all-encompassingness. As such we are to understand that the Divine towers over Creation as its controller and master but from the perspective of essence. The Divine is the essence of Creation, composing its dual aspects, underlying these and binding as well as uniting them into one. Thus, the image is to be reverenced, and meditated upon and its teaching realized in order to attain spiritual enlightenment.

There is one more important tantric teaching about the lotus. Smelling the lotus signifies opening to the consciousness of the Creator. Scientific experimentation has shown that the Ancient Egyptian lotus has the effect of the modern day Ginko Biloba herb and the drug Viagra. This opening up of the vascular system and the mental pathways facilitates expansion in consciousness.

EGYPTIAN TANTRIC YOGA

THE TANTRIC SYMBOLISM OF THE ANCIENT EGYPTIAN PYRAMID

The Ancient Egyptian Pyramid represents important tantric symbolism. It provides mystical insight into the nature of numbers and to the relationship between the physical world and the transcendental Self. The mystical symbolism of the number four refers to the four sides of the pyramid (d-e-f-g). Four is the number of time and space, the physical universe. The single side of the pyramid, being a triangle, represents the number three as well as the Trinity of existence which manifests both as a Divine Trinity of Gods and Goddesses in the form of Father, Mother and Child such as Asar, Aset and Horus or the Divine Trinity of Amun, Ra, Ptah, who refer to the triad of human consciousness (waking, dream and deep sleep) and the essence of existence (witnessing consciousness, mind and the physical universe (see the book *The Hymns of Amun* by Dr. Muata Ashby. The number four is an emanation of the number three and the number three is an emanation of the number two and the number two (duality) is an emanation of the one, singular and non-dual essence (God). Thus, the multiplicity comes together at the top (h) into one point, known as the *Eye of Horus* which represents universal consciousness. Thus, the pyramid is a Tantric symbol which shows how creation and the Divine are inseparably related.

The pyramid as viewed from above.

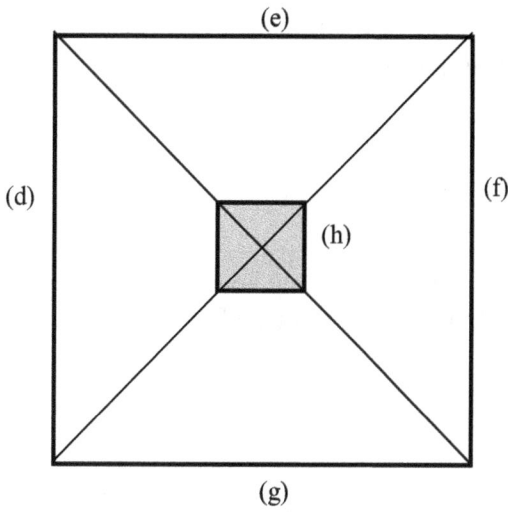

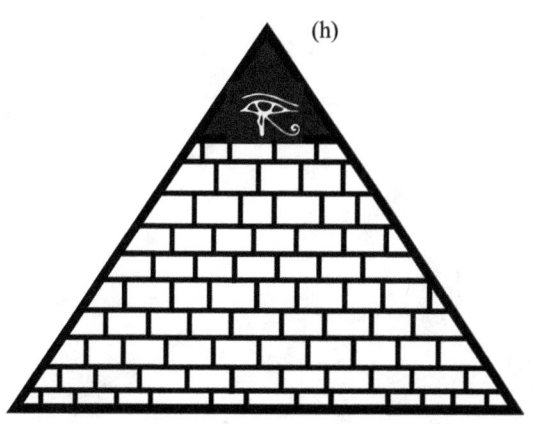

Mystical Philosophy of Universal Consciousness

Tantric Symbolism of the Spinx

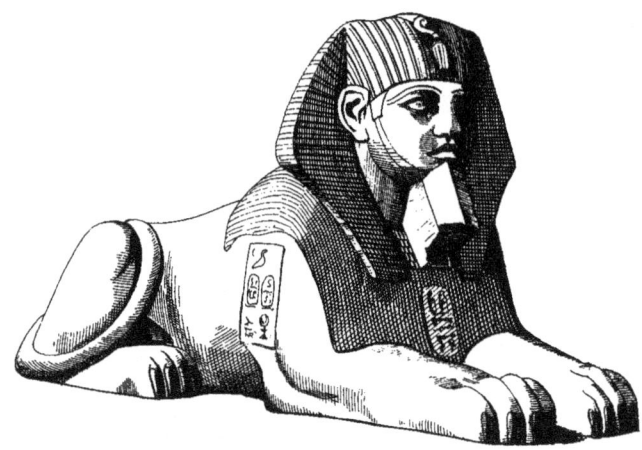

In many ways the Hormakhet (Sphinx) represents the ultimate conception of the Kemetic Tantric ideal. Composed of a human head and a lions body, the symbolism turns us towards the notion of a united higher and lower Self, the spirit and matter are connected, i.e. "tantrasized." Again the tantrism of the sphinx makes use of the serpentine symbolism, with the arat (serpent) at the forehead.

Below- the Ancient Egyptian Hor-m-Akhet (Sphinx).

The archeological and geological evidence surrounding the great Sphinx in Giza, Egypt, Africa, shows that it was created no later than 10,000 B.C.E. to 7,000 B.C.E. This gives us the understanding that Kamit, Ancient Egypt, produced the earliest known artifacts, which denotes civilization. Thus, the Kamitan or Ancient Egyptian civilization is the oldest known civilization in our history.

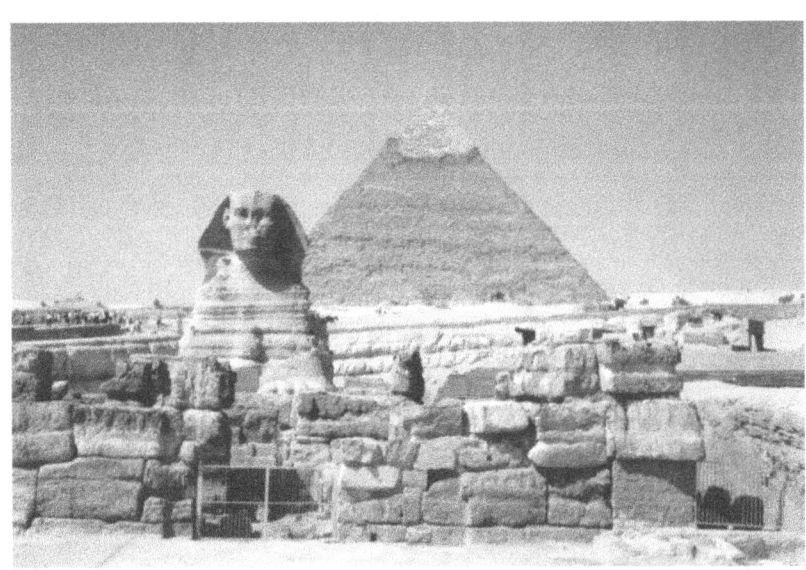

EGYPTIAN TANTRIC YOGA

It is important to understand that what we have in the Sphinx is not just a monument now dated as the earliest monument in history (based on irrefutable geological evidence). Its existence signifies the earliest practice not only of high-art and architecture, but it is also the first monumental statue in history dedicated to religion and tantric philosophy. This massive project including the Sphinx and its attendant Temple required intensive planning and engineering skill. Despite its deteriorated state, the Sphinx stands not only as the most ancient mystical symbol in this historical period, but also as the most ancient architectural monument, and a testament to the presence of Ancient African (Egyptian) culture in the earliest period of antiquity. Further, this means that while the two other emerging civilizations of antiquity (Sumer and Indus) were in their Neolithic period (characterized by the development of agriculture, pottery and the making of polished stone implements), Ancient Egypt had already achieved mastery over monumental art, architecture and religion as an adjunct to social order, as the Sphinx is a symbol of the Pharaoh (leader and upholder of Maat-order, justice and truth) as the god Heru. The iconography of the Sphinx is typical of that which is seen throughout Ancient Egyptian history and signals the achievement of the a culture of high morals which governs the entire civilization to the Persian and Greek conquest. The Sphinx is the oldest known monument and it relates to the solar mysticism of Anu as well as to the oldest form of spiritual practice known. From it we also derive certain important knowledge in reference to the antiquity of civilization in Ancient Egypt.

The Great Sphinx and its attendant monuments as well as other structures throughout Egypt which appear to be compatible architecturally should therefore be considered as part of a pinnacle of high culture that was reached well before the Dynastic age, i.e. previous to 5,000 B.C.E. The form of the Sphinx itself, displaying the lion body with the human head, but also with the particularly "leonine" headdress including the lion's mane, was a legacy accepted by the Pharaohs of the Dynastic Period. In the Ancient Egyptian mythological system of government, the Pharaoh is considered as a living manifestation of Heru and he or she wields the leonine power which comes from the sun, Ra, in order to rule. Thus, the Pharaohs also wore and were depicted wearing the leonine headdress. The sundisk is the conduit through which the Spirit transmits Life Force energy to the world, i.e. the Lion Power, and this force is accessed by turning towards the Divine in the form of the sun. Hence, the orientation of the Sphinx towards the east, facing the rising sun. All of this mystical philosophy and more is contained in the symbolic-metaphorical form and teaching of the Sphinx. Thus, we have a link of Ancient Egyptian culture back to the Age of Leo and the commencement of the current cycle of the Great Year in remote antiquity.

Heru-m-akhet or "Heru in the Horizon" or "manifesting" in the horizon, the "Sphinx," actually represents an ancient conjunction formed by the great Sphinx in Giza, Egypt and the heavens. This conjunction signals the beginning of the "New Great Year." It has been noted by orthodox as well as nonconformist Egyptologists alike, that the main symbolisms used in Ancient Egypt vary over time Nonconformist Egyptilogists see this as a commemoration of the zodiacal symbol pertaining to the particular Great Month in question. What is controversial to the orthodox Egyptologists is the implication that the Ancient Egyptians marked time by the Great Year, and this would mean that Ancient Egyptian civilization goes back 12 millenniums, well beyond any other civilization in history. This further signifies that all of the history books and concepts related to history and the contributions of Africa to humanity would have to be

Mystical Philosophy of Universal Consciousness

rewritten. Also, since it has been shown that the Ancient Egyptians commemorated the Zodiacal sign of Leo at the commencement of the Great Year it means that the knowledge of the precession of the equinoxes, the Great Year and the signs of the Zodiac proceeded from Ancient Egypt to Babylon and Greece and not the other way around. The twelve zodiacal signs for these constellations were named by the 2nd-century astronomer Ptolemy, as follows: Aries (ram), Taurus (bull), Gemini (twins), Cancer (crab), Leo (lion), Virgo (virgin), Libra (balance), Scorpio (scorpion), Sagittarius (archer), Capricorn (goat), Aquarius (water-bearer), and Pisces (fishes).

One striking form of symbolism that is seen from the beginning to the end of the Ancient Egyptian history is the Sphinx/Pharaonic Leonine headdress.

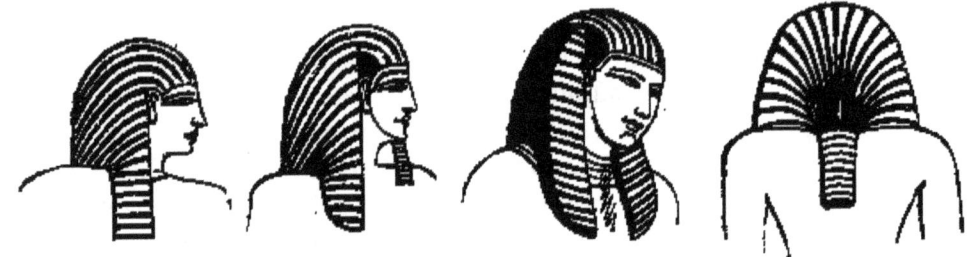

Figure: Above- The Heru-m-akhet (Sphinx) Pharaonic headdress.[19]

Figure: Below- Drawing of the Sphinx from a sculpture in Egypt

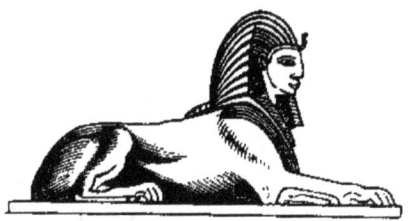

For more on the teaching of the Heru-m-akhet see the book Anunian Theology by Muata Ashby

The Tantric Teachings of The Egyptian Book of Coming Forth By Day

The *Egyptian Book of Coming Forth By Day* is indeed the ritualization of the myth of Asar, Aset and Horus. It is the means by which the deeper mystical implications of the myth are to be understood and practiced. Therefore, it represents the stage in which the teachings of the myth are to be practiced and lived. If a myth is simply read and looked upon as entertainment or as an amusing form of diversion it will not have a profound effect on the mind and it will not cause a transformation leading to enlightenment. However, if it is correctly understood and *lived*, then its teachings will be understood and the truths within them will be realized. This is the goal of any true mystical philosophy.

There are several examples of Tantric symbolism in the ancient Egyptian *Book of Coming Forth By Day*. Many times they are references which refer to the "Eye" which represents the eye of intuitional spiritual wisdom at the sixth spiritual energy center at the forehead. At other times,

---

[19] These illustrations appeared in the book *The Ancient Egyptians: Their Life and Customs*-Sir J. Garner Wilkinson 1854 A.C.E.

they are references to the back or the spine-vertebrae, signifying the four upper spiritual centers which comprise the higher levels of development which are also related to the Djed Pillar (back-vertebrae) of Asar. The following are some of those references.

> I filled Asar, the scribe Ani, triumphant, for thee the *Utchat* after it had failed on the day of the battle of the two Fighters.
> What then is it?
> It is the day of the fight between Horus and Set. Set throwing excrement in the face of Horus and then Horus carrying off the testicles of Set, for Djehuti did this with his fingers himself. I raise up the hair in the time of storms in the sky.
> What then is it?
> It is the Right Eye of Ra in its raging against him after he had made it depart. Djehuti raises up the hair there, and he brings the eye, living, healthy and sound, without defect to its lord;
> Otherwise said, it is the eye when it is sick, when it is weeping for its fellow; Djehuti stands up then to wash it.
> **Egyptian Book of Coming Forth By Day - Ch. 17, 65-74**

Here the scribe Ani is identified with Asar and there is an allusion to the battle between Horus and Set where at one point Set got the upper hand over Horus because Horus' *Eye* was temporarily incapacitated. The point is once again plainly made, that it is through Djehuti, that Horus is able to finally prevail over Set. By taking control of himself through reason and self-control (Djehuti), Horus is able to activate his *Eye of intuitional vision,* which is the eye of reason that burns up the impurities of the mind (ignorance, anger, hatred, greed etc.)

The "storms" represent confusion, frustration and conflict in the mind. The storm dishevels the hair and causes it to fall down over the forehead. This is a subtle reference to the "third Eye" or the sixth psycho-spiritual energy center which represents intuitional vision. It's mystical location is at the forehead. When there is a storm of emotions, ignorance, passion and desire, intuitional vision, that is perceiving the spiritual reality, becomes blocked. Djehuti (reason) uncovers the eye and allows the spiritual vision to emerge again. It is also Horus (as an aspect of Djehuti) who emasculated Set. This means that Set's sexual power was taken away and placed under the control of reason. Thus, when sexual energy and emotion are controlled and channelized, spiritual wisdom and victory in the battle of life (struggle of Horus and Set), which leads to spiritual enlightenment, can occur.

"Like is He unto that which he hath made, and became his name."

Egyptian Book of Coming Forth By Day
17:20

The hekau above is a profound exposition of Tantric philosophy. It imparts the wisdom that He (God) is like unto what He has made (the universe). There is no separation between God and creation that can be detected or inferred in his statement. It is a perfect and concise understanding of the wisdom we have already studied and it is the basis of the Theologies of

Mystical Philosophy of Universal Consciousness

Asar, Ra, Amun, Ptah and Aset. Creation itself is *The God* (Neter). This is a most important point which a spiritual aspirant should reflect on at all times. From the smallest sub-atomic particle to the most gigantic heavenly body, all is the Divine. All is the Self. Through your studies of the teachings you have learned that what your senses present to you has been and is illusory. You have learned that everything that exists has the same substratum or source and sustenance. Now you must begin to understand that this entire universe is not different from the Divine. Think about it. Think about all of the people you know, are they not composed of elements? Are those elements not composed of atoms? Are those atoms not composed of energy? Is this booklet you are reading not composed of the same material? How about the earth, the sun, the stars? How about your own body, the air you breath, the food you eat, are these not the same substance? They are! Go even further, what is the substance of your thoughts, your dreams? It is all an expression of the same essence.

Remaining quiet in a closed place, close the booklet here. Take a comfortable seated position and close your eyes and reflect on this.

Now think of your relationships, your family members and everyone you have ever known. They have the same source which is also your source. Right now do not focus on their outer appearance, their ethnic origins or their actions. Simply look into their deeper essence and realize that this is the same source, the same substratum from which all is given existence. Deep down we are all the same but also we are the same on the surface as well. Consider the skin, consider the outer surface of any person, object or thing in creation. Is it not made of elements, atoms and energy? This is Tantric thought. This is the unifying force of mystical awareness and when this way of thinking is practiced it counteracts the thoughts of separation and ignorance because this way of thinking is based on truth and reality and reality leads to enlightenment, the spiritual resurrection of the soul.

Remaining quiet in a closed place, close the booklet here. Close your eyes and reflect on this.

From the perspective of the mystical teachings of Tantrism, every act which occurs in the realm of time and space is sexual. In the spiritual scriptures before creation, it is said the Self (God) was alone and devoid of form. This is the Primeval Ocean. As soon as the Self or Soul interacts with thoughts, feelings or physical objects through the mind and senses and the body there is a duality which must be present, the Self and the other. In reality only the Self exists and the "other" objects (anything other than the Self - thoughts, feelings, desires, physical objects, human beings, animals, plants, planets, stars, etc.) are like emanations which have come out of The Self. This is likened to a person's mind when they dream. When there is a dream, an entire world system arises seemingly out of nowhere and when the person awakens that world recedes back into "nowhere". That nowhere is the deep unconscious mind. In the same way, this world has arisen out of the cosmic mind (God) and this physical world is considered as the "other" or opposite to the Self. As soon as there is an "other" there is duality and as soon as there is duality there is interaction. In tantric symbolism this interaction is portrayed as a sexual union wherein the male principle (the Self) infuses the female (Creation) in the same manner as a person having a dream infuses his/her own consciousness with thoughts, objects, desires and feelings in order to create an entire universe within the mind.

EGYPTIAN TANTRIC YOGA

The danger in going from the principle of one (non-duality) to the principle of duality is the danger of forgetting the original oneness and falling into the delusion that duality is the true state of being. This is the predicament of human embodiment, which is experienced by the soul. Despite the higher reality of oneness, people believe that all objects in creation are separate and unrelated. This causes a state of delusion which gives rise to egoism and other negative qualities of the mind (anger, hatred, greed). If there is awareness of truth, there cannot be negativity and ignorance. This is the goal of tantric philosophy.

The Role of Sexuality in Human Relationships and Society

Modern society and mass culture promote sexuality as a means to experiencing pleasure and feeling good about oneself. As an externality, sexuality cannot be depended on just as one cannot depend on the weather. Therefore, on a very basic logical level, the dependence on sexuality as a means to feel wanted, youthful or vital is in reality a profound farce into which the human mind has fallen. As old age sets in those who have based their life on the premise above begin to feel lost because they cannot keep up the activities of the past. This is the source of mid life crAset as well as adultery and many other problems in relationships.

Relationships which are based on sex, demands, and expectations are doomed to experience strife because none of these are stable factors even in ordinary relationships which do not include sexual intercourse. The source of the problem lies in the ignorance of the higher purpose and destiny of the human soul. Sexual energy is the driving force of life and its purpose is to assist the soul in carrying out the goals of a lifetime, specifically to gain knowledge and wisdom of the Self which leads to enlightenment. This is accomplished through promoting a process which leads to development and integration of the intellectual and emotional elements of one's psyche through the relationships, occupation and life ambitions. If the relationships, occupation and life ambitions have as the main goal to provide pleasure, then they are doomed to failure. A person with this goal will experience constant need to pursue activities in the hope of achieving pleasure, like a drug addict must continually get drops to experiencing a high only to find that the high is diminishing and the body is gradually being destroyed. However, if the relationships, occupation and life ambitions are based on the understanding that they are tools which the soul has been given to promote spiritual advancement then they can be as a ladder to heaven.

So relationships based on spiritual principles should not be demanding or promoting expectations from others. Many people develop the idea that if a partner does not want to engage in sex that this means the partner is losing love or having an adulterous affair. There is no trust in the relationship because "love" has been equated with sex. Therefore, the absence of sex means an absence of love. Often times the feeling of being wanted and appreciated has been equated with sex and so people seek sexual relations as a means to feel wanted and appreciated. Many people set conditions for their love and impose demands on others: "If you do this I will do that for you", "If you don't do this then that means that you don't love me". These statements are based on ignorance, immaturity and dependence and will inevitably lead to strife, disappointment and unrest in a relationship.

Mystical Philosophy of Universal Consciousness

A true relationship will not be based on sexuality, demands or conditions. However, through understanding, forgiveness, control of the sexual urge and the development of higher goals in life, sex and vows can be a means to discover a greater connection in a relationship. True love and friendship is an open door. There will be no conditions or demands. When a relationship is based on these principles each partner can feel secure and not need to search for comfort elsewhere. As old age sets in, both have set into motion a process wherein the sexual feelings have been sublimated into a spiritual union with each other as well as with the higher Self within. This leads to frustration and bitterness in old age. When life is based on selfishness, personal desires, demands and fear, it leads to sorrow and contraction in consciousness leading to intensification of egoism and all of the negative qualities in human nature. When life is lived based on the principles of mystical spirituality (Tantric Philosophy) it leads to expansion in consciousness and the unfoldment of universal love in the human heart. Therefore, peace and harmony are promoted and enhanced as life goes on. While true love is universal, this should not be taken to mean that the mystical teachings promote a philosophy commonly referred to as "free love". In reality, the modern free love movement which promotes promiscuity and multiple partners is an escape from the true necessity of life which is sexual restraint. It is an attempt to justify and promote sexual indulgence with multiple partners in an attempt to achieve greater sexual gratification. In the end this movement leads to depletion of the vital forces, diseases, and it promotes mental unrest and disappointment in relationships as well as the inability to discover true love and caring. Universal love, from the mystical point of view, implies discovering that all life is an expression of the Divine and that one's very self, the innermost reality within the heart, is filled with boundless love and peace. Therefore universal love refers to a caring that encompasses the entire universe. It is a vision which comes from living a life of selflessness, public service and sex sublimation. When these principles are promoted, the desire for expressing sexual feelings give way to the higher purposes of life, a sexual communion with the universe. When this occurs, great inventions and advancements in all areas of society are brought forth from the men and women who are able to control, sublimate and transcend the gross level of sexual expression. In this context, those who act for the benefit of others, those who work for the benefit of humanity, are to be considered as advanced souls. Their legacy is the light of knowledge, peace, harmony, virtue and love which inspire others to achieve great heights in life. Universal love is the promotion of universal peace and justice for all. It implies sharing one's skills and expertise for the purpose of lifting others up so that they may experience the elevated levels of human existence and spiritual glory. It implies an understanding that even those who do evil deeds have the same divine basis as everyone else. However, they are misguided due to ignorance. Therefore, universal love implies forgiveness and the willingness to chastise others when they commit evil acts in order that they should learn the proper way to live based on truth. Universal love is a most advanced development in human evolution and at its height it leads to universal consciousness and spiritual enlightenment, in effect, communing with the universal source of love, the Supreme Self (God).

"When opulence and extravagance are a necessity instead of righteousness and truth, society will be governed by greed and injustice."

Ancient Egyptian Proverb

When society bases its values on sex and material wealth, there develops a process wherein young people become misguided as to the purpose of life and set out to satisfy the urges of the lower self as soon as possible. Oblivious to the higher spiritual reality, young people confuse love with sex, money and fame and thus travel the self-destructive path wherein their actions lead to detrimental situations and the decay of society. An example of this is the growing numbers of teen-age mothers who desired to become pregnant in order to "have somebody to love" and or to "get a boy to love and stay with them" or for the pursuit of pleasure, not thinking about the consequences. The boys on the other hand feel that "sex is a pleasure tool and that if the girl got pregnant it is her problem", and so they shirk any responsibility. Others feel that females are objects to be used and so treat them as possessions to be controlled against their will. Others profess to be devoid of sexual misconduct simply because they do not say or do things which are considered evil by society. However, in their thoughts they harbor desires, longings and other secret expectations and these inevitably lead to gross expressions in the form of disapproval, hatred, lust, resentment, etc. against others.

Procreation is a tool of nature which is used to bring about the possibility for spiritual evolution by providing a place for the soul to gain human experiences. If it is used for the purpose of personal pleasure it will lead to pain and sorrow. However, if it is used as a part of life when a relationship is ready to produce offspring then it is a source of inspiration, greater closeness and spiritual awareness. An advanced society should not promote sexual intercourse before the age of 25 and outside of a situation wherein the parents will be responsible for the child. Also the society should be ready to assist in caring for the child.

Every member of society should be expected to promote justice and righteousness by chastising and educating any child wherever he or she may be acting in a negative way. This principle follows an ancient African tradition embodied in the proverb: "It takes a whole village to raise one child". Therefore, the society is also responsible for the development of children and it will be the recipient of the positive or negative development of every member of society. In modern times people are more interested in their own lives rather than the community so they do not care when others are in trouble or threatened by the negative elements. So the "village" is in need of spiritual upliftment as well. It cannot survive if its citizens are selfish, deluded, weak, and frustrated. These are the conditions which breed criminal behavior and self-destruction in society.

All of the aberrant behaviors which have been outlined above, that are in contradiction with the precepts of MAAT (righteousness, order, truth), developed out of the ignorance of the true meaning and purpose of life. The soul uses the body in order to progress spiritually. In reality it is neither male nor female but chooses one of these in order to gain specific forms of knowledge and experience. In general, when the soul needs to experience and grow in the area of emotions it incarnates as a female personality; when it needs to develop in the area of reasoning it incarnates as a male personality. However, through the process of reincarnation it has experienced many male and female lifetimes. Therefore, the egoism and vanity of maleness or femaleness, the pride, conceit and indulgence in sexuality in gross as well as subtle ways, is in reality an expression of ignorance of the truth of the soul.

The level of maturity in an individual may be gauged by the values which are held. If an individual values that which is transient, ephemeral and superficial this is clearly a sign of spiritual immaturity. If the values given more importance are those things which are lasting and

Mystical Philosophy of Universal Consciousness

abiding, and which lead to truth, wisdom, inner peace and justice, then the individual is moving toward spiritual maturity and emancipation from the world of human pain and suffering. In the same way, societies may be measured as to their level of development. If a society promotes that which is superficial it is considered to be immature. In Ancient Egypt, the tallest and largest buildings were the temples. In fact, the largest structure, known to the ancient world was the Temple known today as the Great Pyramid at Giza. At the top of this structure was a depiction of the *"Eye of Horus"* representing spiritual vision. This shows that Ancient Egyptian society placed spiritual values above those of the lower nature. In modern times, society placed the greatest value on sex, money, and fame. Spiritual wealth in the form of mental peace and self-discovery are abiding principles which are carried forth after death which leads to spiritual expansion and union with God. Sex, money and fame are only useful when there is a body to experience these with. After death they engender restlessness and ignorance in the deep unconsciousness. Therefore, the predilection (a disposition in favor of something; preference) toward the superficial, egoistic values of life denotes immaturity as a civilization and foreshadows future disharmony in society.

The predilection toward material values produces progeny who become the embodiment of Setian feelings, emotions and desires (anger, greed, unrest, egoism, selfishness, conceit, vanity, pleasure seeking, personal gratification, etc.) which lead to callousness, hardheartedness and predatory behaviors towards others. With these feelings it becomes possible to desecrate all that is good even while professing to be righteous and upstanding, while insidiously engineering the destruction of others for personal gain. Examples of this are to be found not only in the ordinary criminal ranks of society who openly engage in violence, stealing and selling substances which promote physical and mental deterioration and suffering (poisons such as drugs, alcohol and tobacco) but also in society at large. Some examples include medical doctors who tell patients that they must have operations even when they don't need them, lawyers who promote litigation in order to gain more fees, business people who sell products which are not good for society (items which promote pollution, do not work as advertised, promote the prurient interests (pornography), promote vanity and self-centeredness, etc.).

The sublimation of the sex drive is the mother of all sublime thoughts and aspirations in human consciousness as well as the source for the will power to carry those visions to completion. Thus, procreation as well as the creative expression of consciousness in the form of inventions and social advancements, both have their proper place in the scheme which has been set for by the Divine, through the medium of nature and human existence. Therefore, Tantrism, is the practice of studying the teachings related to understanding the nature of creation which expresses as pairs of opposites (male and female) that have a common source in the Supreme Self, who is without sex, form or any kind of conditioning. Tantrism is the study of sexuality and its influence on human consciousness as well as the wisdom it holds as a symbol of the Divine. It is not an excuse to indulge in sexuality, but a profound study and mystical practice of discovering the underlying oneness behind all creation.

EGYPTIAN TANTRIC YOGA

Kemetic Tantra Yoga and the Serpent Power

As mentioned earlier, the form of yoga which concerns the development of the latent Life Force energy within all human beings is a part of Tantric philosophy. In Ancient Egypt it was presided over by the goddesses Arat, Uadjit and Nekhebet. In India it is presided over by Goddess Kundalini, thus it is known in India as Kundalini Yoga. The inner Life Force is likened to a serpent because its movements are likened to the coils of a serpent.

The Life Force energy lies dormant at the base of the spine awaiting the time when the human being is pure in mind and body so as to manifest the higher spiritual dimensions of consciousness. Otherwise it remains dormant at the lower levels of psycho-spiritual consciousness as long as a person lives according to the lower nature (ignorance, lust, greed, etc.) As spiritual development unfolds it moves upward through seven psycho-spiritual energy centers until it reaches the pinnacle at the crown of the head and unites the individual's consciousness with the cosmos. This union symbolizes the joining of the individuals awareness with that of the universe (God), thus it is known as cosmic consciousness. Expansion in consciousness is a factor of sublimated sexual energy. Those who create in the plane of elevated thoughts and philosophical ideals are using the same energy which others use to conceive children on the physical plane. However, the conception of progeny on the physical plane is limited and perishable while the conception in the form of one's own conscious expansion is limitless and infinite. This is the highest vision of sexuality within the Tantric ideal, the union of opposites which begets expanded consciousness, supreme harmony, peace and bliss.

The Life Force energy is a drive toward expansion. Whenever the energy is blocked or obstructed the result is negativity and disease. When there is expansion there is health and bliss. Negative emotions, and delusions about where to find true happiness constitute the source of blockages in the movement of the Life Force energy. Therefore, Tantric philosophy encompasses a program for cleansing the mind and body so as to propitiate the positive movement of the Life Force energy. This can be accomplished by living according to the teachings of Tantric Philosophy described in this volume.

The Greenfield Papyrus, the Papyrus of Kenna and the Pillar of Asar contain three of the most striking symbols of the life Force energy and its movement. Within Ancient Egyptian iconography they detail the psycho-spiritual evolution in a human being. The scenes in the Greenfield and Kenna papyruses presented here come from the portion known as the "weighing of the heart." The scene presents the heart of the spiritual aspirant being weighed against spiritual truth (Maat). The heart of the initiate is composed of seven centers of psycho-spiritual consciousness depicted as circles or rings. The picture from the Papyrus of Kenna shows Ammit, the monster who devours the unrighteous. Notice that he is biting the scales of MAAT between the third and fourth circles. These circles indicate levels of spiritual evolution or psycho-spiritual consciousness. The Greenfield Papyrus shows the centers as a chain with seven links at the end of which the heart hangs down. These centers refer to the judgment of the heart of the initiate. Centers 1-3 indicate immature human beings who live to seek sensual pleasures (food, sex, control or competition with others) and centers 4-7 indicate individuals who are progressing on the spiritual path (selfless love, self-control, intuitional vision, expansion in consciousness). The symbol of the serpent at the level of the brow which is so well-known in Ancient Egypt indicates

Mystical Philosophy of Universal Consciousness

the energy consciousness at the level of the sixth energy center and the serpent on the top of the head refers to the energy center at the crown of the head. (For more information on the serpent power and the Serpent Power Yoga see the book *The Serpent Power* by Muata Ashby)

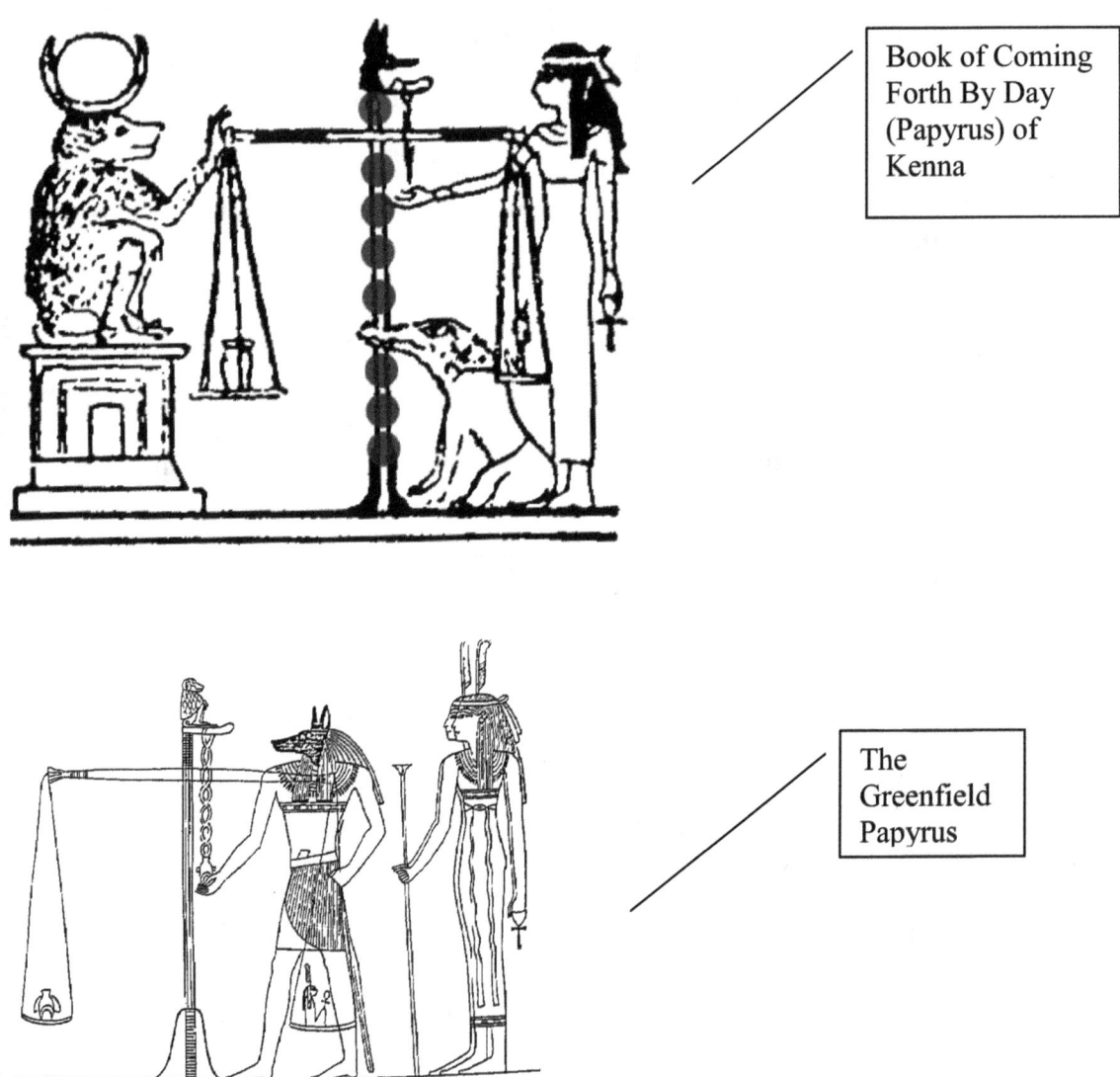

Book of Coming Forth By Day (Papyrus) of Kenna

The Greenfield Papyrus

The Pillar of Asar indicates the four upper levels of psycho-spiritual evolution which represents higher metaphysical attainment in the form of expanded awareness of the underlying unity of all creation as well as the expanded awareness of the innermost Self within. Therefore, these symbols contain important Tantric teachings about the transcendental reality and are to be considered as visual meditations which can be used for the study and reflection upon the teachings.

EGYPTIAN TANTRIC YOGA

The mystical Caduceus symbol is a primary example of the mysticism of the Serpent Power in the Asarian Tradition.

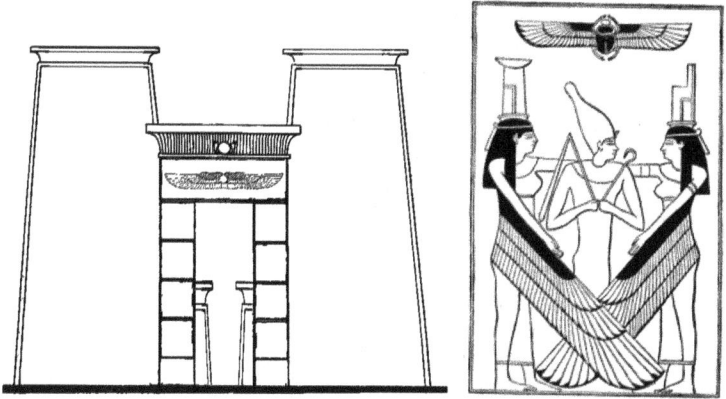

Above: The Ancient Egyptian temple entrance is an important Tantric symbol. The schematic drawing above shows the two Pylons or large structures at either side of the Ancient Egyptian Temple symbolizing Aset and Nebethet and the single opening, symbolic of Asar.

The single opening symbolizes non-duality and singularity of consciousness. Thus, on entering into the Temple, there is a symbolic ritual-meditation leading toward a spiritual movement out of the world (duality - ASET AND NEBETHET) and into the shrine wherein the underlying oneness of the universe (Asar) is to be explored and discovered. Thus the Supreme Spirit (oneness) expresses in creation through the principle of duality.

Mystical Philosophy of Universal Consciousness

The Teaching of the Caduceus

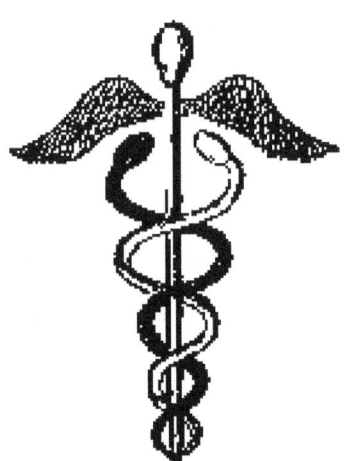

The caduceus is one of the oldest human symbols for the concept of the trinity of soul and dual consciousness. The soul of God uses two opposing forces which are actually aspects of the same one force, to create the Creation. Everything in Creation is infuces with these opposite forces and as long as they remain separate, in varying degrees of opposition and motion they appear as duality. If these were to be controlled and balanced they would merge and become one. If they become one they reunite with the source that gave rise to them. This in brief is the concept of the Serpent Power Yoga. It is related to the Tantric philosophy because these same two opposing forces are the same male and female opposites of Creation, manifesting as gods and goddesses and human beings. If a human being seeks to unite, to have a Divine Marriage with god then that person is actually seeking to reunite the male and female opposites of the life force as well. Therefore, the serpent power disciplines are actually extensions of the Egyptian Tantric Yoga philosophy and disciplines.

The Ancient Egyptian god Djehuti (A) holds the caduceus (from the Temple of Seti I-Abdu, Egypt). The caduceus is the symbol of the life force power wielded by the god, which sustains life and leads to spiritual enlightenment. The Greeks adopted the teaching of Djehuti and called him Hermes. (B)

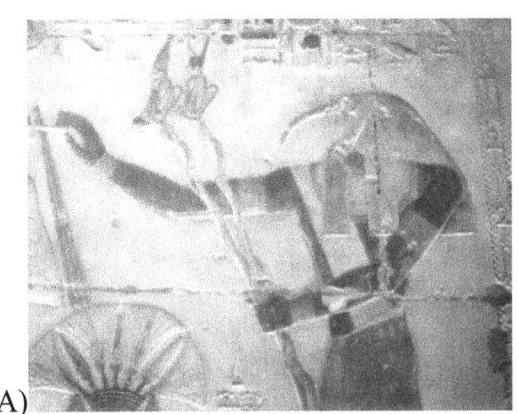

(A)

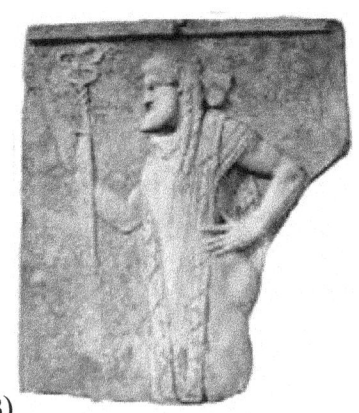

(B)

Mystical Philosophy of Universal Consciousness

Below: The God Ptah in the form of a dwarf stands on crocodiles while the same two goddesses (Aset and Nebethet) stand at his side- another example of the Kemetic Caduceus.

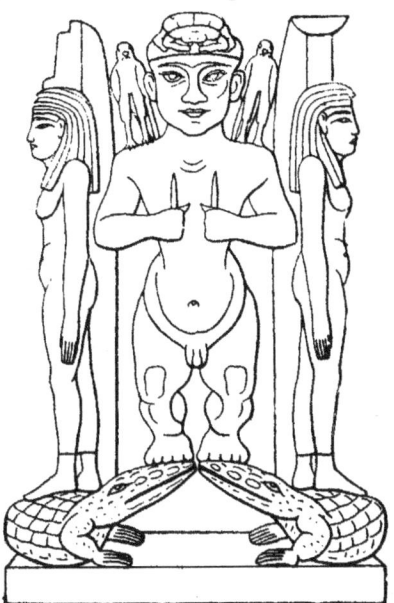

The Serpent Power and Tantra Yoga

Arat Sekhem is the Ancient Egyptian-African name for the Serpent Power. Kundalini is the east Indian term for the Serpent Power. The east Indian concept is discussed here because of its notoriety and because it has some important similarities to the Ancient Egyptian practice. However, some of the teachings and techniques and iconographies are different. Kundalini and Tantra Yoga are known as the forms of yoga which bestow liberation and enjoyment at the same time. This is because the union of the personal life force with the universal life force bestows upon the practitioner a unique form of experience which transcends the ordinary orgasm experienced in the sexual union between two human beings. With the force of a storm, as if containing countless orgasms, it engulfs the soul (individualized consciousness) and carries it to experience union with the Self and in so joining, the soul and the Self transcend the consciousness of opposites. Joy incomparable and unparalleled ecstasy is the fruit of consummated Tantra. The path of Arat-Kundalini opens the door to reunify Geb and Nut and in so doing, Shu dissolves and the original state before their separation becomes reality. In their union there is non-duality, oneness of consciousness, the primordial state, male and female as one.

There is a mystical teaching called the *unmoved mover*. The Self is the unmoved mover and the Life Force energy is seen as the "female" moving energy. This is why the Uraeus serpent of Ancient Egypt and the Kundalini Serpent of India are both female deities. Also, this is why Christian mystics view the soul as the "female" essence which travels up to the altar in the Christian Mass to meet God the "Father" in the form of the "host."

EGYPTIAN TANTRIC YOGA

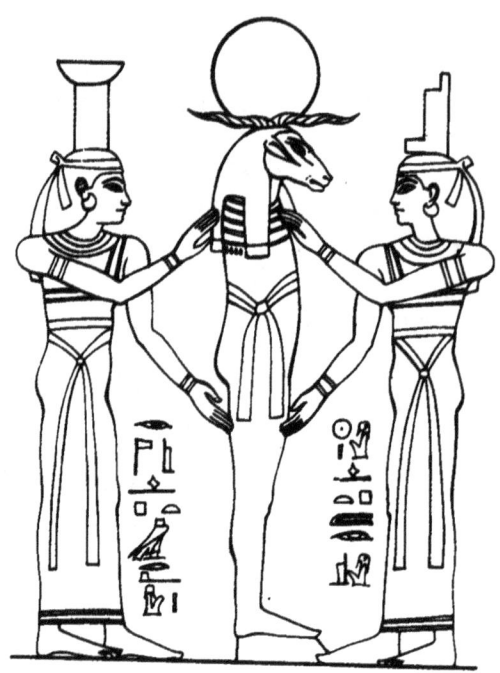

Figure: (above right) Another example[21] of the Kamitan Caduceus, with Atum-Ra

The underlying theme of non-duality occurs across the panorama of the Neterian theologies and as the image and scripture above shows, there is an understanding of the essential nature of all divinities as being expressions of the same single and transcendental, primary divinity. In the above figure, the two great goddesses Nebethet and Aset attend on Atum-Ra as he stands on the pedestal of Maat. Once again, the image of the Trinity is given with one male aspect and two female aspects, symbolizing non-duality (one God, one Spirit) and duality (two goddesses), respectively. Further, this image essentially links three High Gods (Asar, Ra and Atum) into One. This presentation points to the highly advanced philosophical view that the Ancient Egyptian Sages were putting forth, that the gods and goddesses (Neteru) are merely images for worship, and are not to be seen as ultimate or absolute realities in and of themselves. Actually they are aspects of the same transcendental reality. The main image presented in the center is of Atum, whose name means "completion," or "totality." They are to be understood as windows into the transcendent, avenues by which the energies of the mind and body may be channeled towards a higher, spiritual goal in life. Not until Vedanta philosophy emerges in India, is there another form of mysticism like it in the world.

This means that essentially, Asar and Ra are actually one being. This is most clearly demonstrated by the depiction of Asar, in a Divine Boat (Neshmet). It is said that Ra has the Moon and Sun as his eyes, and either works as a passageway to the deeper transcendental Self, just as the eyes of a human being act as a window into the inner Self. Also, it is the sun that is responsible for both daylight (sunlight) and moonlight (a reflection of sunlight). The moon is a symbol of Asar, while the sun is a symbol of Ra. So there is a being who encompasses and transcends them and it is known as Heru. This idea of the oneness of the Supreme Being is stated again directly in the image above which reads: *This[22] is Asar resting in Ra, Ra resting in Asar.*

---

[21] See other examples in the sections entitled "Kabbalism, Ancient Egypt and the Mysticism of the Tree of Life" and "The Early Practice of Yoga in India and the Connection to Ancient Egypt"

[22] The Creator, *Atum-Ra*

Mystical Philosophy of Universal Consciousness

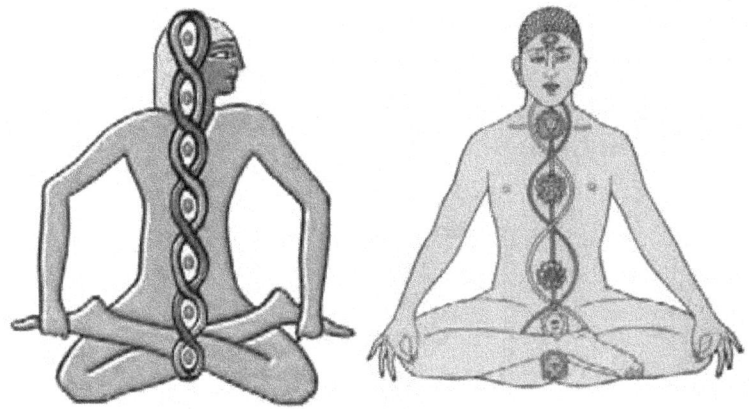

Above right: Indian artistic representation of the yogi seated in the lotus posture displaying the three main channels of the Kundalini Shakti (Serpent Power) and the 7 Chakras (Life Force energy centers) 19th century A.C.E.

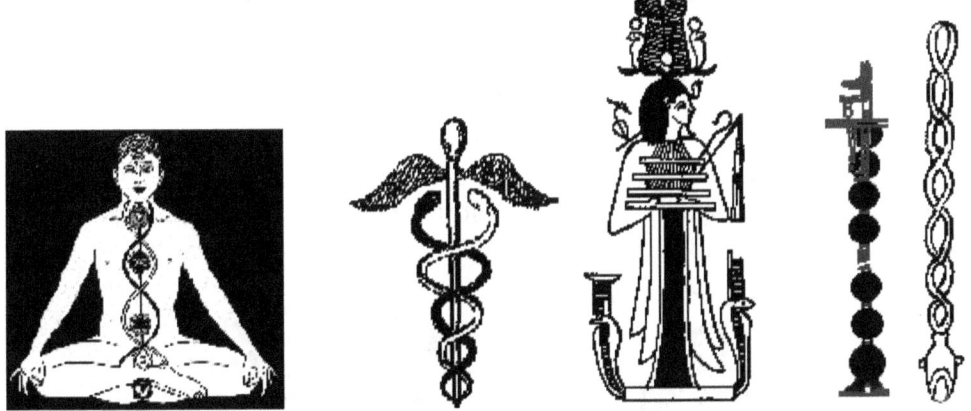

Figure: Left-An East Indian depiction of the Chakras with the Sushumna (central) and Ida and Pingala (intertwining conduits).

Figure: Two Center images- left - the Hermetic[20] Caduceus with the central Shaft (Asar), and the intertwining serpents (Uadjit and Nekhebit, also known as Aset and Nebethet); right-Ancient caduceus motif: Asar with the serpent goddesses.

Figure: Far Right- The Kamitan Energy Consciousness Centers (depicted as Spheres-Chakras or serpentine chains)

---

[20] Late Ancient Egyptian motif.

EGYPTIAN TANTRIC YOGA

Below- the Ancient Egyptian concept of the caduceus appears not just as the staff of Djehuti but as the Supreme Divinity with two serpents at either side or two goddesses on either side. The following depiction of the god Asar with the two serpent goddesses in the form of a Caduceus, symbolizes the Serpent Power (Arat Sekhem (Ancient Egyptian name, Kundalini Yoga (East Indian Name).

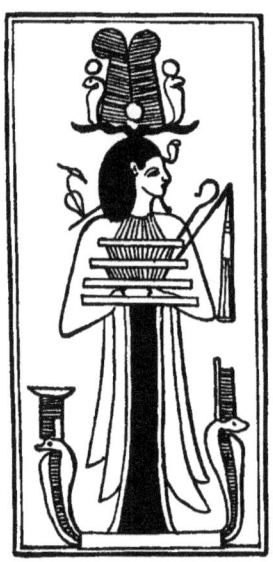

The modern day caduceus symbol (below left) represents the same ideal of the two opposing forces coming together, meeting at the head and allowing the consciousness to take flight into spiritual realms of higher consciousness.

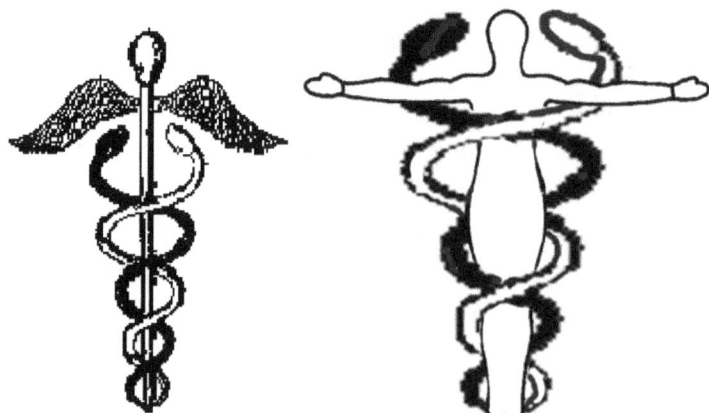

Below left: Ancient Egyptian artistic representation of the yogi seated in the lotus posture displaying the three main channels of the *Arat Shekhem* (Serpent Power) and the *Sefech Ba Ra* (7 Life Force energy centers) 5th dynasty (4th millennium B.C.E.)

EGYPTIAN TANTRIC YOGA

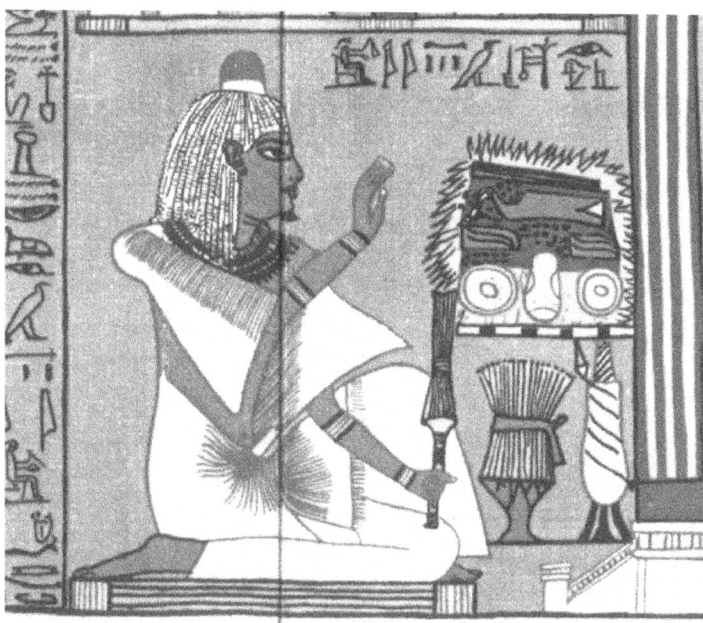

Above: Scene from the inner shrine in the Papyrus of Ani, showing the anointing of the spirit upon meeting face to face with God.

Ani, as a glorified-living soul, holds the sekhem scepter while worshipping Asar.

Ani is making an offering with two hetep tables (one being out of view). They include the male and female symbols. Thus Ani is offering his individual consciousness (which manifests as maleness and femaleness) in order to become like Asar who is androgynous. This is the true nature of the inner self.

The ritual of the Christian mass is symbolized by the movement of the Serpent Fire up the ethereal spinal column to the crown of the head. In Ancient Egyptian mystical symbolism the movement of the Serpent Power Energy to the crown of the head is symbolized by the grease cone at the crown of the head which oozes down to the body. The ritual of anointing was pictorially depicted in the Ancient Egyptian Books of *Coming Forth By Day* at the stage when the initiate would reach the inner shrine which signified coming face to face with God. This anointing was symbolized by the change into gleaming vestments and the *"grease cone"* on his head. The term "Christ" used in Christianity originally conveyed this tantric message. Christ means "anointed one" or a person who has attained spiritual enlightenment (Christ Consciousness).

As stated earlier, you must strive to control your urges in any form they may arise. If you strive to control the sexual urge the desire for compulsive shopping may arise, you may develop a desire for parties, or you may indulge in eating. You must strive for balance and moderation in every aspect of life. This is the Maatian practice of ***Keeping the balance.***

Mystical Philosophy of Universal Consciousness

In this way, Tantrism is to be understood as a science of sublimation of the psycho-spiritual energies which uses sexual metaphors which relate to the opposites of creation. When these opposites are united, the opposites cease to be, there are no more separations or differences and consciousness becomes whole. There is no more wavering between one duality to another. There is oneness of consciousness. In this practice you may see your spouse or partner as a deity and then you practice seeing all things as a manifestation of the Supreme Divinity which is neither male nor female but manifests as maleness and femaleness in nature. Having practiced this you will begin identifying yourself with the androgynous Supreme Being which is your true nature. In this practice control of the sexual urge and the lower desires is of paramount importance. You cannot progress in spiritual life without controlling the worldly desires. Therefore, you should practice abstaining from indulging in egoistic whims and fancies of the mind. For example, if you are sexually active you should begin with short periods of celibacy of 2 weeks to 30 days and building from there according to your capacity in a balanced manner. In this practice you must pay close attention to all of the other aspects of the spiritual discipline: Study of the teachings, reflection on them, reciting the words of power, physical exercises and especially the Kundalini-Uraeus serpent power meditation exercises. If you do not practice in an integral fashion you will develop uncontrolled urges and develop psycho-physical problems in your spiritual program or you may not be able to keep the goals you have set and fail in your program. You must set realistic goals, they should not be extreme but should challenge you. However, never go to extremes with any facet of the program. Let it develop from a spark to a raging fire in its own time. Thus, when the practice of Tantrism is complete you have extended your vision from solely human awareness with individual body consciousness to encompass not only your body but the entire universe as your self.

The soul is neither male nor female. Therefore, the union between a man and a woman is only a temporary development. Those who see this union as a means to experiences sensual pleasures are bound to be disappointed and frustrated eventually because at some point the body will not sustain these activities. The pressure from modern society to be sexually active and physically vital belies the ignorance of modern culture. A culture which promotes youth as the ideal and old age as the undesirable is actually placing that which is ephemeral and superficial over that which is in accordance with nature. The lust for pleasure has blinded societies view of reality. Sex is a means to procreation as well as a means to gain a deeper experience of partnership in a relationship and to aid the person to develop patience, understanding and deeper love for others. Any relationship, be it marital, parental, friendly, etc. requires increasing understanding, patience and love in order to survive and prosper. In order for these qualities to develop in a relationship there must be sacrifice. One must sacrifice one's greed, anger and lust because these cannot be sustained by one's partners in a relationship in perpetuity. If selflessness, understanding, forgiveness and sacrifice do not increase in a relationship, the personal desires, opinions and expectations hold sway over the mind and one sees only one's own feelings and then the other becomes the source of ones unfulfilled needs. The relationship becomes bitter and opens the way for experiences of hate, betrayal and infidelity. Partners in a successful relationship must help each other to become self-reliant, confident and peaceful. This can only occur when there is increasing trust and expansion of love in a relationship. Mistrust, or the feeling that the other cannot be relied upon are sources of pain in a relationship.

EGYPTIAN TANTRIC YOGA

Most people believe that sex relations bring people closer and opens the way to understanding and love. So they indulge in the pleasures of sex, hoping to develop closeness with others as they seek to "fall" in love. This is one of the greatest follies of human nature. When conflict arises, the misunderstandings and frustrations deteriorate their feeling which once seemed so strong and unshakable. If sex and physical contact really signified true love, why is the divorce rate so high (over 50%)? Why is there so much adultery and why is there so much frustration and break-ups among those who engage in physical relationships? Promiscuity and sexuality are as common or even more so than in ancient times. Should this not mean that this is the most loving society in history? The answer is that physical contact, sexuality and sentimental attachments are not measures of love. This idea is one of the most destructive errors of society. Under these criteria, people equate love with an outward show of sex relations, gifts, praises, etc. But when these fail to come it is viewed as disapproval and lack of love. Whenever someone does not feel like sex or physical contact they are viewed as losing their love for the partner. In reality, what might be happening is that their needs are changing according to the divine plan for their spiritual evolution but modern society views this development as a loss of interest, passion and love for the other. Passion may be understood as an infatuation with form and relationship. You are enamored with a particular person or object and your relationship with that person or thing. You have become passionate because the object or person appeals to your mind and that notion which you have learned to pursue because you believe it will satisfy your inner desire. Love relationships which are based on passionate confirmations of outer displays of affection (gifts, hugs, sex relations, etc.) are in reality not love at all but a hypocritical relationship in which two immature people are afraid to let go of their dependence on passion in order to discover a higher form of love. They are afraid that if they let go of the passionate confirmations their mate will not want them any longer.

The folly of physical attraction is that it is based on ignorance, illusion and engendered by passion. When two people first notice an initial attractiveness, it is in reality a reflection of a deeper sensitivity. This is especially true of young love. However, as relationships develop conflict or if ignorant notions of love are inculcated by society, the original spark of love is lost and the relationship leads to pain and eventual disillusionment. It turns into an empty relationship based on habit or fear of separating. The original spark which kindled the spirit was in reality a recognition of the spirit in the other person. What kills this recognition and the feeling of interest in the other person is the emergence of and inordinate pressure of self-centeredness and egoistic desires, demands and passion which cannot be fulfilled by the other person. The error was in becoming enamored with the externality of a relationship, the superficial physical pleasures and not discovering its deeper basis. Most people love what they like and discard what they do not like. They like people when they perceive those people are beautiful, witty, famous or wealthy but not when the luster has been lost. Therefore, becoming attached to externalities in the world is a grievous error which has dire consequences in human life.

The external appearance of a person is dictated by the particular energy pattern they are projecting from the deepest level of their consciousness, the soul. These patterns are a form of energy which the senses of others can perceive. This is why even though the body is constantly changing throughout life, as modern science has shown, it retains the same pattern even through old age and thus it is possible to recognize someone even when the features of the body have changed dramatically. This is also why two or more different people who come from totally

Mystical Philosophy of Universal Consciousness

different parts of the world may look alike or have certain qualities or ways of being that you have recognized in someone else. They are expressing the same kind of energy pattern because they have had the same kind of feeling and have had the same kind of thoughts as other people. In this manner, the spiritual energy from the soul works with the DNA of a particular, group and family and produces a similar and yet unique appearance. Most people have learned to react favorably to certain patterns and not to others. So when someone looks a certain way it is "pretty" or "sexy" or "smart" and other ways are "ugly" or "dumb" or "flashy", etc. These learned responses are mostly learned from society and family and some have been brought forward from one's previous life experiences.

These learned responses are what constitute the basis for the likes and dislikes within your personality and they lead you to certain associations, circumstances and experiences. So in order to change the course of life it is necessary to discover and understand the unconscious tendencies of the mind and then to consciously work on discovering a deeper, more substantial basis within yourself and your relationship. In this manner, you as an individual as well as your relationships, will grow beyond the superficial and create an unshakable love which is based on truth and the sublime goal of discovering the Self in the other person. This is extremely important because when the Self in the other person is discovered, it is the same as discovering the Self in one's very own heart. Demanding and expecting one's egoistic desires to be met by others is in reality demanding and expecting of oneself, that which one cannot provide through egoistic means, satisfaction and true contentment. In order to practice true tantrism it is necessary to break down the barriers of ignorance and the egoistic desires for self-satisfaction. Only in this manner is it possible to release the soul and your relationships from the pressure of ignorance which drives you and your relationship to be un-satisfying and disappointing.

Thus, based on the ignorant and limited vision of love, popular culture and sex therapists promote the idea that a healthy relationship is equated with healthy sex relations and healthy sex relations means regular passionate sex encounters. According to this view, if there is no sex there is no passion, happiness or love in a relationship or at least these factors are wanting in the relationship. However, the ideal of mystical spirituality provides a more exalted vision for those who choose to engage in relationships. This vision is based on spiritual wisdom, the sublime goal of universal love and cosmic consciousness.

In a maturing relationship, as spiritual understanding, sacrifice of egoistic desires, independence and harmony are promoted in a relationship, there is an increasing experience of true love which goes beyond physical sex or outward shows of passion. Nature has decreed that sex cannot be performed in old age. Therefore, it is an activity, like others in life, which must be transcended, just as a child transcends toys. Further, when increasing understanding of others and of one's own true nature increases, the need for physical contact with others becomes trivial. At this stage, sex relations are no longer needed as a means to feel loved or to experience affection because one's expanded consciousness reaches out and recognizes the unity with all humanity. Therefore, there is no need to have relations on the gross physical plane. Just as the soul is neither male nor female, love is in reality not fully experienced in its complete form through a male and female relationship or through friendships and associations of various kinds.

EGYPTIAN TANTRIC YOGA

Chapter 137A of the *Book of Coming Forth By Day* states:

And behold, these things shall be performed by one who is clean, and is ceremonially pure, a man who hath eaten neither meat nor fish, and who hath not had intercourse with women (applies to female initiates not having intercourse with men as well).

Through celibacy, right action and spiritual study, a deeper feeling can be discovered wherein the very source of one's true being can manifest. This is why the ancient spiritual texts of all faiths exhort all followers to keep chaste and devoted to the Divine. Celibacy is not giving up happiness or pleasure, but a means to discover greater happiness, pleasure and true love. Celibacy allows the mind and nervous system to develop to its full capacity and it allows a higher manifestation of creativity to occur in the form of thoughts and ideas rather than as lustful feelings and misguided physical attachments which keep the mind distracted, deluded and bound to lower thoughts, feelings and experiences. The practice of celibacy allows spiritual energy to flow into an elevated process of mental development rather than the degraded thoughts of lust which rob the mind of its peace, contentment and inner creative ability.

True celibacy implies more than abstention from sexual activity. The desire for acquiring, possessing and experiencing worldly objects is an expression of sexual desire or the need to unite with something in order to feel whole. True celibacy implies abstention from all feelings of desire for worldly pleasures, be they those which are experienced through the company of others or through the acquisition of physical objects (car, toys, computer, food) or by means of entertainment (parties, shows, television) or other enjoyments of the senses (music, fragrant smells, soft surroundings, etc.). The advanced practice of celibacy implies the abstention from coveting that which is not rightfully yours. This means anything that is not acquired through your own work and merit according to the precepts of Maat (truth, justice, order, harmony, etc.). Otherwise, infidelity and depravity can exist even if there is no adultery or outer expressions of desire. This internal form of craving and longing leads to fantasies, imaginations about objects of desire. The result is mental agitation and the inability to develop higher forms of spiritual awareness in one's own spiritual journey as well as in one's relationships. It is a subtle mental form of delusion which engenders discontent and aversion for one's partner, leading to dislike and hatred. So even if people stay together they may not commit adultery but the original spark of love which brought them together lost the chance to evolve into sublime love. Instead it dies and becomes a source of pain and sorrow, a pathetic existence. They commit infidelity and develop anger and hatred in their minds. So true celibacy is celibacy of thought, word and deed and not just relating to the sex act.

When true celibacy (abstaining from egoistic and carnal desires) is practiced in its advanced stages, peace of mind can be experienced in any surroundings and under any conditions. It will not require the presence of others, the presence of some particular objects you like or the occurrence of some particular situation in order for you to feel happy or content. When the mind is curbed from its incessant movement toward the world it is then possible to discover the inner treasure of boundless energy and peace within, which cannot be discovered anywhere in this world through any kind of activity. The peace and joy derived from worldly activities is only a refraction of the bliss of the Self which is experienced through the body. When the body is removed as a medium of enjoyment the Self is experienced in the full and unhindered form. It is

Mystical Philosophy of Universal Consciousness

an indescribable kind of bliss which arises when the energies of the body are conserved and the mind is devoid of ignorance, negative thoughts and feelings. The teachings of celibacy are to be developed gradually, with spiritual understanding, and should not be forced on anyone. Those who choose married life and who decide to have offspring will be better prepared to deal with the demands of married life if they practice a measure of celibacy prior to and during the relationship because the quality of their physical nature will produce healthier children and the quality of their minds will allow them to provide a better environment for a family to develop in. Also, they will be better prepared to mature in a relationship when it is not based on demands from the partner. Immature people demand and expect of others in order to experience self-worth, happiness and pleasure. A maturing individual is someone who is growing in independence, peacefulness and fortitude. Therefore, a truly spiritual relationship is composed of people who are helping the other to grow in peace, independence and understanding rather than those who maintain expectations and impose conditions on others as requirements for their love and approval. It involves giving other the support to pursue their life's work and not holding onto them or holding them back from realizing their dreams by forcing them to meet unreasonable standards to constantly prove their love.

When people have no avenue to create in their life's work there is a stunting, stagnating movement in the mind, which seeks satisfaction through procreation or other gross means. Society is in need of caring, loving souls who will give of themselves for the good of humanity (selfless service) and not in need of more people who will burden society with egoistic desires, delusions, ignorance and greed. It is not in need of more people who will come into the world with no one to take care of them or into broken homes or to teen mothers.

The misunderstanding and misuse of sexual energy leads to licentiousness and delusion. For example, many women feel happy when men look at them, not realizing that they are accepting negative energies of lust from that man. Likewise, men feel the desires arising in women and feel compelled to "let nature take its course." This behavior causes depletion of the psycho-physical energies of the mind and body as well as reduced will. What is needed here is to develop a mental barrier against such unwanted intrusions through the practice of correct thinking and the various disciplines of sex sublimation.

Yoga physical exercises are designed to balance the psycho-physical energies and to enable a person to channelize them towards positive work. All of these methods should be used in an integral fashion to develop a healthy psycho-physical constitution which will be able to discover the mysteries of the inner self.

EGYPTIAN TANTRIC YOGA

The Mystical Implications of the Djed

The *Djed* pillar, is associated with the Ancient Egyptian Gods, Ptah as well as Asar. It is part of a profound mystical teaching that encompasses the mystical Life Force energy which engenders the universe and which is the driving force that sustains all life and impels human beings to action. In the Ausarian Resurrection myth it is written that when Asar was killed by Set, his body was thrown into the Nile and it came ashore on the banks of Syria. There it grew into a tree with a fragrant aroma and the king of that land had it cut into a pillar. The pillar of Asar-Ptah refers to the human vertebrae and the Serpent Power or Life Force energy which exists in the subtle spine of every human being. It refers to the four highest states of psycho-spiritual consciousness in a human being with the uppermost tier symbolizing ultimate spiritual enlightenment. Also, the Djed refers to the special realm of the Duat (astral Plane) wherein Asar or spiritual resurrection can be discovered in much the same way as the Christian *Tree of Life* refers to resurrection in Christian mystical mythology.

The Duat or Ancient Egyptian concept of the *Netherworld* is a special place of existence. This is the abode of Asar-Ptah as well as the ultimate destination of those who become spiritually enlightened. It is the realm of Supreme Peace. It is known as *Sekhet-Aaru* or in other times *Amentet*. Amentet is a reference which unites the symbolism of Asar and Ptah with that of Amun, thus relating the deities of Ancient Egypt into a singular essence and dispelling the notion of polytheism. This is an important tantric theme. The Djed symbolizes the awakening human soul who is well "established" or "steadfast" or "stability" in the knowledge of the Self. *Djeddedu*, refers to the abode of Asar within the Tuat.

Djeddu was the name of two towns in Ancient Egypt. In mystical terms it refers to being firmly established in the Netherworld. The Ancient Egyptian word Djeddu also refers to "steadfastness" or "stability" as well as the pillar of Asar. This is the principle being referred to in the following verse from the *Egyptian Book of Coming Forth By Day*, Chapter I: 13-15:

nuk Djeddy, se Djeddy au am-a em Djeddu Mesi - a em Djeddu

"I am Djeddi (steadfast), son of Djeddi (steadfast), conceived and born in the region of Djeddu (steadfastness)."

Mystical Philosophy of Universal Consciousness

A spiritual aspirant is urged to become "established' in truth and spiritual awareness. Thus the verse above acts as a mantram or hekau to enlighten the mind to the spiritual truth.

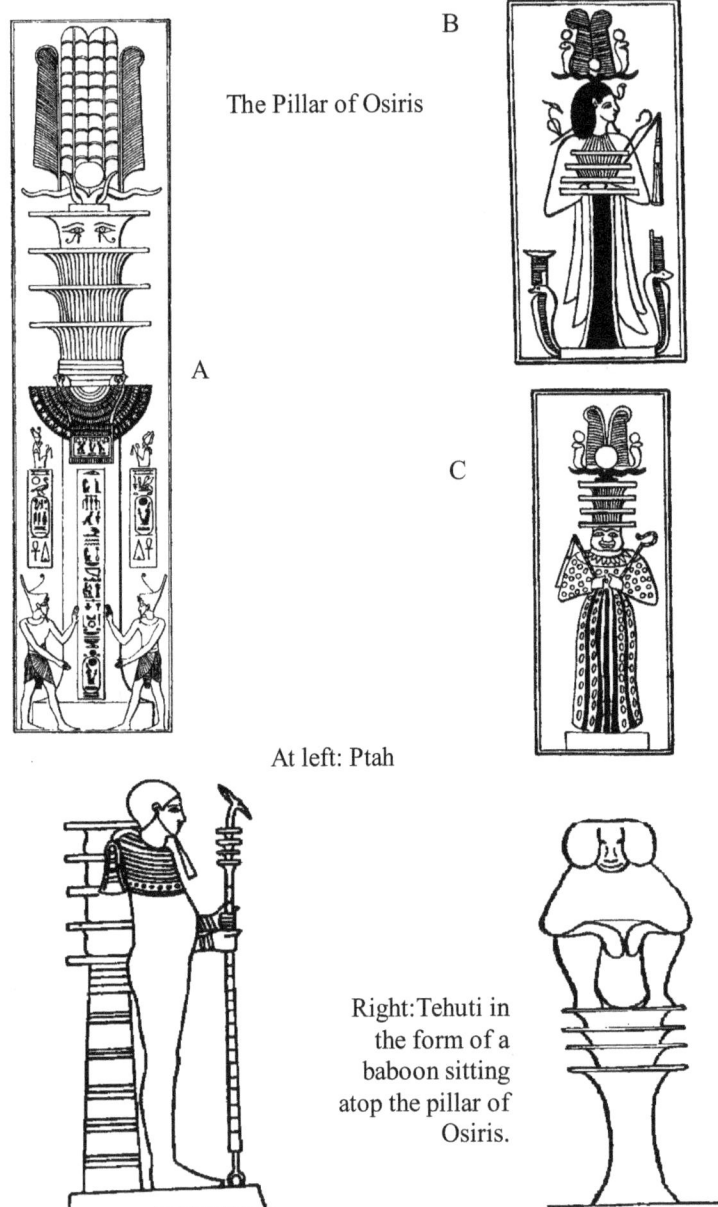

The Pillar of Osiris

At left: Ptah

Right: Tehuti in the form of a baboon sitting atop the pillar of Osiris.

The Ancient Egyptian concept of creation includes three realms. These are the TA, ⎯𝕀𝕀 (Earth), Pet, ⎕□△ (Heaven), and the Duat ★🐦☐ ⌇𓂭 (the Underworld). "Ta" is the gross physical plane. The Duat is the abode of the gods, goddesses, spirits and souls. It is the plane of thoughts and subtle nature devoid of gross physicality. It is the realm where those who are evil or unrighteous are punished (Hell), but it is also where the righteous live in happiness (Heaven). It is the "other world", the spirit realm. The Duat is also known as Amenta since it is the realm of Amen (Amun, The Hidden Supreme Being). The Duat is the realm where Ra, as symbolized by the sun, traverses after reaching the western horizon, in other words, the movement of Ra between sunset and sunrise, i.e. at night. Some people thought that the Duat was under the earth since they saw Ra traverse downward and around the earth and emerged in the east, however, this interpretation is the understanding of the uninitiated masses. The esoteric wisdom about the Duat is that it is the realm of the unconscious human mind and at the same time, the realm of cosmic consciousness or the mind of God. Both the physical universe and the Astral plane, the Duat, are parts of that cosmic consciousness.

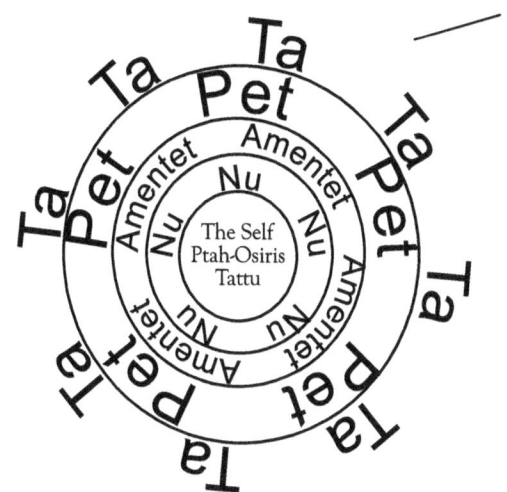

At left: A two dimensional schematic drawing of creation and its relationship to the Self or Soul, based on Ancient Egyptian mystical philosophy.

The Ancient Egyptian concept of creation includes three realms. These are the TA, ⎯⎯ ⅏ (Earth), Pet, ▭ ▫▫ (Heaven), and the Tuat ★ ◣ ▭ ∽◿ (the Netherworld - Amenta, Astral plane).

All realms originate from the Self and are created by temporarily (period of billions of years in human terms)

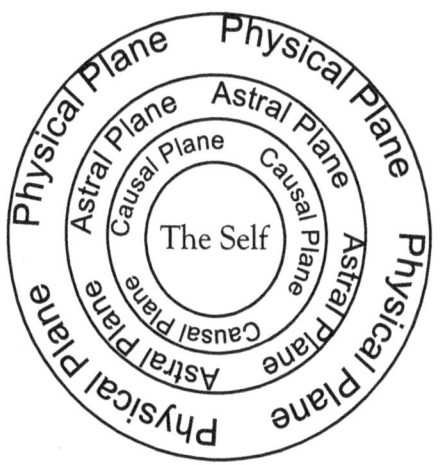

At left: A two dimensional schematic drawing of the Self and Creation.

The Self (God) emanates the Causal plane, the Causal plane emanates the Astral plane and the Astral plane emanated the Physical plane.

Thus, the mystical reading of the symbolism above shows that the self symbolizes the Life Force energy which engenders life within creation. The self is the root of all creation.

Mystical Philosophy of Universal Consciousness

The Mystical Sistrum

There is deep mystical symbolism in the images and teachings surrounding the Triad or Asar, Aset and Nebethet. In the temples of *Denderah, Edfu, Philae and others,* there are sculptured representations of the Mysteries of Asar. These show *The Asar* (initiate) lying on a bier (ritual bed), and Aset and Nebethet, who stand nearby, being referred to as the "two widows" of the dead Asar (see page 141). Aset and Nebethet are depicted as looking exactly alike, the only difference being in their head dresses: Aset ⌓, Nebethet ⌓ or ⌓. However, the symbols of these goddesses are in reality just inverted images of each other. The symbol of Aset is the symbol of Nebethet when inverted ⌓➔⌓. Therefore, each is a reflection of the other, thus, it can be said that both life and death are aspects of the same principle.

The bodies and facial features of Aset and Nebethet are exactly alike. This likeness which Aset and Nebethet share is important when they are related to Asar. As Asar sits on the throne, he is supported by the two goddesses, Aset and Nebethet. Symbolically, Asar represents the Supreme Soul, the all-encompassing Divinity which transcends time and space. Aset represents wisdom and enlightened consciousness. She is the knower of all words of power and has the power to resurrect Horus. Nebethet represents temporal consciousness or awareness of time and space. She is related to mortal life and mortal death. This symbolism is evident in the sistrums which bear the likeness of Aset on one side and of Nebethet on the other, and the writings of Plutarch, the Ancient Greek historian, where he says that Aset represents "generation" while Nebethet represents "chaos and dissolution". Also, in the hieroglyphic texts, Aset is referred to as the "day" and Nebethet as the "night". Aset is the things that "are" and Nebethet represents the things which will "come into being and then die". Thus, the state of spiritual Enlightenment is being referred to here as Aset, and it is this enlightened state of mind which the initiate in the Osirian Mysteries (*Asar Shetaiu*) has as the goal. The Enlightenment of Asar is the state of consciousness in which one is aware of the transient aspects of creation (Nebethet) as well as the transcendental (Aset). This is why Asar is depicted with the two goddesses. Aset represents the transcendental aspect of matter, that is, matter when seen through the eyes of wisdom rather than through the illusions and delusions produced by the ego and spiritual ignorance. So, an enlightened personality is endowed with dual consciousness. To become one with Asar means to attain the consciousness of Asar, to become aware of the transcendental, infinite and immortal nature beyond time and space (Aset) while also being aware of the temporal and fleeting human nature (Nebethet), the practical realities of time and space.

Aset is the true heroine of the epic Ausarian Resurrection story. She not only causes the resurrection of Asar, but the resurrection of Horus as well. The mystical interpretation is that intuitional awareness (Aset) resurrects human consciousness. With respect to her relationship to Set, Aset represents his real nemesis. Even though the struggle of the story seems to manifest as a battle between Set and Horus, in reality it is between Set and Aset. At every turn, Set's schemes and desires are thwarted by Aset as she helps Horus to overcome his schemes (Set's) and in the end, he loses the struggle to be the king, no matter what he tries to do. Thus, it is underlying presence of the Spirit (Asar) and the cunning wisdom of Aset which enables Horus to be victorious over Set. It is this same aspect of intellectual development (as represented by Aset) which enables a spiritual aspirant to discover the increasingly subtle levels of the teachings in

EGYPTIAN TANTRIC YOGA

order to defeat Set in the form of ignorance, selfishness, egoism and brutishness within his/her own personality.

In reference to the iconography surrounding Aset, in the spiritual struggle against Set, there is one important artifact which was used at the time of uttering prayers and meditations. This is the *Sistrum*. The sistrum is commonly known as the rattle of Aset or Hathor (both are aspects of the same goddess principle). The sistrum consists of a handle surmounted by a metal hoop through which four pieces of metal rods are set. When shaken, the rods hit against the loop (see below) and cause a distinctive sound. The sistrum was produced in two forms. The second form incorporated the figure of the *Naos* or shrine (Holy of Holies) of the goddess instead of a loop. Plutarch, the ancient Greek writer, wrote about the sistrum and its spiritual significance:

"The Sistrum also shows that existent things must be shaken up and never have cessation from impulse, but as it were, be wakened when they fall asleep and die away.

For they say they turn aside and beat off Typhon [Set] with sistra, corruption binds nature fast and brings her to a stand. The Sistrum frees her and raises her from death by means of motion. Now the sistrum has a curved top, and its arch contains the four [things]. For the part of the cosmos which is subject to generation is circumscribed to the sphere of the moon, and all [things] in it are moved and changed by the four elements - fire and earth and water and air.

And on the arch of the sistrum, at the top, they put the metal figure of a cat with a human face and at the bottom, below the shaken things, the face sometimes of Aset and sometimes of Nebethet, - symbolizing by the faces generation and consummation (for these are the changes and motions of the elements.

The Ancient Egyptian name of the sistrum is *skhem* or *sesheshet*. The goddess or priestess who holds and plays the sistrum to the Divine is known as *Neter sesheshet*. The *hoop* is a symbol of the *world-encircling* orbit of the moon. The sistrum often has two faces of Hathor. The two faces of Hathor represent Aset and Nebethet or life and death, respectively, the opposites of creation. The four metal rods represent the elements, but also the four spiritual energy centers of the spiritual body known as the pillar of Asar. The human body, the energy which causes it to live and the subtle substance which composes the thoughts in the human mind, are all made up of minute particles of the elements. The mystical meaning of the shaking up of the rattle refers to the shaking up of human consciousness from the evil of ignorance and complacency which leads to spiritual stagnation and the development of evil (sinful-Setian) flaws in the human character (anger, hatred, greed, selfishness, lust, elation, depression, etc.). This process further relates to awakening the mind to the futility of trying to satisfy the desires of the lower nature, the fallacy of vanity and egoism, and the fleeting nature of happiness which is gained through and is dependent on worldly attainments or achievements. Further, the sistrum refers to realizing the transient and relative nature of human existence and the discovery of a higher vision wherein the Divine is to be recognized and experienced. It means, moving from ignorance to true knowledge, and from the pain of human suffering to the glory of divine inspiration and abiding happiness.

Mystical Philosophy of Universal Consciousness

The Sistrum may be likened to the *Conch* in Indian mystical symbolism, and the hand held Buddhist prayer wheel, as they are used for the same purpose, to "churn the ethers" in order to stir up the latent spiritual energies which lead to spiritual enlightenment. Other cultures may use bells, cymbals or other hand held objects to accomplish the same effect.

The Supreme Divinity: All-Encompassing and Eternal

From time immemorial, the symbol of wings has been used to signify freedom and expansion. In the Ancient Egyptian Myth of Asar is it said that Horus defeated Set by becoming *Ur-Uatchit* or "The Winged Sundisk", the all-encompassing Divinity.

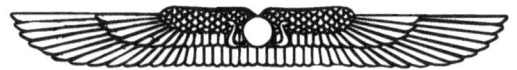

"Horus defeated Set by becoming the Ur-Uatchit. The sacred form of Ur-Uatchit, the winged sundisk with two urei, symbolizes the goddess Nekhebet on the right and the goddess Uatchet on the left. Thus it was decreed by Djehuti that the Ur-Uatchet should be seen decorating every temple as a protection from evil."

From the Osirian Resurrection Myth - Hekau 176b

The teaching above in reference to the all-encompassing nature of God is echoed in the following statement.

It being of such a quality, God, who is author of all generation and production, and of all elemental forces, as being superior to them, immaterial and incorporeal exalted above the realm of nature and likewise begotten and undivided, entire of himself and concealed in himself, is supreme above all these and embraces them all in himself. And because he contains everything and gives himself to all the universe, he is made manifest out from them. Because he is superior to the universe, he is spread out over it by himself, and is manifested as separate, removed, high in the air and unfolded by himself above the forces and elementary principles in the world.

—Iamblichus, Egyptian Initiate
(circa 250-330)

Ur-Uatchit is the epitome of Ancient Egyptian Tantric mystical philosophy. It is the supreme exposition of the understanding of all-encompassing, all-pervasive, absolute existence.

EGYPTIAN TANTRIC YOGA

Therefore, the wings are used by both gods and goddesses in Ancient Egyptian mythology because the Supreme Divinity encompasses both male and female, all opposites and all existence. Thus, in order to overcome evil (the concept of opposites) it is necessary to discuss the all encompassing vision of creation. Within this understanding there cannot be evil since there is no duality (opposites).

The Sekhm Scepter

The Sekhem (Sekhm) scepter is a symbol of the power of the Peraah (Kink). This power is derived from the generative essence of the bull and manifests as the lion goddess in the form of Sekhmit. The bull is a sumbol of the God Asar in his form as the "Moon Bull." However, many other male divinities display this symbol as a reference to the understanding that all the male divinities are in reality aspects of the same one and supreme divinity. Recall that in Kemetic spirituality (Shetaut Neter, Neterianism) the male divinity is the source of the life sustaining essence of creation and it is the goddess who manifests that energy.

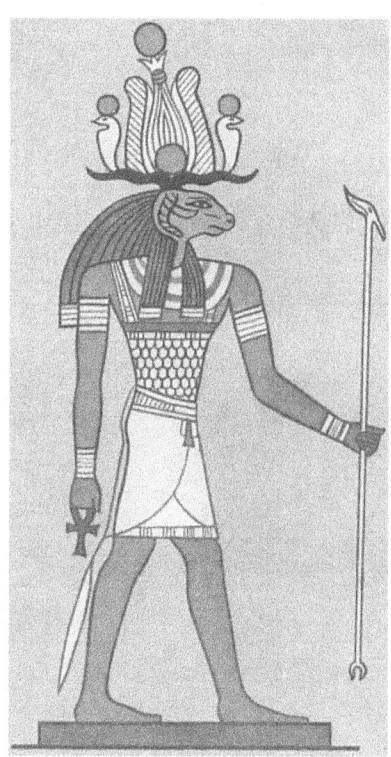

Hery-shaf- god of "manliness- bravery -respect-he on his lake-his land gray." Hery-shaf displays the bulls tail.

Mystical Philosophy of Universal Consciousness

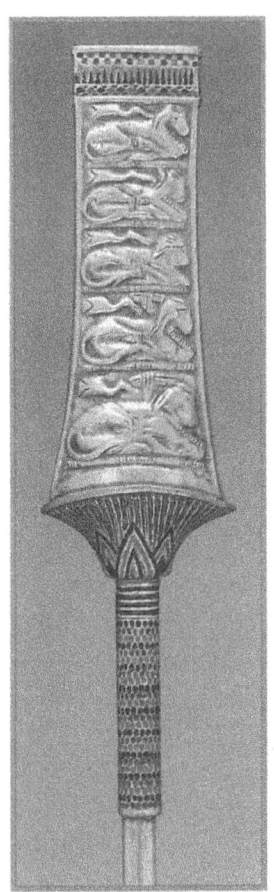

Rear View

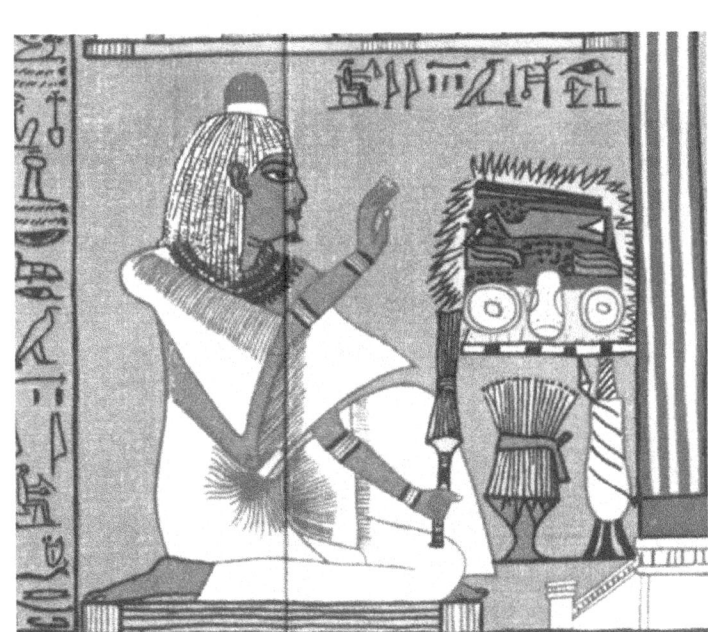

Above: Ani holds a Sekhm Scepter in the Pert M Hru (Book of the Dead) of Ani

The Sekhm Scepter

EGYPTIAN TANTRIC YOGA

That same tail is held in the hand of the nobles and king who wields its power to conduct the affairs of rulership. Below is a drawing from the tomb of Senofer. He is seated with his sister. He holds the sekhm scepter in his right hand.

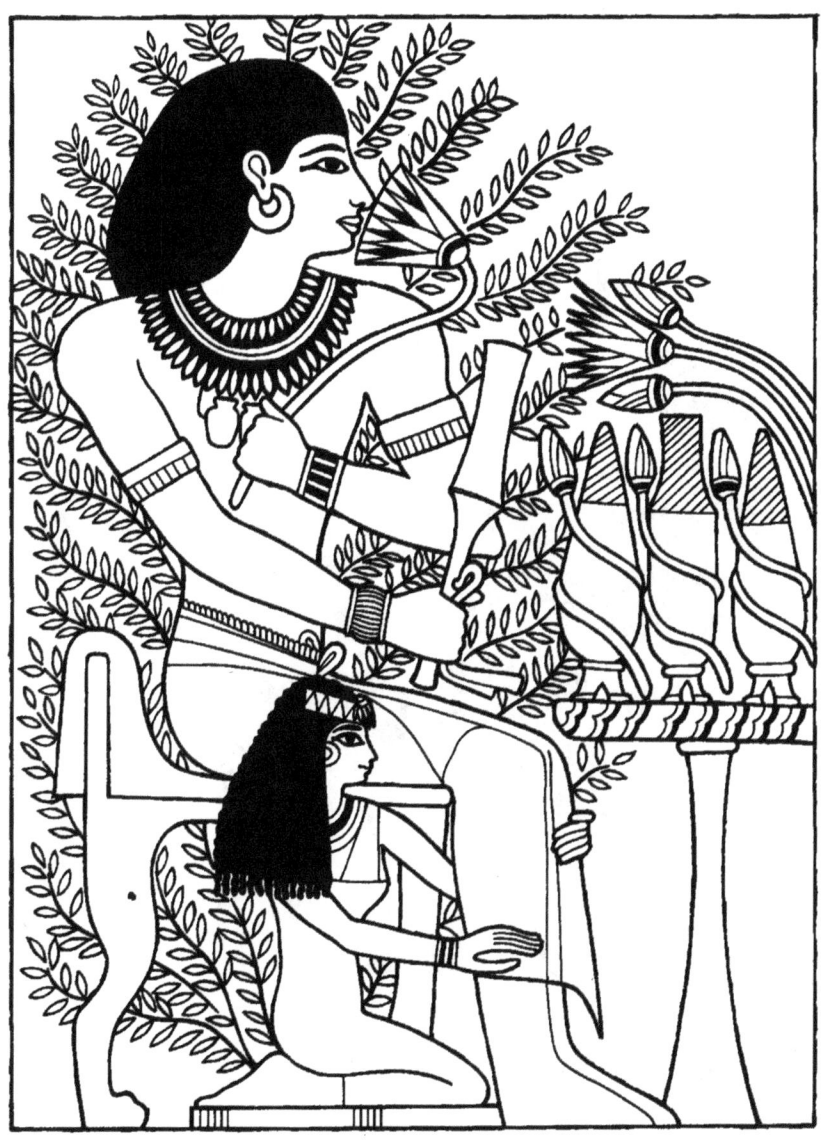

The sekhm scepter is a symbol of the generative power of God which is the male sexual energy. When this energy is transferred to the female (Goddess) it manifests as creation, the generated offspring of the god and goddess. Thus, anyone who holds it is as if holding the phallus in their hand. The right hand is the electric side of the body and it is through this side that the power is wielded. In this manner the male energy is commingled with the female aspect of the personality and the impregnated personality within gives rise to wondrous creations, the arts, magnanimity, the virtuous nature of the personality and most important of all, Nehast, the great spiritual awakening, the goal of life.

# Part 6: The Sublime Vision of Egyptian Tantra Yoga

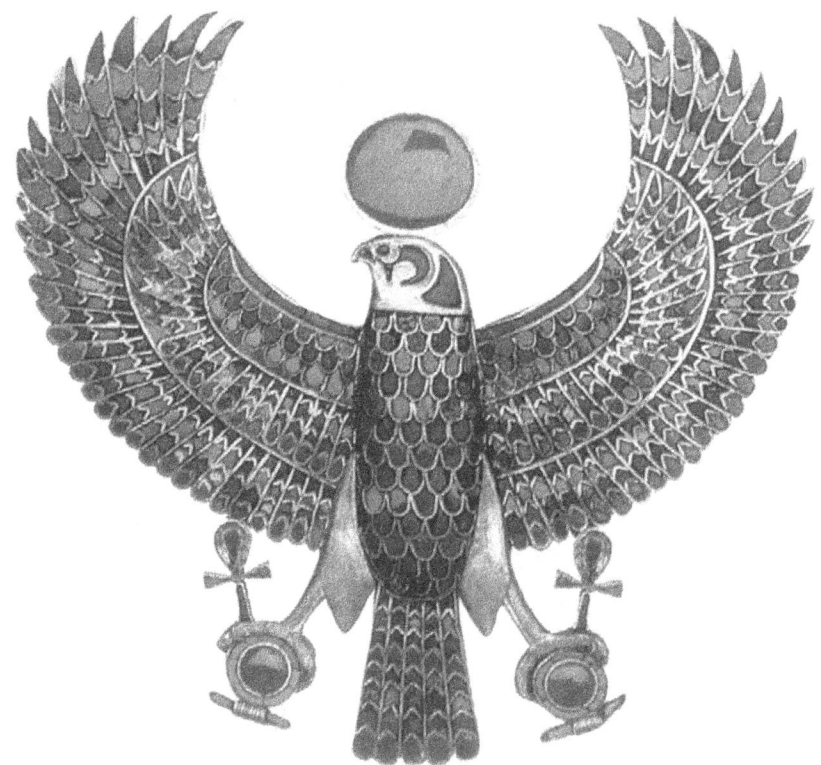

Marriage, Celibacy, Relationships, Conflicts and Spiritual Life

EGYPTIAN TANTRIC YOGA

Marriage, Celibacy, Relationships, Conflicts and Spiritual Life

Many people have misconceptions about spiritual life. They believe that they cannot be leading a "spiritual life" if they are living in the "world." Consequently they develop self-defeating ideas like "I can't do what the teachings are asking of me, that's for saints, I'm not a saint" or "I can't give up sex" or "If everyone in the world becomes celibate what will happen to the world. These ideas are compounded by the strong karmic complexes within partners in a relationship and many times they are used as excuses for avoiding the changes in life which they know deep down are necessary but which they are too weak to do. It is important to understand that spiritual life is not about self-denial or some morbid idea of renouncing happiness and comfort. It is the process of discovering what is truly fulfilling, liberating and meaningful in life and giving up those things which lead to bondage and pain..

A typical situation in life is a young couple coming together due to mutual attraction. They begin a relationship wherein they are inseparable. They cannot bare to be away from each other and they are even engaging in sexual relations. Over time, they begin to mature and they discover that they have other interest along with their interest in each other. However, they both develop jealousy which sometimes escalates into anger, shouting and cursing at each other. They develop a pattern of continually making up and swearing they will not do this again but inevitably, they fall into the pit of frustration which leads to anger. If they are not careful this anger will develop into hatred and they will begin to say and do things which they will later regret. However, at the time of their negative actions they cannot control themselves because the pressure they feel from their desires and frustrations renders their will power and self control weak. Also it dulls their ability to reason and therefore understand each other. Instead of growing up together they are becoming more entrenched in their childish behaviors (tantrums when they cannot get what they want) and they are growing apart.

Sometimes people in a relationship become jealous. Jealousy stems from the feeling of possessiveness and attachment. Under the influence of sentimental attachment people want to feel that they "belong to each other" and this feeling escalated into a notion of ownership. Therefore, ideas like "You belong to me." When this error intensifies one partner may seek to exert his or her control over the other: "If you love me you will not leave me or go anywhere without me," etc. Of course this development will lead to all kinds of disastrous outcomes.

Oftentimes people enter into relationships to satisfy their own desires. Unable to see a higher ideal in life a woman may discover that she can use her body (attractiveness) to lead men on in order to get things out of them. The relationship boils down to "If you really love me you will do this for me" or "If you want some of this you know what I want." Men on the other hand may see the opportunity to get what they want out of women so they may do things with the expectation of receiving a reward in the form of pleasure. They may get flowers, presents or money and then expect to be pampered, sexually satisfied, etc. Both ways there is folly here. Believing that someone can satisfy you is like believing that the oceans of the world can be contained in a cup and held in one's hand or trying to evaporate the ocean with a matchstick. The ocean of desires can never be quenched by indulging in the pleasures of the world or through any attempt to satisfy the desires of the mind and body through objects, people, wealth, etc. They only multiply

Mystical Philosophy of Universal Consciousness

and the entanglements reproduce like wildfire on a dry summer day in a forest full of petrified trees. Yet people strive every day to win a lottery or to beautify their bodies so as to gain popularity, fortune, etc. only to be frustrated regardless of their efforts in life and only to give up whatever they will acquire throughout their life at the time of their death.

In a lesser degree these egoistic desires and feelings manifest in relations which are considered as "normal." Ordinary married people engage in competitions to see who can get more out of a relationship. Others may feel the need to be selfless but will still expect something in return. There will be statements like "I did this and this and this and you have done nothing" and so on. Under these conditions the marital roles become associated with how a person can render service to the other, to the relationship or the family and the persons needs and aspirations are many times overlooked, creating resentment and frustration. I woman may feel that her mate is useful to the extent that he makes money or can fix things or provide for her while the male may feel she is worthwhile to the extent that she looks good or can cook or can satisfy him in bed and so on. She might hold sex as an incentive for getting him to do what she desires and if he does not submit to her she will curse him with her weapons of angry words and hurtful, humiliating remarks. He may bring flowers, candy and expect to have sex only to find that she is not in the mood or that she is punishing him for something he did that she did not appreciate. Unable to handle his ego with its emotions and desires there is frustration and anger which will eventually turn into hatred. She will eventually lose respect for him and develop disgust with the relationship. He may also curse her and if the negativity escalates there will be violence. The civil courts are full of these cases but it is amazing how many more situations like this exist in the general society which do not even get to court. The frustration and misunderstanding engenders a desire to look elsewhere for satisfaction "since you only live once" so therefore, there will be adultery and infidelity. If they stay together as time goes on when the sexual attraction wears off due to old age there will be disgust and regret over time wasted.

Of course these are pathetic developments in a relationship especially when you consider that the Soul is degrading itself to the extent of associating with a limited form, the body and its ignorance, desires and frustrations. Further, the ignorant soul is submitting to the whims and desires of not only another personality but of nature itself. Creation is only a reflection of the absolute and transcendental Self. Therefore, from an egoistic point of view it is imperfect and changeable as well as transient and perishable. Unenlightened personalities are also whimsical, transient and willful. Is it logical to base your life on something that is whimsical, transient and willful? What would you advise someone who is digging for gold in a coal mine to do? Would you advise them to continue searching in the coal mine, to "follow their dream" because they will find what they are looking for if they "work hard"?

Popular culture has much to blame for the disastrous nature of relationships. In the Western countries marriages end in divorce in over 65% of all cases. The divorce rate for second marriages is even higher. If adultery and infidelity were considered in this number it would be clear that marital relationships are in extreme crAset. However, the culture extols the glory of marriage and is unable to face the truth about relationships. This failure leads to untold miseries and sufferings as children are born into broken homes or homes wherein negative values are promoted. These environments will pollute their minds and render them incapable of carrying on positive relationships. Also this failure leads to the degradation of society as the inability to deal with this problem causes people to sink deeper into despair, ignorance and debauchery in the form of mental dullness and negative emotions (anger, hatred, greed) and indulgence in superficial sexual pleasures (recreational sex, pornography, prostitution, drugs) as a means to compensate from the inability to provide for the higher needs of the Soul.

Most relationships are based on ulterior motives and animal desires. The human body is susceptible to the desire to procreate and to experience sexual pleasures. When overcome by these feelings human being secretly (unconsciously) seeks to fulfill these desires through all relations. An ignorant person does not realize that this is nature's goal and not theirs. Nature engenders the sexual desire in all creatures as a means to perpetuate life. However, people (the Soul) identify this desire as their own and thus seek to pursue this goal by any means and this indiscriminate movement to fulfill the sex desire leads to unwanted pregnancies or pregnancies which are wanted but which people are not ready to handle. This is all possible because the sex desire has not been understood and it has gained control over a person's personality, their emotions, will and intellect. Thus, they are incapable of controlling their actions, thoughts or feelings and they become the slaves of nature instead of being its master. Animals have no choice. They MUST obey the calls of nature to fight, procreate, hunt, etc. Human beings have a higher potential of reasoning and intuition. These abilities, when developed, can allow a human being to go beyond their animal instincts. This is one of the wisdom teachings embodied in the Ancient Egyptian Sphinx. The lion body symbolizes the animal self, the lower self in a human being. The human head symbolizes the higher potential or the possibility to attain spiritual enlightenment. Those who are caught in the snare of nature get bogged down in the myriad troubles and concerns of married life, the endless pressure to act in some way which will get what is desires or to please others or to take care of the needs of others (spouse, children). They may even believe that they are "enjoying life" because "isn't this what life is all about, having kids, raising a family to see them grow up and have pride to see the family line go on?" and so on. What is life, where do I come from, why should I marry, why should I bring anyone into the world, who is the person coming into the world anyway, where do they come from? None of these questions enter the mind. people just live on without being reflective, just blindly acting without examining the wisdom of their actions. All of this renders a person incapable of thinking on higher levels because they are constantly distracted by their own needs and desires as well as the needs and desires of those around them as well as the psychological pressure they feel due to the ignorant ideas and principles which they live by.

It was stated earlier that the female constitution is a vehicle in which the soul can experience and learn about emotion while the male constitution allows it to learn more about reasoning. Generally speaking, it must also be understood that females are more passionate than males and also that they are more emotional. However, in many ways they can control their sexual desire better than males. Thus, the male will be less able to resist temptations from the female due to weaker will power. Generally speaking, it will be easier for women to follow the spiritual path of devotion towards the Divine. Generally speaking, for men the spiritual path of studying the wisdom teachings will be easier. However, as a man or woman practices all of the paths of the Yoga of Devotion for channeling the emotions and directing them towards the Divine, the Yoga of Righteous action for developing the ability to act correctly in order to promote spiritual awareness, the Yoga of Meditation to develop the will power and the yoga of Wisdom to develop wisdom about the nature of creation and the nature of the Divine they will rise above the mire of

Mystical Philosophy of Universal Consciousness

the lower self. However, these disciplines are not easy but their result is real and abiding peace, contentment and happiness.

Conflict in a relationship arises due to the clashing of egos with their divergent desires. One partner wants their feelings or ideas satisfied to the exclusion of the other partner. Thus, egoistic desire is the deeper cause of all conflict in a relationship. How can this problem be alleviated? First there must be an understanding of the dynamics of the principle of opposites in creation and how it operated in men and women and consequently in their relationships. Everything in creation exhibits a polarity, a maleness and or femaleness. Human beings also exhibit maleness or femaleness in accordance with the situation, the thoughts in the mind, the balance of hormones and life force energies, etc. An aspirant of Yoga must learn to become aware of these changes and know how to remain detached from them at all times. An aspirant must study the opposites of creation and then practice them. This means that they must act male or female in accordance with the situation. Men and women have this ability because half of the chromosomes in every cell of the body are male and the other half female. Also, the human mind, being beyond gender, can control gender in the personality when it is separated from the ego level of consciousness. Therefore, an aspirant should practice acting like the androgynous spirit within but when confronted with worldly situations an aspirant should act either male or female to promote harmony whenever it is appropriate. What does this mean? Maleness and femaleness is a principle that goes beyond sexuality. Maleness in the world refers to the emissive aspect of human relations, the giver or one putting out or speaking. The female aspect refers to the receiving or taking in. The nature of creation is a constant give and take. This teaching is embodied in the Ancient Egyptian concept of Heru-Set and the Chinese concept of Yin and Yang. Sometimes the giving movement may be violent, such as a storm, but as the storm moves across the land it will blow down all the trees except those that are supple and flexible. This suppleness or flexibility is the female aspect and the storm is the male aspect in this example. The storm here also symbolizes anger and fighting. A man can receive and a woman can give, but if two people are angry at the same time they are givers of negative energy and a conflict ensues.

A wise aspirant should realize that since creation is designed to be calm sometimes and stormy at others. This is a very important point. The world is not designed to be harmonious all the time. Things change, sometimes for the better but most often for the worst. This is so because God does not souls to become stagnant on earth, but to spur them on towards self-discovery through the adventures of life.

Since unenlightened human beings are caught up in the movements of matter, due to the fact that they have not discovered their androgynous self beyond gender and its movements, sometimes they will become angry (the storm) and at these times when confronted with such a personality who is being male one should act female, flexible, by not yelling back or fighting back. When the energy of maleness wanes the balance will be restored. If you fight back at that time when the person is irrational and caught up in the egoistic gender energy it will be more difficult to restore harmony. However, if there is understanding (silence, giving space to the other person and allowing the energy to flow instead of accusing, recriminating, etc.) during times of anger, the reconciliation will be easy. Further, this practice will prevent the mind of an ago doctors said "we know all there is to know" and then stopped experimenting and learning? What will the doctors of the future say about the knowledge of today? What make a person become prideful and deluded? Ignorance, distraction are the causes. The cures for these problems are humility, virtuous living and study of the teachings. In reality, all of your ideas exalting your own sex or denigrating another, the boosting of the ego, etc. are based on ignorance and delusion due to the absence of the knowledge of the Self. They are like believing that the world is flat or that the sky is blue, etc. Ignorance is sustained by the pressure of egoistic desires, expectations, distractions due to mental agitation caused by disharmony and unrest in relationships and worldly entanglements. Ignorance can only be countered with knowledge and the best course for spiritual aspirants who seek or are already in relationships is to understand and practice the teachings of tantric mystical wisdom. The wisdom teachings will open the door to transcendence, engendering the faith that there is a higher vision of life, and the practice will allow you to realize (experience) the deeper meaning of the teachings through your relationships.

Eventually, if a higher understanding does not occur a relationship will not grow and the initial desire which spawned a superficial form of love will not grow into real love. The relationship will degrade. In nature animal species survive by learning and adapting to new conditions and circumstances. If an animal runs into a trap and escapes from it the animal will know to avoid the trap in the future. If the trap kills the animal there is no opportunity for the animal to learn anything. Similarly, if people in trouble divorce they are killing their relationship and they cannot learn how to resolve the problems and then to transcend them. They are dooming themselves to experience the same problems with other partners no matter how much they try to change things. All the while they have distracted themselves from discovering the true source of happiness, inner peace and contentment.

Some people believe that life is to be accepted as it is. If you end up in a bad situation that's your lot in life so live with it. They use religion as something to hold over others, to force them into staying in bad relations" because God said so" and many times they trap themselves in their own snare. Others believe that a good relationship is a situation where problems arise and are dealt with in a mature manner and this is certainly a beginning. But what is the ultimate purpose of the relationship, to live in some manner of peace and harmony only to reincarnate and do it again? This teaching of mystical spirituality is not for everyone. Certainly most people are unable to control their urges and marriage serves as an arrangement in which they can begin to channelize their urges and emotions towards positive ends. Therefore, there is no need to worry about if the world will go on or not if people begin to practice celibacy and so on. Similarly there is no need to hide behind the excuses of not being able to follow the teachings because every human being has the innate potential to achieve the highest spiritual enlightenment. This has been proven by sages and saints all over the world throughout history.

If the ideal of tantric mystical spiritual is kept in view the Soul expands from the constricting bonds of the ego and it begins to enjoy the freedom and peace of the Higher Self. As this movement goes on a human being internally detaches from all relationships while at the same time developing a higher form of love which transcends the superficialities of the ego. A human being is not like a lower form, an animal or other creature. A human being has the potential to rise above the urges of nature while an animal must obey the call of nature. However, in the state of ignorance the human being is worst off than an animal because an animal does not have all the

Mystical Philosophy of Universal Consciousness

cares and worries of a human being nor the fears, inadequacies and failings. The goal of life is to reach a state of consciousness that transcends life itself and not to end up in the pathetic situation of sobbing at one's deathbed regretting the loss of life and the opportunity to pursue the fleeting sense pleasures, not remembering all the pain and sorrow which they have wrought. Instead, a mature personality should grow in wisdom and spiritual experience to such an extent that they are looking forward to assuming their place as the monarch of eternity, the master of Creation.

THE KEMETIC PRINCIPLES OF MARRIAGE

"When thou find sensibility of heart, joined with softness of manners, an accomplished mind, with a form agreeable to thy fancy, take her home to thy house; she is worthy to be thy friend, thy companion in life, the wife of thy bosom."

"Remember thou art man's reasonable companion, not the slave of his passion; the end of thy being is not merely to gratify his loose desire, but to assist him in the toils of life, to soothe him with thy tenderness, and recompense his care and like treatment with soft endearments."

"If you take for a wife a good time woman who is joyful and who is well known in the town, if she is fickle and seems to live for the moment, do not reject her. Let her eat. The joyful person brings happiness."

"When you prosper and establish your home, love your wife with ardor. Then fill her belly and clothe her back. Caress her. Give her ointments to soothe her body. Fulfill her wishes for as long as you live. She is a fertile field for her husband. Do not be brutal. Good manners will influence her better than force. Do not contend with her in the courts. Keep her from the need to resort to outside powers. Her eye is her storm when she gazes. It is by such treatment that she will be compelled to stay in your house."

In Ancient Egypt marriage was considered a stabilizing aspect in society. This is evident from the hieroglyphic text, which denotes the word for marriage in the Ancient Egyptian language itself. These hieroglyphs provide important keys to understanding the Kemetic culture as it relates to the concepts of male-female interrelations and the purpose of marriage.

EGYPTIAN TANTRIC YOGA

The following Ancient Egyptian hieroglyphs about the concept of marriage give insight into its nature as a social institution and human relationship.

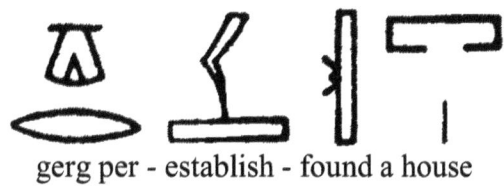

gerg per - establish - found a house

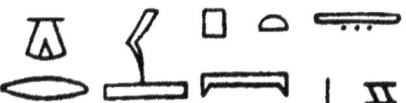

gerg pe-ta - establish - found heaven and earth (The Divine Marriage-Union of the Opposites)

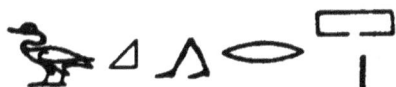

ak er per - to enter a house in marriage

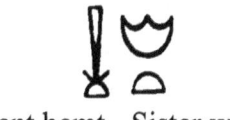

Sent hemt - Sister wife

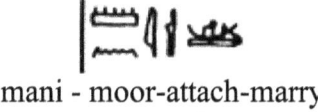

mani - moor-attach-marry

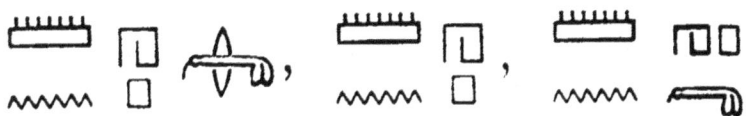

menhep-copulate-marriage-spouse-sexpartner

Mystical Philosophy of Universal Consciousness

Marriage, Sexuality and Celibacy for Neterian Priests and Priestesses

In Ancient Egypt marriage was considered a stabilizing aspect in society. This is evident from the hieroglyphic text, which denotes the word for marriage in the Ancient Egyptian language itself. These hieroglyphs provide important keys to understanding the Kemetic culture as it relates to the concepts of male-female interrelations and the purpose of marriage.

These are guidelines based on the teachings and they are meant to be adjusted in their application for the present day conditions. The main objective of marriage from the perspective of society is to engender the continuation of humanity. From the perspective of the ignorant soul its purpose is to provide a framework through which the soul can have certain experiences in time and space within a marital context. Two people of the opposite sex come together to make a household wherein they can cooperate to raise a family. The man enters the house with his sister and the woman enters the house with her brother (not blood relative – metaphorically all men and women are brothers and sisters).

It is important to understand that in ancient times the priests and priestess discovered the best arrangement for human beings who want to practice advanced spirituality, that is, pursue the path of spiritual enlightenment and immortality. It is to serve humanity by serving God. The instructions given in the Neterian texts provide guidelines for that service. Human beings should study the mysteries, participate in the temple rituals, become virtuous and give drink to the thirsty, food to the hungry, clothes to the clotheless and shelter to the homeless.

One way to serve humanity is to promote peace and prosperity for society. Marriage is a means to achieve that peace in a well ordered and mentally balanced society. Marriage allows the wild tendencies of the personality to be chanellized into productive endeavors. Marriage allows the desires for companionship and procreation to be expressed in an orderly manner in such a way that these endeavors lead to eventual sublimation of those desires into fulfillment in insight and love of the transcendental Divine. If they are allowed to run free society will degrade to chaos, with rampant promiscuity, divorce, children born without responsible parents to take care of them, disease and many other problems. So those human beings who are at a level of consciousness that they desire the experience of worldly human romantic and sexual relationships should be encouraged to follow the householder life. Through such a relationship a person with worldly tendencies and egoistic notions can develop into a caring and insightful personality. If the worldly tendencies of the personality are controlled the egoism and selfishness turns into caring and service through love of someone other than self. Actually that is a lower mystery of life. When a person is through with the lower mysteries of human interrelationships they can also gain higher knowledge from interacting with the Neteru through myth and ritual. That knowledge allows a person to grow to the capacity of having the divine marriage, the marriage with the Neter, the Divine itself.

In ancient times since population was low and society was well ordered along agrarian lines it was possible to have children freely and then look forward to old age and greater time spent at the temple. In the present day, the chaos of society does not allow for such freedom. Another issue is that due to economic concerns and the limited number of suitable partners, it is very difficult to find elevated members of the opposite sex to enter into a Neterian marriage. Most people in the general society are ignorant of the Neterian culture and have been inculcated with orthodox western religious beliefs or western secular ideals. Therefore, it is very unlikely for a person practicing Neterian spirituality, especially at the level of the priesthood, to be married to someone who is of a different faith or philosophy and to develop a relationship that can promote peace and prosperity and the service of Neter. It is even less likely to work out a relationship between a person who practices Neterianism or some other mystical religion and a person who practices or believes in orthodox religion. Further, the unprecedented level of social psychosis, and frustration has generally reduced the pool of reasonably well-integrated human beings even by worldly standards of normalcy. Therefore, sexual and marital as well as close business relationships and partnerships with members of other traditions that are not compatible with the Neterian culture are to be discouraged.

The Neterian marriage is an agreement made by two individuals to come together to make a home and produce a family. However, for priests and priestesses the discipline is different than that of the masses. The higher purpose of spiritual living is to grow in patience, forbearance, nonviolence, self-control, detachment, and cosmic love, love beyond family, community and country.

Priests and priestesses may be married or unmarried. If they are married they must practice ritual cleansing before entering the temple if they have engaged in sexual intercourse. So whether married or not the discipline of celibacy is to be observed by all who work as priests and priestesses. Celibacy allows the energy of the sexual encounter to be dissipated and the personality will be able to apply itself to the worship of the Divine. Also, realize that in ancient times there was not the pressure to have sex, which is so prevalent in modern culture. Therefore, an aspirant needs to control the sensory input of the world, avoiding company with those who are lewd, vulgar or of degraded culture as well as those forms of entertainment that promote lewdness, profanity and vulgarity.

The ideal of marriage in Neterian culture is not the same as the modern culture. Partners are not forced to stay together if they do not want to be married nor are they forced or coerced to marry in a temple. They unite by choice and they can separate by choice. Also, unions are not arranged by the parents. However their relationship is not based on externalities such as sex or unnatural pleasure-seeking. Those things will always lead to frustration and eventual divorce because a mind that is in a relationship for pleasure only, seeking externalities such as sex-appeal and good looks will be constantly engaged in adulterous thought processes that will eventually compel the mind to act impulsively and promiscuously with the senses, and eventually with the genitals. Marriage is to be based on Maat, righteousness. Any relation that is based on truth will be fruitful and will lead to the evolution of all concerned. In such a relationship there is a greater capacity to grow and a greater capacity for forgiveness and selflessness. So if a Neterian follower wishes to marry in order to experience the householder life they may do so but that should not interfere with the work at the temple and the practice of control of the sex urge. Due to economic reasons and other social strife reasons it is more difficult in the present day to have the householder-priesthood lifestyle. If a conflict would be there and a choice is to be made between the two the aspirant should reflect on what is most important to them and follow that.

Mystical Philosophy of Universal Consciousness

Those who are married and cooperating with each other to follow the path of advancing spirituality should continue in their partnership but with the ideal of growing in independence and greater devotion to the temple work which they may or may not work in the same projects (temple) together. Those who are ready to be unmarried and dedicate themselves fully to the path of Neterian spirituality should do so.

The important thing to understand is that in order to have positive spiritual evolution there can and should be "some" strife in a relationship. But if there is sufficient strife to interfere with the practice of the teachings or if there is unrighteousness (one person acting in contradiction with the precepts of maat) that interferes with the proper practice of the spiritual disciplines and rituals those in the relationship should consider separating if the conflicts cannot be resolved. It should be understood that there is no abiding happiness in the world and no abiding sorrow either; however, both can be a trap if encountered in excess. Too much happiness can lead to stagnation in the spiritual life because things are seen as good and there will be no impetus to seek a better answer to the mysteries of life. Too much strife does not allow the movement of spiritual inquiry to proceed properly because there will be too much stress. (for more details see the book *Egyptian Tantra Yoga* by Sebai Muata Ashby)

Vegetarianism, Celibacy and Self-Control of the Neterian Clergy

The teachings of vegetarianism and control of the sex urge of the clergy are well documented. If there is no control in these areas the higher aspects of the teachings and their practices will not be understood easily or correctly. Therefore, it is enjoined that aspirants should gradually turn towards a live of self-control, discipline and purity in order to allow the mind and body to settle so as to be able to peacefully enter into higher states of consciousness.

Teachings from the Temple of Aset (Isis) on Vegetarianism for the Initiates (Spiritual Aspirants): "Plutarch, a student of the mysteries of Aset, reported that the initiates followed a strict diet made up of vegetables and fruits and *abstained from particular kinds of foods* (swine, sheep, fish, etc.)..."

Teachings from the *Egyptian Book of the Dead (Pert EM Heru Text)* on Vegetarianism. Note: Chapters numbers refer to Chapters in the text. (translated text by Dr. Muata Ashby) In Chapter 36, of the *Pert Em Heru*, the chapter of "Entering the inner shrine, making the offering and becoming one with Asar:"

"Henceforth, this chapter shall be recited by a person who is purified and washed; one who has not eaten animal flesh or fish."

Chapter 10, Verse 11:

"...And behold, these things (mysteries of the temple) **shall be performed by one who is clean and pure, a person who has eaten neither meat nor fish and who has not had sexual intercourse."**

EGYPTIAN TANTRIC YOGA

Chapter 31:69:

> **"This Chapter can be known by those who recite it and study it when they see no more, hear no more, have no more sexual intercourse and eat no meat or fish."**

From Herodotus:

> It was the Egyptians who first made it an offence against piety to have intercourse with women in temples, or to enter temples after intercourse without having previously washed. Hardly any nation except the Egyptians and Greeks has any such scruple, but nearly all consider men and women to be, in this respect, no different from animals, which, whether they are beasts or birds, they constantly see coupling in temples and sacred places-and if the god concerned had any objection to this, he would not allow it to occur.[23]

The practice of vegetarianism may be considered both a discipline and also a lifestyle. There are several references to the practice of vegetarianism in Ancient Egypt. The cow was revered there since ancient times, well before the emergence of Hinduism as we have seen, and the general diet of the Ancient Egyptians included a mostly vegetarian diet and fasting. The dietetic concept adopted by Hippocrates, that improper foods are the cause of disease, was espoused by the Ancient Egyptians in the early Dynastic Period. The initiates were required to keep a much more restrictive dietary regimen than the general populous, which excluded not only meats, but also alcoholic beverages and carnal indulgences. These austerities constituted an advanced form of ascetic lifestyle which allowed the Ancient Egyptian initiates to pursue the paths of spiritual development, unhindered by the proclivities of the lower nature. Ancient Egyptian Temple practices led to the development of Western Monasticism in Christianity, Judaism and Islam. The following ancient texts are instructive in these disciplines.

> "The priests (of Ancient Egypt), having renounced all other occupation and human labour, devoted their whole life to contemplation and vision of things divine. By vision they achieve honour, safety and piety, by contemplation of knowledge, and through both a discipline of lifestyle which is secret and has the dignity of antiquity. Living always with divine knowledge and inspiration puts one beyond all greed, restrains the passions, and makes life alert for understanding. They practiced simplicity, restraint, self-control, perseverance and in everything justice and absence of greed.... Their walk was disciplined, and they practiced controlling their gaze, so that if they chose they did not blink. Their laughter was rare, and if did happen, did not go beyond a smile. They kept their hands always within their clothing. . . . Their lifestyle was frugal and simple. Some tasted no wine at all, others a very little: they accused it of causing damage to the nerves and a fullness in the head which impedes research, and of producing desire for sex."[24]

Plutarch outlined the teachings of the Temple of Aset (Isis-Ancient Egypt) for the proper behavior of initiates in his writings about his experiences as an initiate of (Aset) Isis. In the

---

[23] De Selincourt, *Herodotus*, 154 (= *Histories*, II, chap. 64).
[24] *Porphyry*, On Abstinence from Killing Animals, trans. Gillian Clark (Ithaak, 1999). (= *De abstentia*, Book IV, chap 6)

Mystical Philosophy of Universal Consciousness

following excerpts Plutarch describes the purpose and procedure of the diet observed by the initiates of Aset, and the goal to be attained through the rigorous spiritual program.

> "To desire, therefore, and covet after truth, those truths more especially which concern the divine nature, is to aspire to be partakers of that nature itself (1), and to profess that all our studies and inquiries (2) are devoted to the acquisition of holiness. This occupation is surely more truly religious than any external (3) purifications or mere service of the temple can be (4). But more especially must such a disposition of mind be highly acceptable to that goddess to whose service you are dedicated, for her special characteristics are wisdom and foresight, and her very name seems to express the peculiar relation which she bears to knowledge. For "Isis" is a Greek word, and means "knowledge or wisdom,"(5) and "Typhon," (Set) the name of her professed adversary, is also a Greek word, and means " pride and insolence."(6) This latter name is well adapted to one who, full of ignorance and error, tears in pieces (7) and conceals that holy doctrine (about Asar) which the goddess collects, compiles, and delivers to those who aspire after the most perfect participation in the divine nature. This doctrine inculcates a steady perseverance in one uniform and temperate course of life (8), and an abstinence from particular kinds of foods (9), as well as from all indulgence of the carnal appetite (10), and it restrains the intemperate and voluptuous part within due bounds, and at the same time habituates her votaries to undergo those austere and rigid ceremonies which their religion obliges them to observe. The end and aim of all these toils and labors is the attainment of the knowledge of the First and Chief Being (11), who alone is the object of the understanding of the mind; and this knowledge the goddess invites us to seek after, as being near and dwelling continually (12) with her. And this also is what the very name of her temple promiseth to us, that is to say, the knowledge and understanding of the eternal and self-existent Being - now it is called "Iseion," which suggests that if we approach the temple of the goddess rightly, we shall obtain the knowledge of that eternal and self existent Being."

The practice of vegetarianism is important because non-vegetarian foods intensify the physical experience of embodiment and distract the mind by creating impressions in the subconscious and unconscious, which will produce future cravings and desires. This state of mind renders the individual incapable of concentration on significant worldly or high spiritual achievements. Secondly, control of the sexual urge leads to control of the sexual Life Force energy,[25] which can then be directed towards higher mental and spiritual achievement. Further, overindulgence in sexual activity tends to wear down the immunity as it wears down the mental capacity and one becomes a slave to sensual passions and susceptible to sexual and non-sex related diseases. Sexuality also has the potential to entangle a person into relationships which may not be conducive to the proper conduct of spiritual life and may draw the aspirant away from their studies and disciplines. The following verses from the Ancient Egyptian Book of Enlightenment show the practice of vegetarianism and celibacy.

---

[25] The concept of the Life Force will be explained in detail later.

EGYPTIAN TANTRIC YOGA

Chapter 30B of the Ancient Egyptian mystical text *The Book of Coming Forth By Day (PertmHru-Book of the Dead)* states:

> *This utterance shall be recited by a person purified and washed; one who has not eaten animal flesh or fish.*

Chapter 64 of the *Book of Coming Forth By Day (Book of the Dead)* states:

> *This Chapter can be known by those who recite it and study it when they see no more, hear no more, have no more sexual intercourse and eat no meat or fish.*

Chapter 137A of the *Book of Coming Forth By Day (Book of the Dead)* states:

> *And behold, these things shall be performed by one who is clean, and is ceremonially pure, a man who hath eaten neither meat nor fish, and who hath not had intercourse with women* (applies to female initiates not having intercourse with men as well).

(for more details see the books *Egyptian Tantra Yoga* and *Kemetic Diet* by Sebai Muata Ashby)

Mystical Philosophy of Universal Consciousness

CLOTHING AND SEXUALITY IN ANCIENT EGYPT

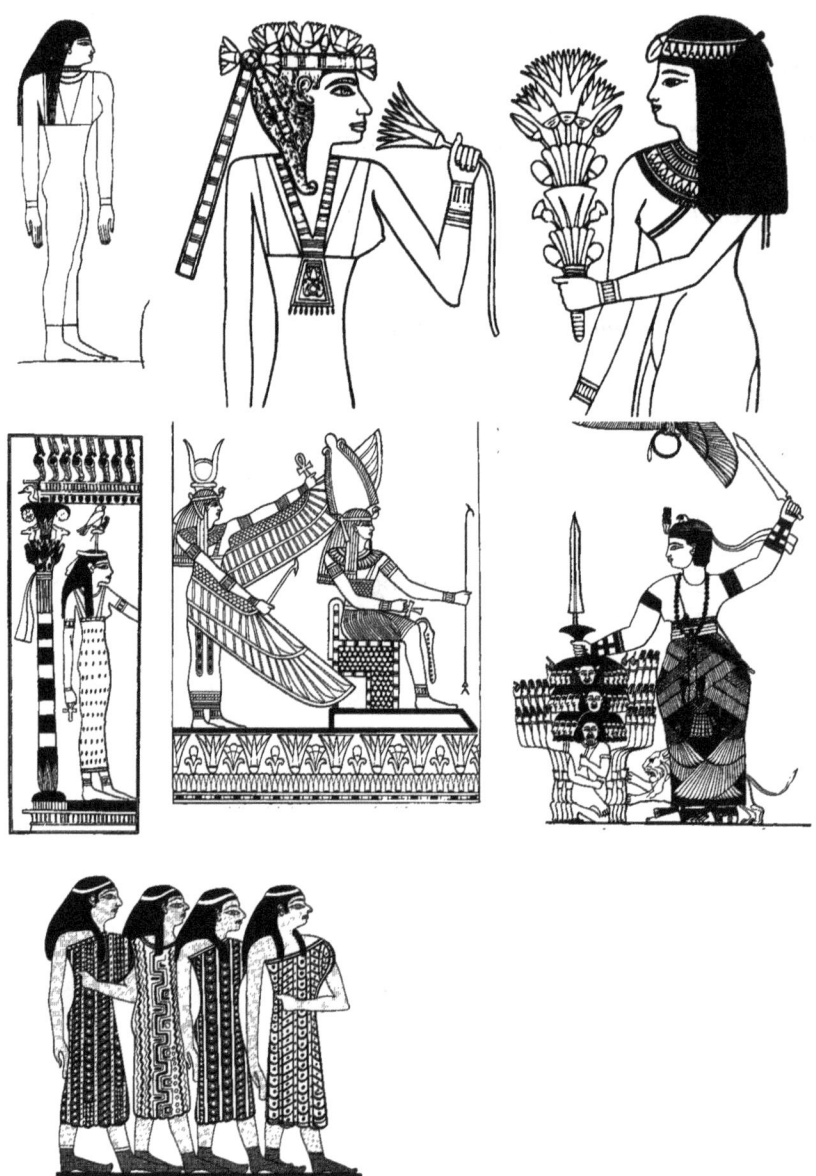

Top Left: Typical garment of the Old Kingdom.
Top Center: Garment with straps and breast exposed.
Top Right: Sari-like-garment with one breast exposed.
Center Left to right: Goddess Waset, Goddess Aset, Queen of Nubia with Garment from below the breasts down.
Bottom left: Semitic visitors to Ancient Egypt.

EGYPTIAN TANTRIC YOGA

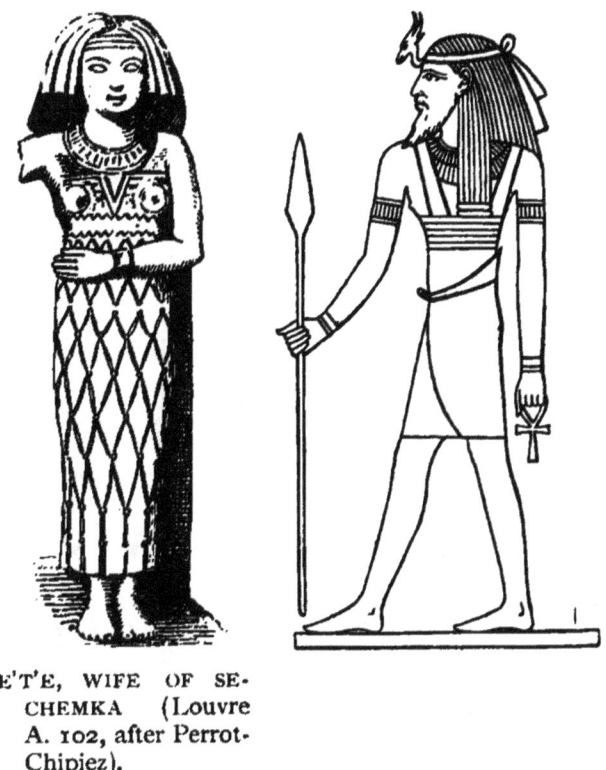

E'T'E, WIFE OF SE-CHEMKA (Louvre A. 102, after Perrot-Chipiez).

Above left: Typical female garment exposing both breasts.
Above right: typical male garment with straps, exposing both breasts.

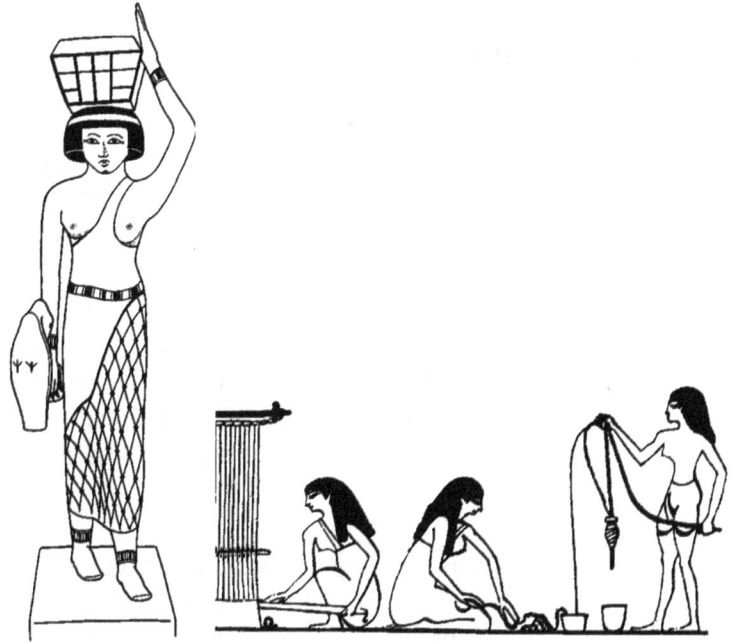

Above left: Ancient Egyptian displaying a common garment exposing both breasts.

Above right: Working women of ancient Egypt displaying common garments of the era, garment with straps and at the far right one woman wears only a skirt and is completely topless.

Mystical Philosophy of Universal Consciousness

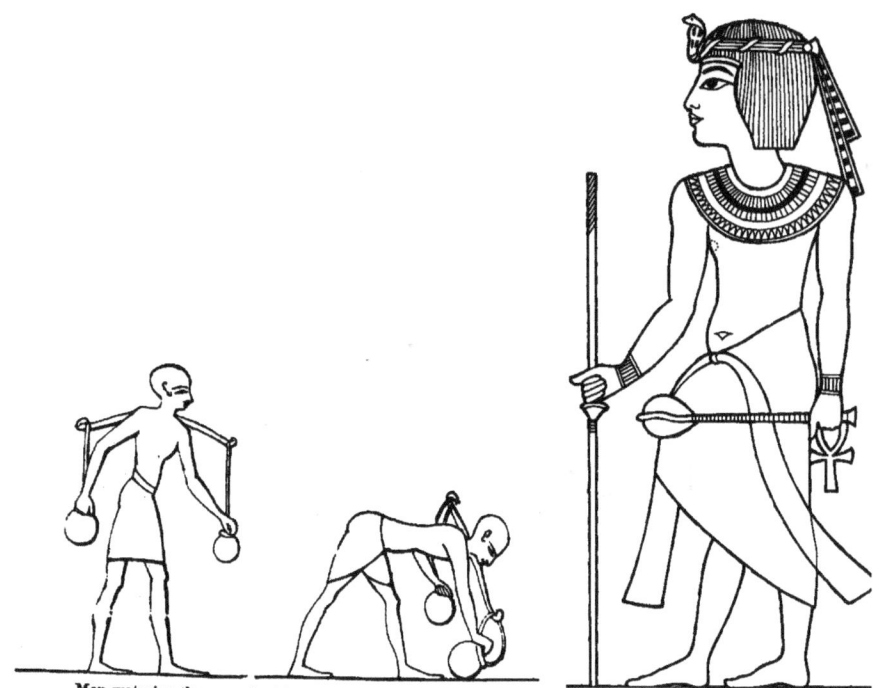

Above: working men of ancient Egypt, displaying a common garment, a kilt skirt, leaving them topless.

Right: Young King Tutankhamon wearing a kilt, bracelets and a collar.

CLOTHING AND SEXUALITY IN ANCIENT EGYPT

The pictures displayed in the previous pages show that the ancient Egyptians lived in a society that did not place undue importance on clothing or think of it as a sexual instrument. Common folk as well as the nobility and including the gods and goddesses wore the same types of clothing. There was no double standard, even between the genders. Men and women wore the same types of clothing with minor variations. Clothing was used not as a means to indiscriminately allure or entice the opposite sex but more as an adornment of that which is already a work of art. Sexuality was reserved for one's spouse who was generally to be one person. Adultery was strictly prohibited although divorce was allowed. Ancient Egyptian men and women thought little of the exposed chest in terms of sexual objects. It would be impossible for a woman in modern times to walk around topless, yet men do this all the time. This double standard did not exist in Ancient Egypt.

The objectification of female breasts as sex objects is an unfortunate byproduct of a sexually dysfunctional society. This mental disorder is a modern development (beginning from the end of the Roman Empire (400 A.C.E.) to the present). Many reasons can explain this; the orthodox practice of religion is one of the most important factors behind the pseudo-prudish behavior.

prude (pro͞od) *n.* One who is excessively concerned with being or appearing to be proper, modest, or righteous.

EGYPTIAN TANTRIC YOGA

The word pseudo-prudish is used here because while modern society claims to be civilized and content and to shun lewd and licentious behavior, it is the most sexually dysfunctional society in the known history of humanity. Prostitution, pornography and sex in the general entertainment media and advertising are unprecedented in history. The scene of a mother nursing a child has become an embarrassment in the eyes of most people due to the association of the breast as a sexual object. In ancient times such a site would have been regarded as an expression of the miracle of life and even as a living reflection of the incarnated spirit in the form of the goddess Aset (Aset) and her son Heru (Horus) which later came to be known as Mary and Jesus (Madonna and child). Such degradations of what was originally an innocent and even spiritual icon, are the hallmarks of cultures, which are spiritually immature and sexually repressed. The word "repressed" here does not refer to the inability to experience physical sexuality but to the inability to experience the true meaning of sexuality.

lewd (lōōd) *adj.* **lewd·er, lewd·est. 1.a.** Preoccupied with sex and sexual desire; lustful. **b.** Obscene; indecent.

li·cen·tious (lī-sĕn′shəs) *adj.* **1.** Lacking moral discipline or ignoring legal restraint, especially in sexual conduct.

The inability to confront the problems of society and the human desires, including sexual ones as well as the higher spiritual needs of life, and to live in accordance with righteous principles has given way to egoistic philosophies of life. Due to the search for a diversion from the harshness of life, the violence, survival pressures, fears, etc., sex came to be used as a means to relieve stress and a diversion from reality as well as a means to control the opposite sex. People became more interested in personal pleasure and greed, and these led to insatiable sexual lust and sexual greed. Also, the misunderstanding of religion along with the ability to physically enslave women led to repudiation of female sexuality due to the male weakness in resisting it; a weakness which arose due to the excesses and lack of self-control of the male dominated members of society. Many men came to believe that women are objects to be controlled for producing sex pleasure and as domestic slaves. Many women have come to believe that men are lusting beings who can be controlled by means of sexuality so they saw sexuality as their only weapon against the tyranny of men, thereby the female idea of men came to be degraded just as men's idea of women was degraded. Even though most men and women do not realize it, underlying most relationships is a seething cauldron of resentment and hatred as well as mistrust which has brewed over a period of many lifetimes as individuals as a factor of thousands of years of partaking in the growing unrighteousness of modern culture and society. Since every human being has an inner voice of the spirit, their conscience, deep down, they know that their degrading actions and concepts of others are in contradiction with truth. Deep down a human being feels guilty and hates him or herself because of the unrighteousness and this self-hatred expresses itself in the form of anger, resentment, intensified mistrust of self and other, culminating in self-destruction of the same relationship which they seek to perpetuate.

In every downfall of a society sexual depravity can be observed. The sexual depravity of ancient Egyptian society (especially in the period of its control by the Persians and Greeks) led to its ultimate destruction. The sexual depravity of ancient Persian society led to its ultimate

Mystical Philosophy of Universal Consciousness

destruction. The sexual depravity of ancient Greek society led to its ultimate destruction. The sexual depravity of ancient Roman society led to its ultimate destruction. The sexual depravity of the Catholic Church led to its disintegration. The sexual depravity of government leaders even in modern times continues to degrade modern society and will ultimately lead to its downfall just as it caused the downfall of over 60% of all first time marriages and an even greater percentage of second marriages which in turn leads to broken homes and children who will grow up to be more dysfunctional than their parents, further compounding the problems of society. Yet modern society marches ahead into the future without stopping to take a look at what is happening, egoistic and overconfident in technology. But the signs are there in the divorce rate as well as in the degree of dissatisfaction in peoples life which is reflected in the levels of crime, drug abuse, suicide, violence, etc. History has shown that when societies as a whole do not take up the cause of truth and righteousness they will be faced with the backlash of pent up psychoses, frustrations and resentments of its populations as well as those whom they are in contact with. Societies, are composed of people and people rarely seek to confront embarrassing issues or problems which require them to change, especially when it involves giving up ideas and concepts (particularly religious ones) or the perception of giving up what they believe to be pleasures of life (especially sense pleasures).

psy·cho·sis (sī-kō′sĭs) *n., pl.* **psy·cho·ses** (-sēz). A severe mental disorder, with or without organic damage, characterized by derangement of personality and loss of contact with reality and causing deterioration of normal social functioning.

The Ancient Egyptians had a healthy outlook on life, sexuality and the opposite sex. It was governed by the principles of Maat (Righteousness) set down by the Sages, priests and priestesses. The kinds of sex crimes so common in modern society such as rape, sodomy, child molesting, pornography, etc. where virtually unknown in ancient Egypt. These forms of depravity were commonplace in Roman society and were intensified in the case of the wealthy or the family of the emperors, who raped anyone they pleased under penalty of instant death for anyone who, refused them. Records remain of emperors such as Nero and Caligula, whose sexual depravities were legendary even in their own time. They would have constant orgies and rape the wives of their guests while the husbands would powerlessly wait in the next room. Such injustices led in many cases to their assassinations and the general disorder of society.

To the Ancient Egyptians, the debauchery of the Greeks and Asians was a sign of social and spiritual immaturity to be shunned if possible. Such activities were recognized as degrading to a human being and to society. Thus, even though Ancient Egyptian society fell into crAset and decline due to invasions form foreign countries, Egyptian society was able to rise again by following the path of Maat, balance, virtue, order in all areas of society. Unlike the emperors of Greece, Persia and Rome, the Ancient Egyptian Pharaoh was not allowed absolute power over Egyptian subjects. The power given to individuals in modern society would be regarded as a path to a degraded culture, by ancient Egyptian standards. A society with sexual dysfunction of epidemic proportions cannot reach out towards righteous worldly goals or uplifting spiritual goals because the mind of its people, which is agitated by lust, greed and the pursuit of sense pleasures is not capable of right thinking or understanding the true meaning and purpose of life. The personal (egoistic) desiring skews the thought process in such a person and this is the underlying cause for inequality between the sexes.

EGYPTIAN TANTRIC YOGA

The process of desiring and lusting renders the mind weak to temptations of all kinds and to greed for more pleasure, leading to an endless and increasing lust which cannot be satisfied and will lead to frustration, mental anguish and confusion about what constitutes virtue and vice. In this mindset people have come to believe that the desiring and lusting process is normal and that it should be promoted at every chance. This has given rise to a media and culture which is generally in a constant state of fixation on sex and sense pleasures, fame and fortune. Under these conditions people are not able to rise above the low state of mind since the pressure of constantly craving and coveting is constantly being reinforced through family interactions, friends, the media, the arts, etc.

However, it should be understood that the problem of sexual dysfunction in modern society is not due to men alone but also to the subservient position that women have been forced into and which most accept. Even men and women who honestly feel caring can also have superiority-inferiority complexes. If this problem is not addressed seriously and constantly it drags on for many years, like a cancer, until every once in a while society experiences an upheaval of some kind in the form of protests, riots etc. Mostly it is experienced as violence between the sexes and general discontent in relationships. By accepting the role of objects and assisting in the perpetuation in the culture, which sees a woman's worth as being based on outer physical appearance, women have allowed themselves to be objectified. While, the most intense examples of this dysfunction in women may be found in prostitutes or exotic dancers, or participants in pornography, for example, this problem affects women generally, as they submit to the culture of male dominance by seeking to look and act like those women who seem to be adulated by the masses of sexually dysfunctional males. Most women use make-up, wear tight fitting clothes, jewelry, etc., and some even use plastic surgery in order to hold onto the illusion of youth and beauty. This is all self-objectification and degradation from a yogic perspective as if saying "Look at me, I am this sexual object, adorned and made up for your attraction and not an immortal spirit, beautiful in my own right." This is a trading of one's real identity for that of a dream. They are all brainwashed as it were, to some degree, with the idea of make-up, personal adornments and clothing as a means to appear sexually attractive and thus accepted. Even those women who live the married life seek to remain attractive to their mates even up to the time of old age and death.

Objectification, from a yogic perspective, is the regard of a person or an object as an instrument to be manipulated and used for one's egoistic pleasure without regard for its deeper intrinsic essence. Objectification is an extreme form of degradation and therefore a great movement away from divine consciousness. A man who sees himself as a lusting desiring personality and who judges his worth by the virility of his personality, sexual conquests or desirability from the opposite sex is also actually objectifying himself as well. In this context, objectification is to be understood as a component of mental conditioning which is in opposition to the main goal of Tantric (yogic) philosophy, which is to see the underlying unity behind the objects of Creation; to see God within all objects and personalities. Desiring and lusting and their related mental disorder of objectification (egoistic mental conditioning), constitute a negative process wherein a human being moves farther and farther away from spiritual enlightenment and closer to disorder, confusion, infidelity, and insanity. It is a movement away from truth and towards ignorance and delusion.

Mystical Philosophy of Universal Consciousness

Thus, a man and woman who hold the degraded view of each other are two sides of the same coin, as it were, working towards their mutual degradation while thinking that they are "following their hearts," or that they are following "nature's primal urge." It must be understood that sexual perversion cannot be found anywhere in nature except in Homo sapiens (human beings) who are living and interacting in a degraded manner.

Clothing is only a manifestation of the deeper thoughts, feelings and desires of human beings. From the culture of clothing society beliefs and desires as well as its psychoses can be discerned. It must be clear that there cannot be true love between partners until in their heart of hearts they see themselves as equals, for gender is not a difference between male and female but only a variation in degree of development in certain organs of the body. Ultimately, beyond the body there is only spirit and in the spirit there is no gender. A society, which lives by the philosophy of righteousness, will flourish. A society which does not live by this teaching will be filled with egoism, gender bias, dysfunction, psychosis, depression, anxiety, drug addicts, unrighteous business people and politicians, sexually transmitted diseases, people who cannot discover peace and contentment or satisfaction no matter how much sexual activity they experience.

The idea of feeling shame or the need to cover the body due to embarrassment or out of fear of rejection or fear of sexual thoughts, etc. are a modern concepts brought into existence by modern culture. They did not exist prior to the Orthodox Judeo-Islamic-Christian movements and the development of Western civilization. Clothing should be used, as a means to promote health and hygiene and not as a sexual instrument just as cars should be designed for efficiency and economy as opposed to egoistic and dangerous thrill seeking instruments or status symbols which are destructive to the environment. Also, clothing should not be used as a means of avoiding issues of sexuality or as a means to run away from sexuality. By forcing social rules like requiring women to not go around topless in an effort to discourage male lewd and lascivious thoughts, the problem of objectification of the breasts and subconscious pent up frustrations and lusting continues because the illness of lewd and lascivious is not being dealt with either in men or women. A society, which follows this principle, will be well ordered and spiritually uplifted.

Part 7: The Art of Kemetic Sex Sublimation

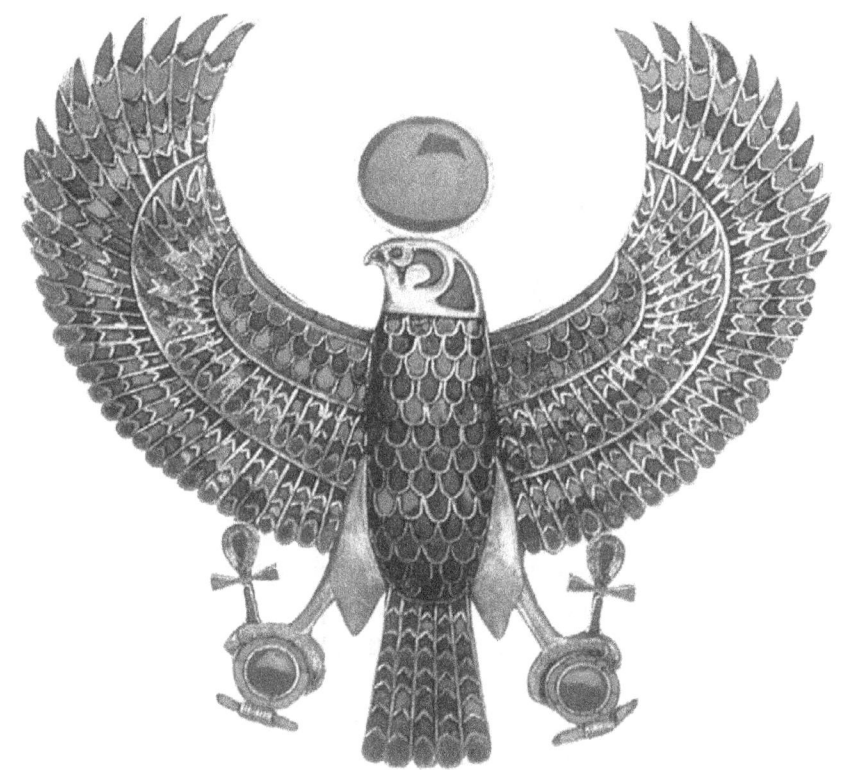

Mystical Philosophy of Universal Consciousness
SEX SUBLIMATION EXERCISES AND MEDITATIONS

Meditation in Egyptian Tantra Yoga: in Egyptian Tantra Yoga the Meditative movement is composed of a culmination of myth, philosophy and ritual in the absorption into the higher, underlying nature of Self through in-depth understanding of the mythic teaching and experiencing it by assuming the characters being united in the teaching.

    d. **Visualization:** based on philosophy: seeing the underlying unity of Creation: Amun-Mut, Asar-Aset, Ptah, Hetheru-Heru, etc. who represent heaven and earth not separated but as aspects of one being.

    e. **Visualization:** based on philosophy: seeing the individual self as becoming one with the Universal Self underlying all.

    f. **Visualization:** sexual symbolism as metaphor of the reunion act of individual initiate and the Universal Self.

NOTE: The transformative effect of the Tantric Meditation will not occur until there exists:
1. absolute faith in the tantric teaching.
2. absolute understanding of the tantric philosophy.
3. absolute absorption in the tantric ritual through repeated practice with devotion, feeling and one pointed concentration (which consequently means a complete letting go of egoistic consciousness.

Tantrism works with the Life Force of Sexuality, to control, harness and sublimate it and employ it towards the goal of raising consciousness to the realization of universal oneness. In this capacity, sex is the ultimate venue not to the fleeting orgasm of the physical plane but to the perennial experience of union with the Divine.

The most important way to control and harness the sexual energies and transmute them into spiritual energy in the form of will-power, righteousness, self-control, universal love, etc. is to develop insight into the nature of the Higher Self through the disciplines of yoga (Study of the Wisdom Teachings, Meditation, detachment, dispassion, etc.).

The physical exercises given here will assist in redirecting the energies which focus and accumulate at the level of the sexual organs and will facilitate the process of controlling the sexual urges and desires. According to the teachings of Serpent Power Yoga (a branch of Tantra Yoga) sexual energy lies dormant at the base of the spine and from there it rises according to the level of spiritual evolution of the person in question. For most people, especially the masses who are ignorant of the spiritual teachings and of their higher spiritual selves, the energy accumulates at the three lower energy consciousness centers and manifests in various forms of egoistic sentiment. These lower centers represent Fear and Survival (level 1), Sexuality and Creativity (level 2) and Power and Control over others (level 3). See the books: *Meditation: The Ancient Egyptian Path to Enlightenment* and *The Serpent Power* by Dr. Muata Ashby.

These three lower levels represent the lower self in a human being. In order to transform consciousness from lower to higher experience it is necessary to have an integral movement in every aspect of one's personality (Emotion, Reason, Action and Will). If this movement is not promoted a person experiences an existence which does not progress beyond the lower experiences of life and there is limited awareness of the divine essence beyond the mundane

EGYPTIAN TANTRIC YOGA

world of time and space. A person who is caught at this level sees him or herself as a sexual being and is oblivious to the greater reality of the soul, which is genderless and supremely fulfilled. Thus, at the lower level, a person is subject to the desires and cravings of the lower nature and the pursuit of sensual pleasures keeps a person engaged in the egoistic conflicts, concepts and feelings which prevent them from discovering real inner peace and contentment. When we speak of sexual energy we are referring to the same Life Force energy which sustains life but which is contaminated with thoughts of duality and separation (egoism). Only when there is duality can there exist the notion of sexual difference and sensual desire. From these erroneous notions the desire to engage in sexual activity arises. When universal consciousness (understanding of the deeper essence of life) arises in the mind, the understanding and experience of non-duality emerges in a person's consciousness and consequently the feeling that all people are human beings and not separate sexual beings arises. This is the form of consciousness which a Sage experiences and it is the source of true fulfillment and inner peace which transcends ordinary human consciousness because there is no longer a burden of sexual desires or insatiable cravings for sensual experiences in the mind.

The following exercises are specifically useful for controlling, harnessing and sublimating sexual energy.

Exercise 1: The Headstand and the Shoulder-stand.

The headstand and the shoulder-stand (page 203) are excellent yogic postures which have the effect of reversing the flow of energy in the body from the lower centers to the higher. (see the *Egyptian Yoga Exercise Workout Book* for more details on how to practice these exercises).

Exercise 2: Serpent Power Visualization.

Another method to sublimate sexual energy is to visualize it being redistributed and transformed into pure Life Force energy (Sekhem, Prana, Chi). The picture depicts and ancient Egyptian youth in the yoga posture known as the Lotus Pose and the rings which are stretched out vertically superimposed on the body represent the seven levels of psycho-spiritual energy consciousness. As you breath in center your attention at the lowest center and visualize the energy as light. See it moving up toward the head and as you do see it nourishing and revitalizing your body as a tree collects water and nutrients from the earth and redistributes them throughout the branches. Breath out and see the energy moving towards the base once more and repeat the exercise. Practice this exercise as many times as you like. You may sit upright or lay on your back.

Mystical Philosophy of Universal Consciousness

SEX SUBLIMATION EXERCISES

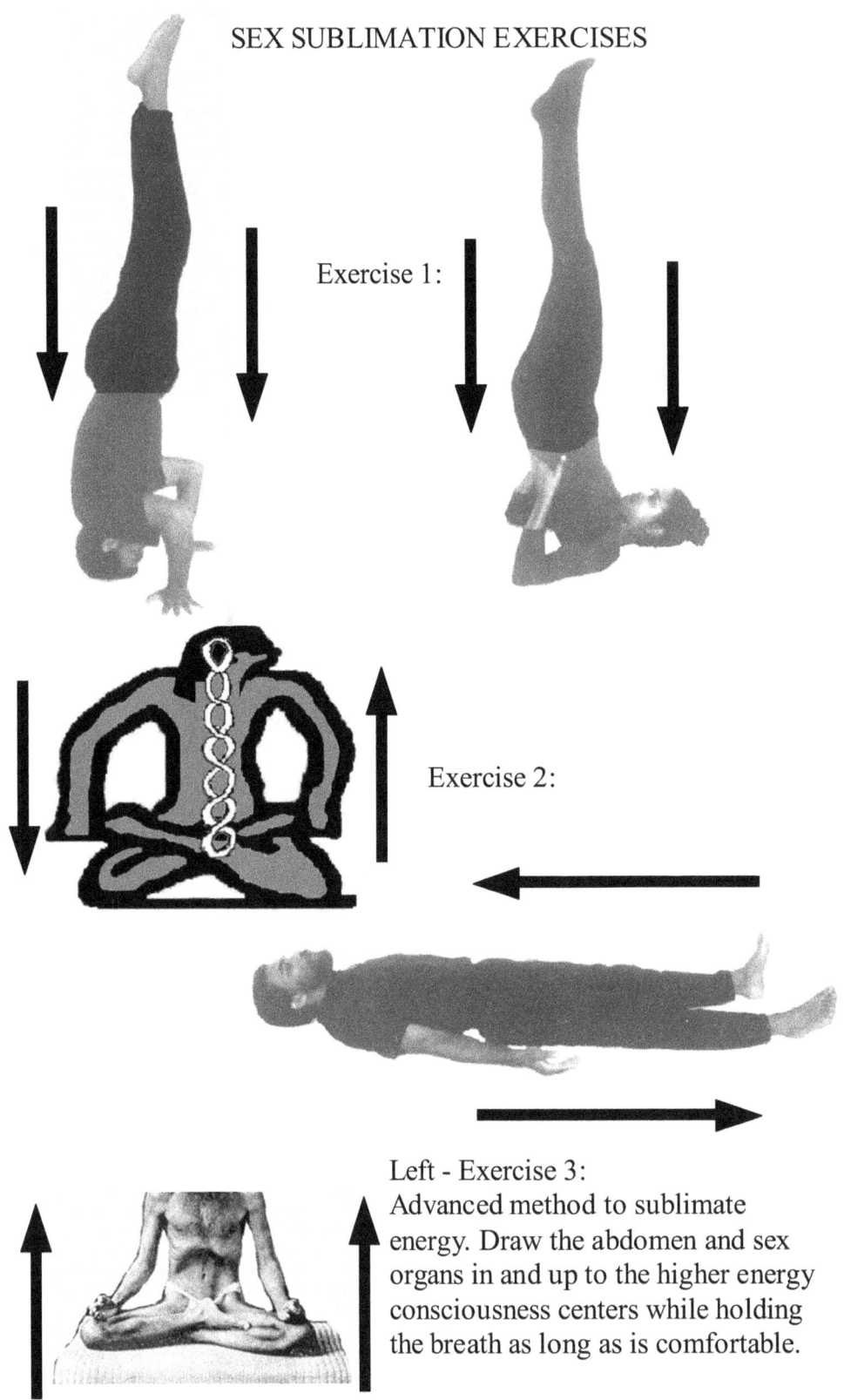

Exercise 1:

Exercise 2:

Left - Exercise 3:
Advanced method to sublimate energy. Draw the abdomen and sex organs in and up to the higher energy consciousness centers while holding the breath as long as is comfortable.

EGYPTIAN TANTRIC YOGA

Kemetic Sex Sublimation Exercise.

It is important to understand that sublimating sex energy, which is actually serpent power, involves more than physical yogic postures. These act to help the personality control the gross energies. However, ultimately, the energy must find its fulfillment, its expression. This may be either in creation of a lower order (in time and space) or of a higher order (in transcendental consciousness). The practice enjoined here is to be done when the personality has begun to be cleansed through the Kemetic Diet system of health, and when the basic program of celibacy has been practiced for some time (sexual intercourse no more than once per month, advanced practice, no more than once per year, more advanced practice 7 years, more advanced practice involves sexual communion with the Divine Self. This requires the highest order of purity of heart, ethical character, and clarity of thought, an increasing knowledge and understanding of the mystical wisdom teaching.

This exercise involves handling sex desire and its accompanying energies in small doses so as not to cross beyond the threshold of the sex climax. In order to do this it is important to work with pure as opposed to impure sexual stimulation. Therefore, pornography, and bestiality and the like are inappropriate for this discipline. Those types of energies will not lend themselves easily to transmutation into a higher form. Fantasies and imaginations about worldly situations, relations or personalities are less detrimental but also less optimal. There is to be no manipulation of genitalia or physical stimulation. Male and female partners can practice with each other in order to stimulate, augment and exchange complementary energies but it is important to choose a partner who is pure. Single people can work with the energies of others without their knowing. This teaching will not be revealed here. Visualizations involving the divinities, especially Geb and Nut, Amsu-min and Asar, Aset and Nebethet are most optimal. The sexuality of these divinities is highly spiritualized and dedicated to creation of life and higher consciousness. This ideal is repeated throughout the mythic and mystic teaching related to them and so it his highly propitious when revealed. It is a shame that in modern times the deeper mystery of these images is not appreciated due to the degradation of society and the ignorance about their deeper meaning. Thus early Christians, Muslims and puritans in modern times sought to destroy or prevent their viewing. The following images come from the temples of ancient Kamit and are provided for the purpose of assisting the practitioner to practice this exercise.

The pictures of the Divine Embrace with Amsu-Min show the initiate pulling the phallus of Amsu into the abdominal region. This is the place where the watery life force of sexuality is transformed into the fire health and the capacity to carry out the divine plan of life. As the divinity acts as a catalyst, infusing the energy it develops into indomitable will, virility and fertility and spiritual love and ultimately spiritual enlightenment.

Work with one image at a time. In the privacy of your room. View for several minutes, examining the detail and recall the teaching of the Myth of Asar, Aset and Heru. Allow yourself to feel the Divine love between Asar and Aset and how their union begets Heru, spiritual aspiration and perfection. Aspire to become this offspring. Allow yourself to assume the role of either Asar (males) or Aset (females). For advanced practice assume both. This is not to be confused with a homosexual experience, but rather the experience of opposites which are to be ultimately united into one whole. When sex desire arises end the arousal visualization. This is the

Mystical Philosophy of Universal Consciousness

homeopathic dose. Do not allow yourself to become over-stimulated. Now enjoin the discipline o visualizing it rising up from the lower energy centers to the higher. Continue with this practice and this may be done at any time whenever there is arousal. However if the arousal is based on the lower stimulation do not attempt to sublimate it. In time the accumulation will lead to ecstasies and expansions of consciousness if all other disciplines are also practiced. Eventually a special glow, a feeling that is a product of this discipline, not unlike the feeling reached after the climax of an ordinary sexual experience will remain perennially and will become intensified whenever there is remembrance of the Divine. This blissful feeling elevates the personality out of worldly affairs and desires as it is a higher fulfillment of those desires that does not require worldly objects, relationships or physicality to experience. This is a higher aspect of Divine Consciousness. There is, beyond this, the expansion of absolute union (ultimate sexual experience) with the Divine. This is the goal for all aspirants to discover. It is complete contentment, satisfaction and happiness that cannot be described.

Begin with one session (experience of one arousal and following with visualization-meditation for sublimation) per week.

Start with the daily chants and invocatory prayers to Asar and Aset or Heru and Hetheru. Light candle, incense, and then unveil image and begin. Following the meditation practice the physical postures enjoined in this book. Do not have physical sexual intercourse for at least 7 days prior or following your Kemetic Tantric sessions.

This exercise will promote the regeneration and cultivation and sublimation of the sexual life force energy. This energy can be used for any creative purpose, begetting physical children, the arts, inspiration, etc. Most importantly it can be used to promote the creation of expanded consciousness and bliss- undifferentiated and unencumbered happiness, termed *awet-ab*, expansion of the heart. Expansion allows the aspirant to spread out, inflate as it were into the extended aspects of higher being, including th astral body (Ka) amd the spiritual body (Sahu), i.e. expanded consciousness.

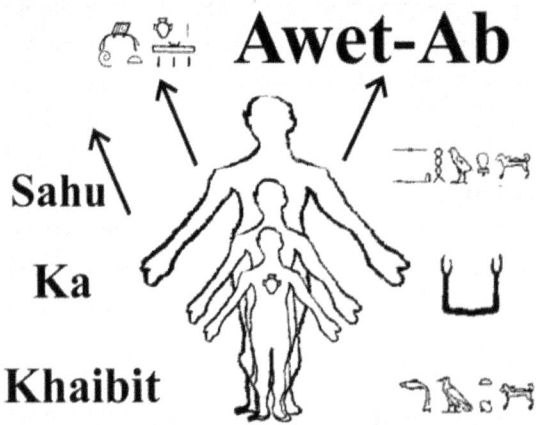

**Expansion of the heart
and
The Three Bodies**

EGYPTIAN TANTRIC YOGA

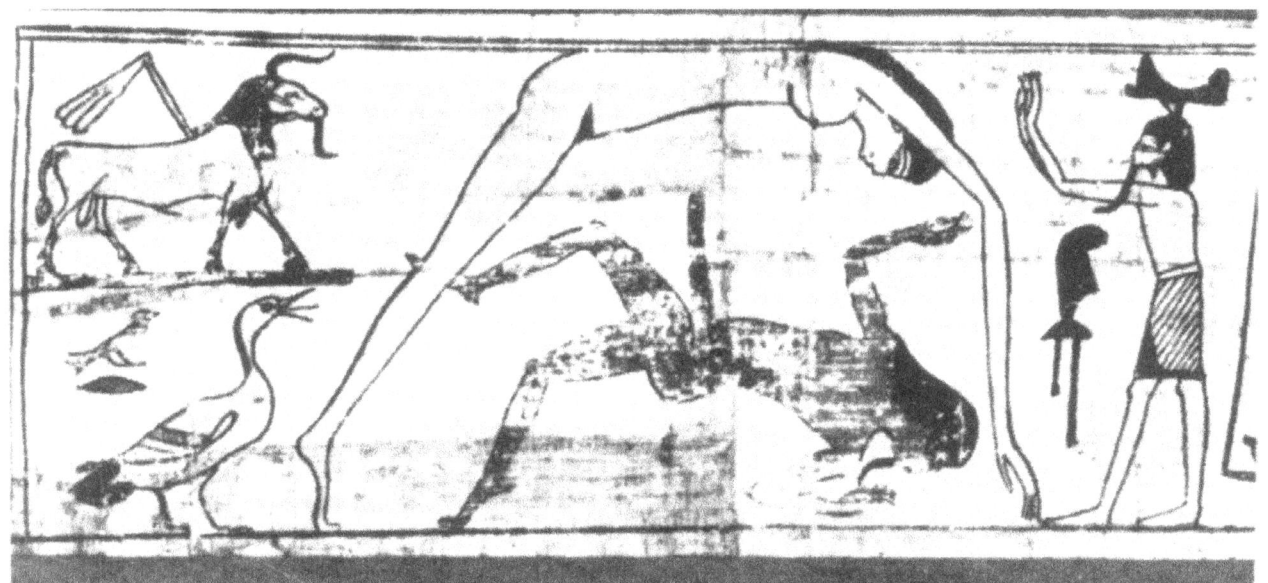

The union of Geb and Nut

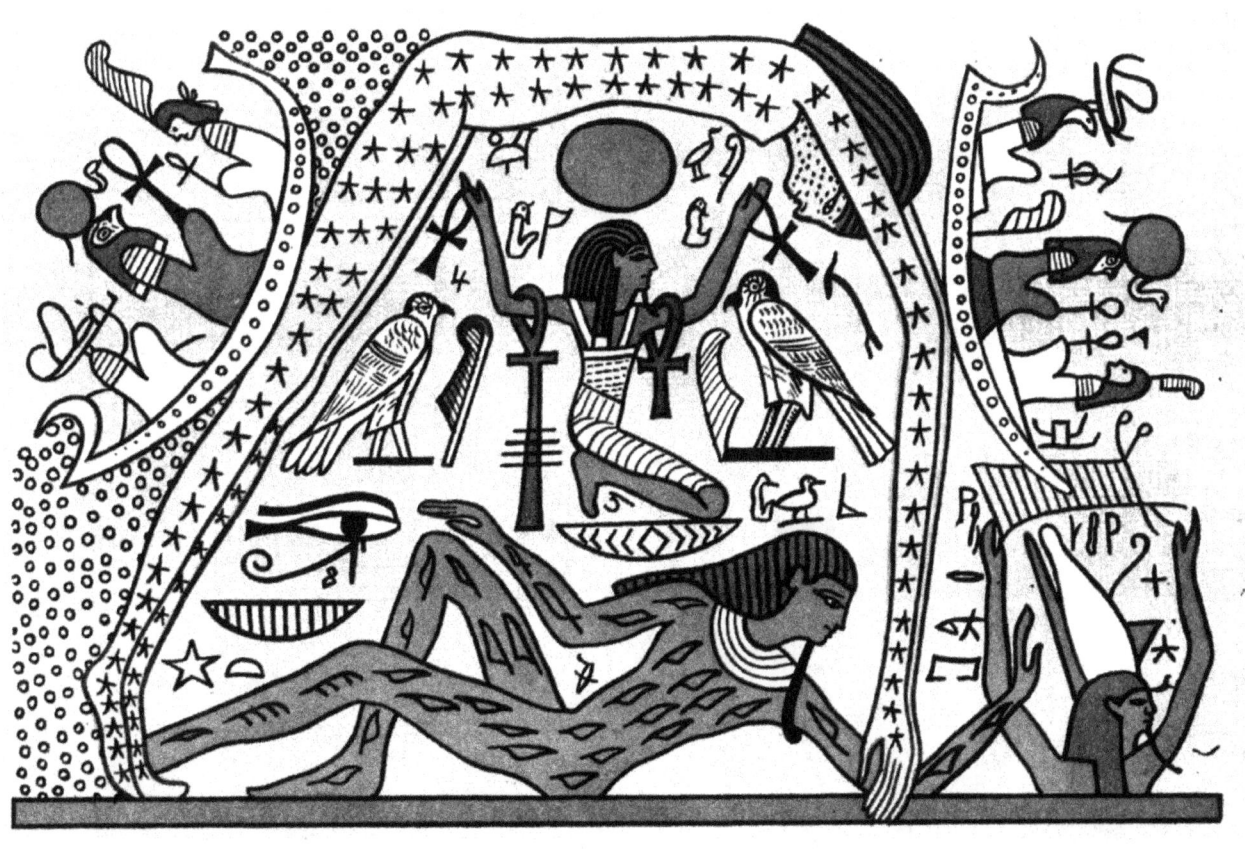

Mystical Philosophy of Universal Consciousness

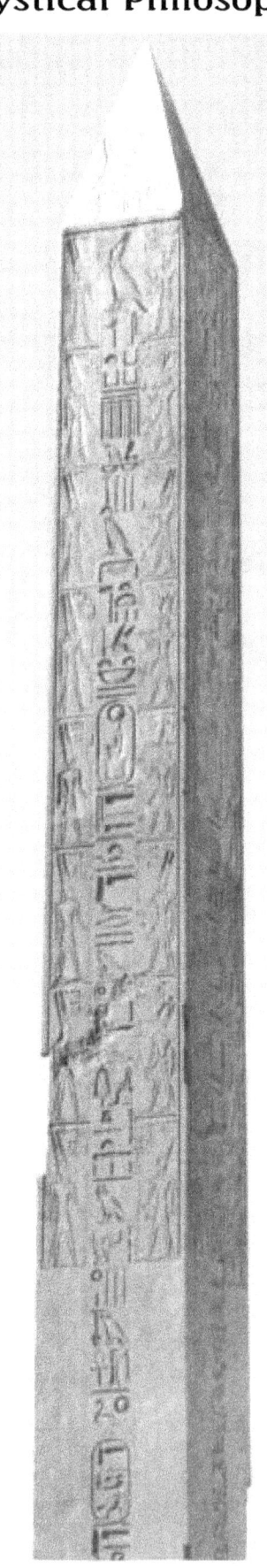

Obelisk Hatshepsut north face (karnak)

EGYPTIAN TANTRIC YOGA

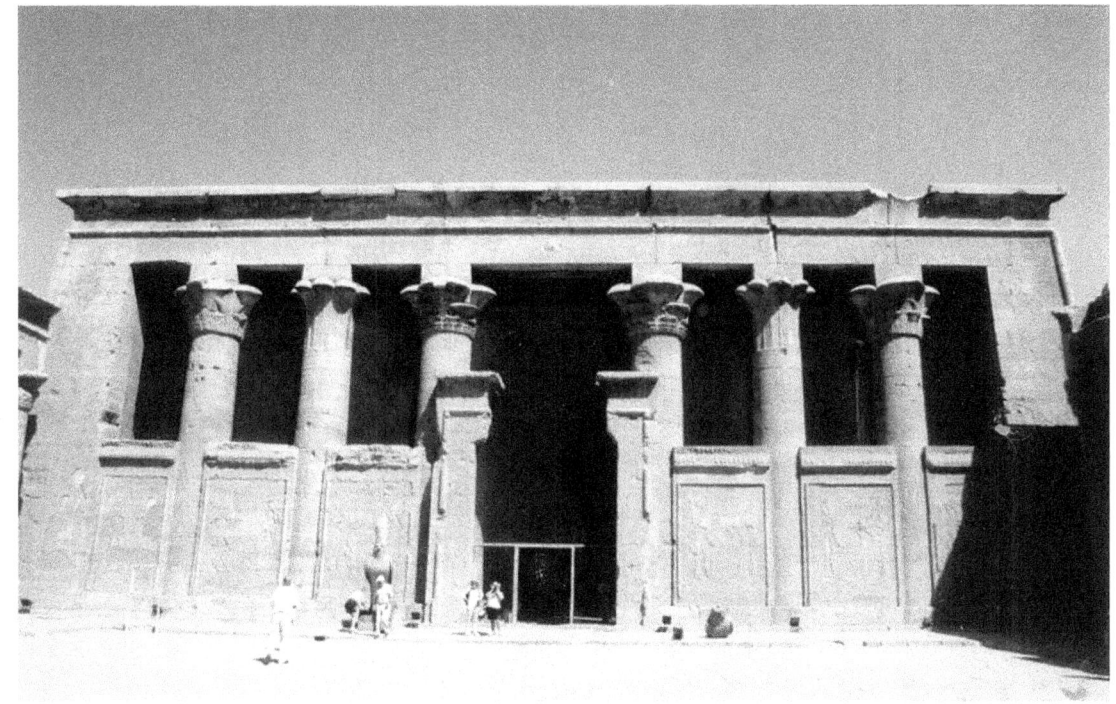

Temple of Heru at Edfu

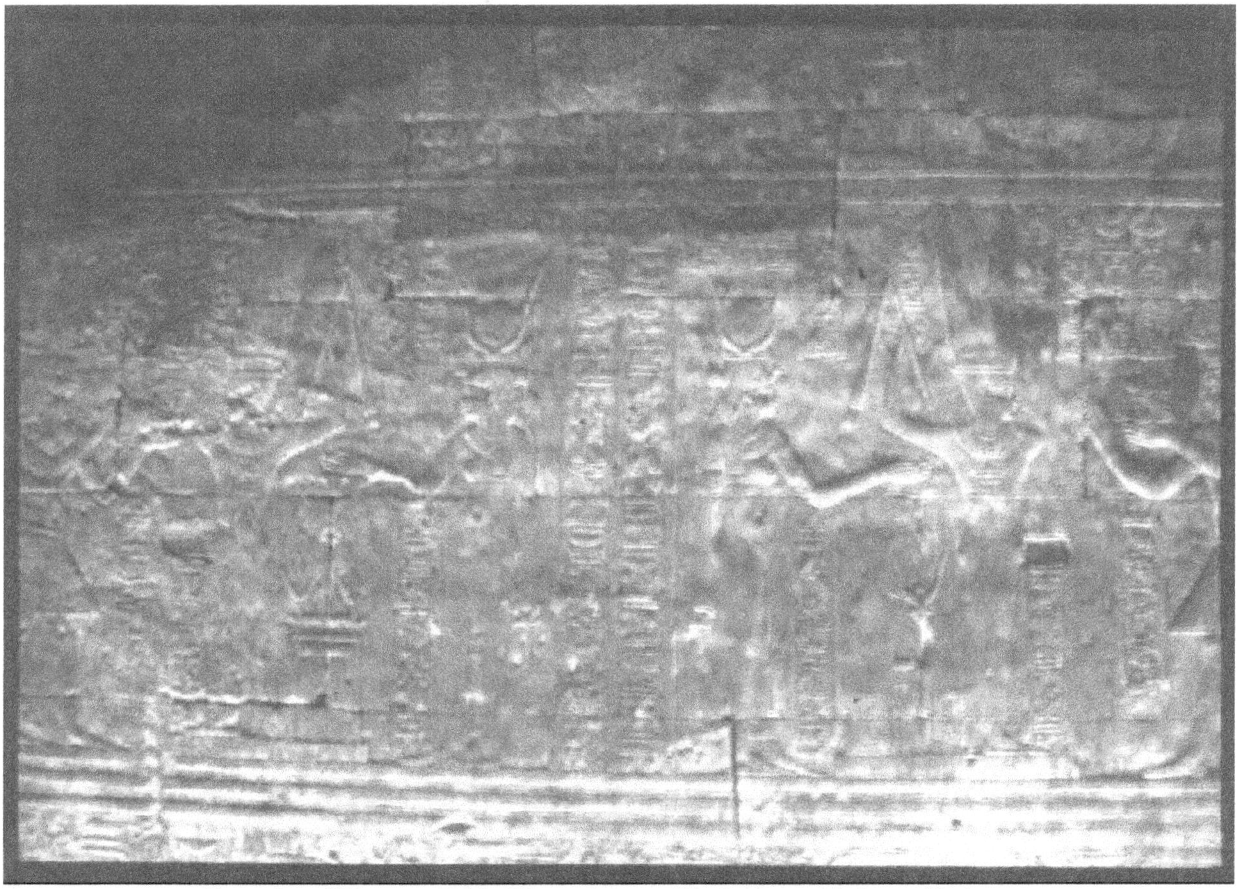

Temple of Heru at Edfu Heru-Amsu--Hetheru receiving offerings

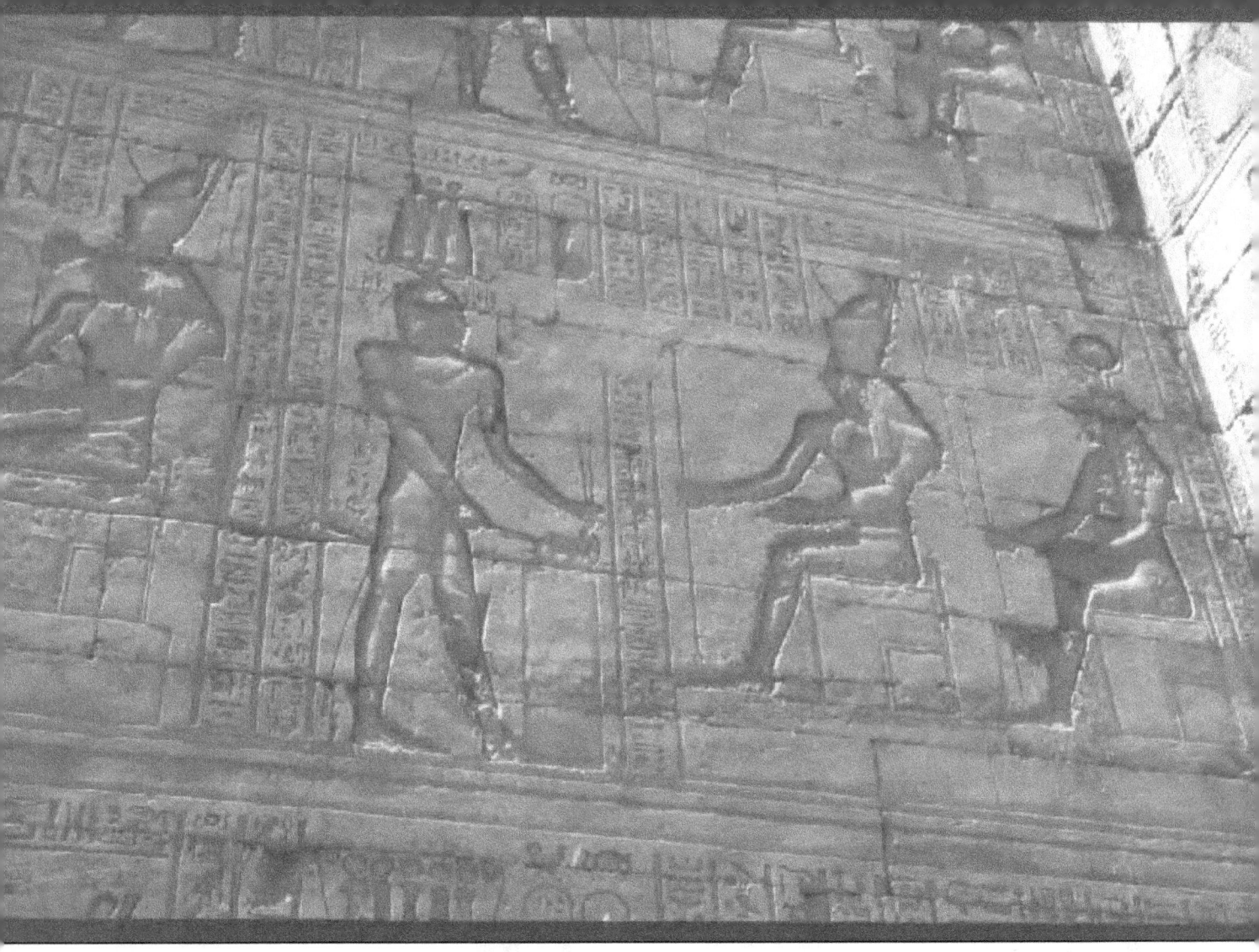

Temple of Heru at Edfu Heru-Hetheru receiving offering

On the following pages:
Temple of Heru at Edfu Divine embrace2
The Divine Embrace with Amsu (Temple of Amun-Karnak, Luxor (Waset-Egypt))
The Divine Embrace with Amsu (Temple of Amun-Karnak, Luxor (Waset-Egypt))
The Divine Embrace with Amsu (Temple of Amun-Karnak, Luxor (Waset-Egypt))

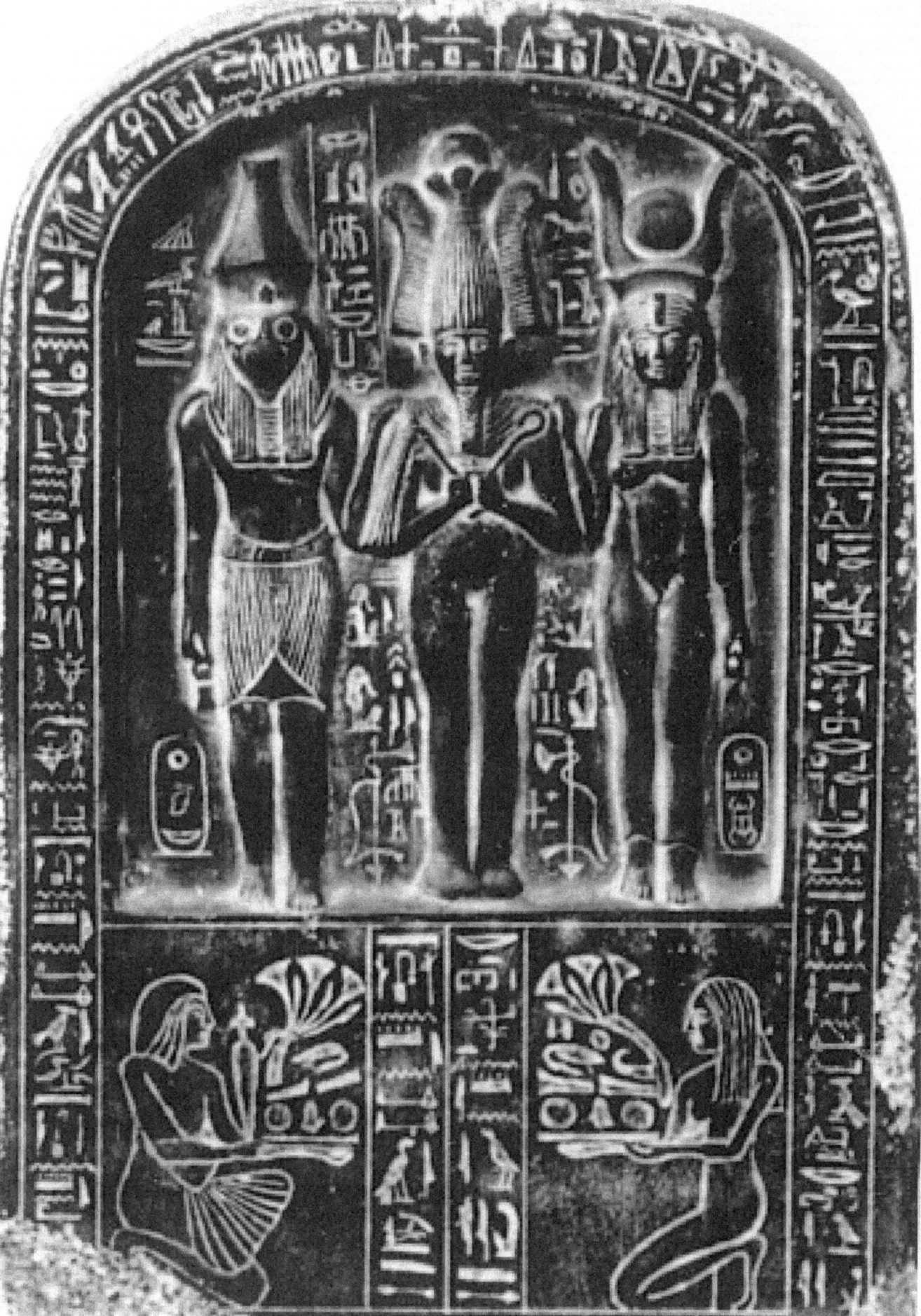

Mystical Philosophy of Universal Consciousness

On the previous page: The Divine Triad: Asar, Aset and Heru

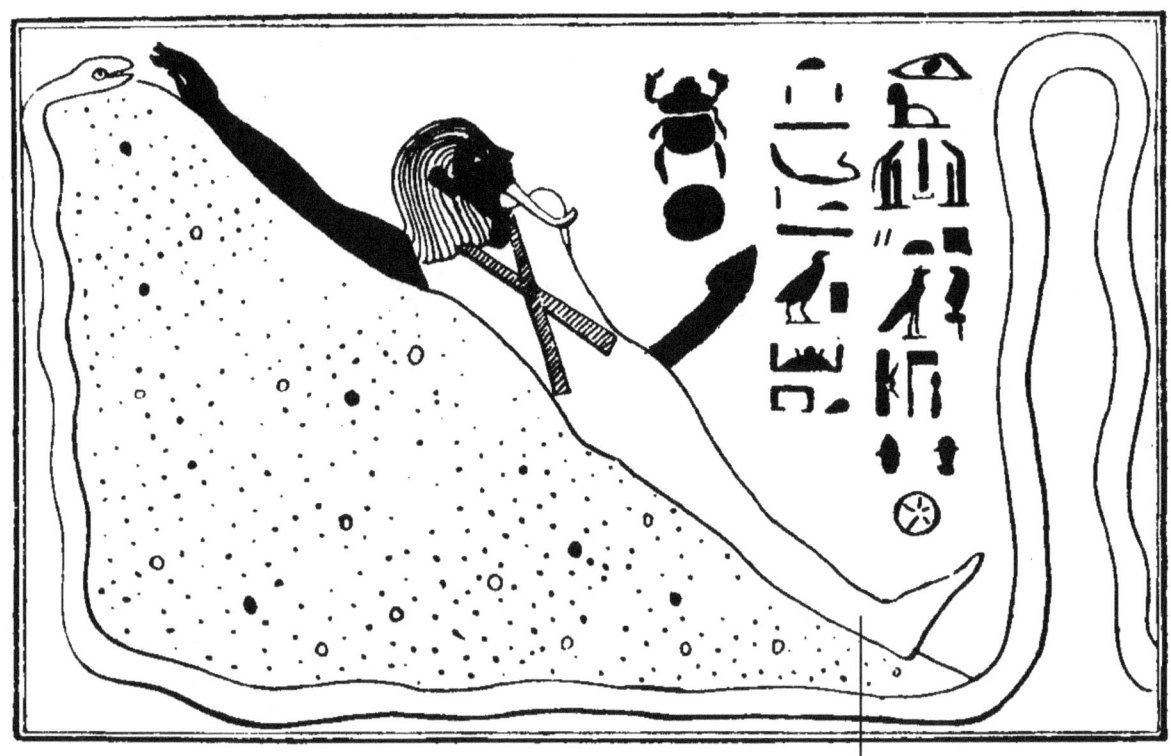

Left: Asar (Osiris) as the creator who engenders Life Force energy into creation through the Mehen Serpent (Power) of the Primeval Waters.

The ejaculate of the god Asar is the essence that sustains and vitalizes all creation. Thus Asar's arousal means creativity and life but mystically it is the nectar of spiritual enlightenment.

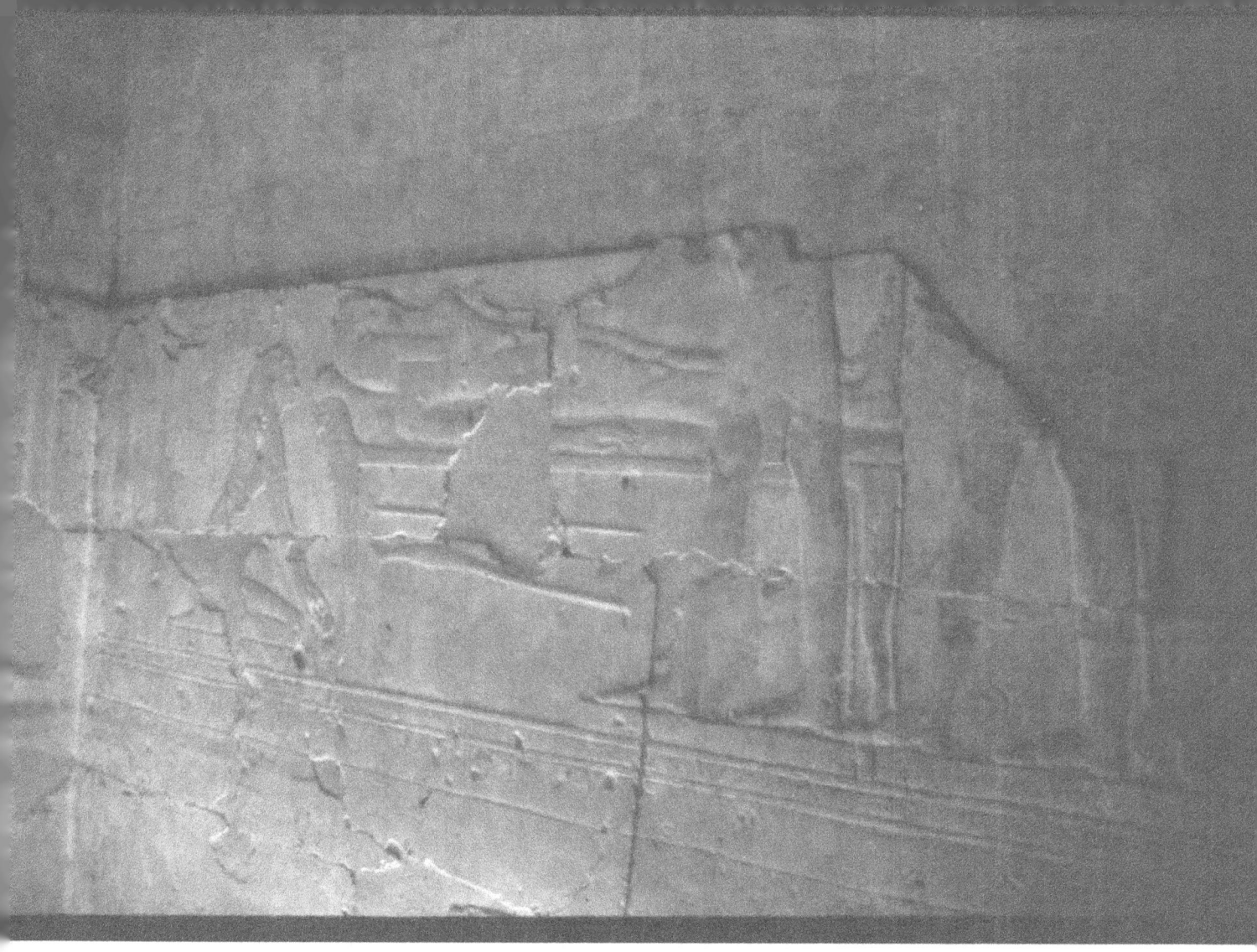

Above: Resurrection scene from the temple of Asar (Abdu, Egypt). Asar impregnates Aset (who is in the form of hawk. For detail see below

Mystical Philosophy of Universal Consciousness

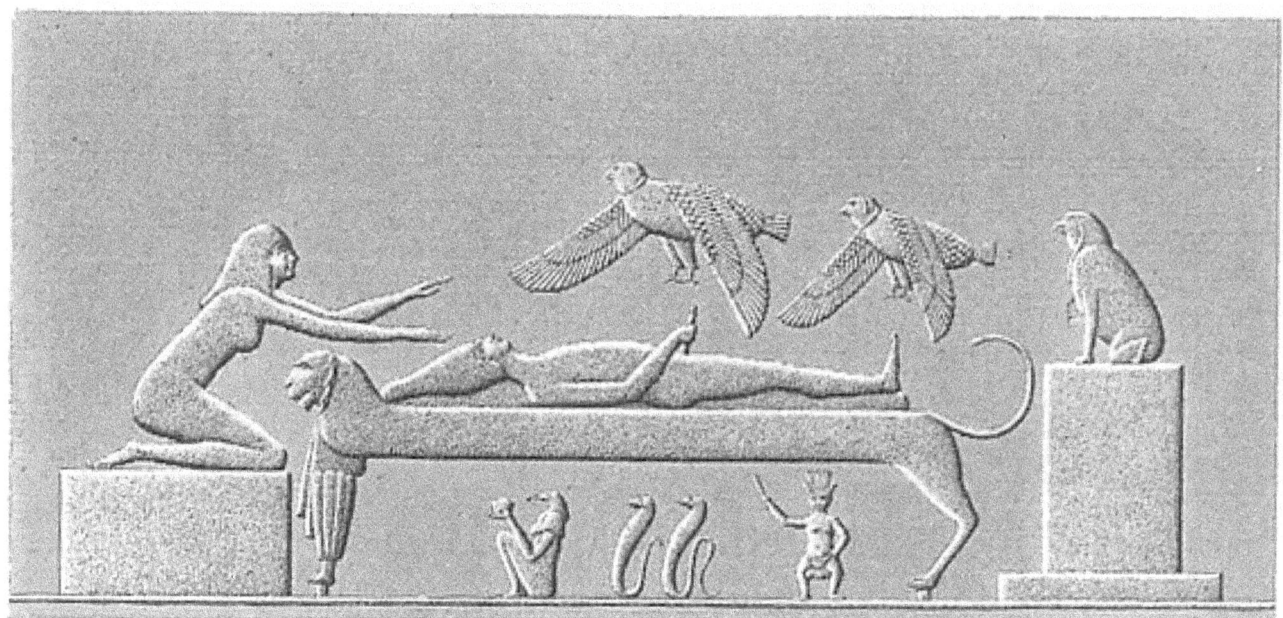

Above: Resurrection scene from the temple of Hetheru (Denderah, Egypt). Asar impregnates Aset (who is in the form of hawk).

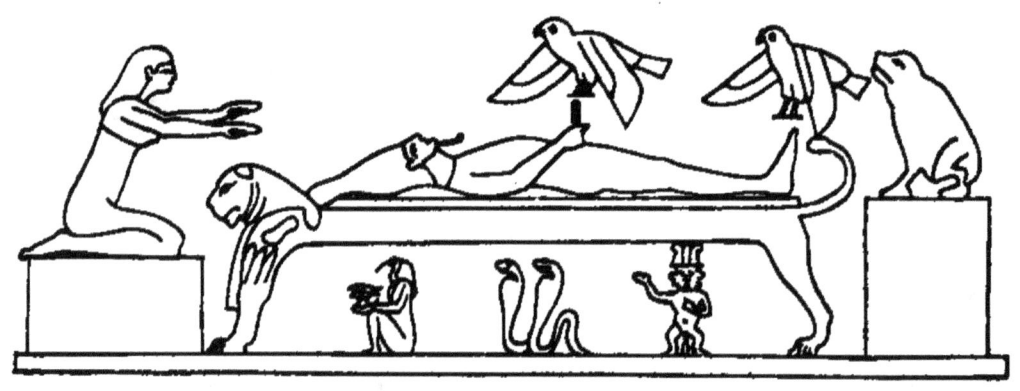

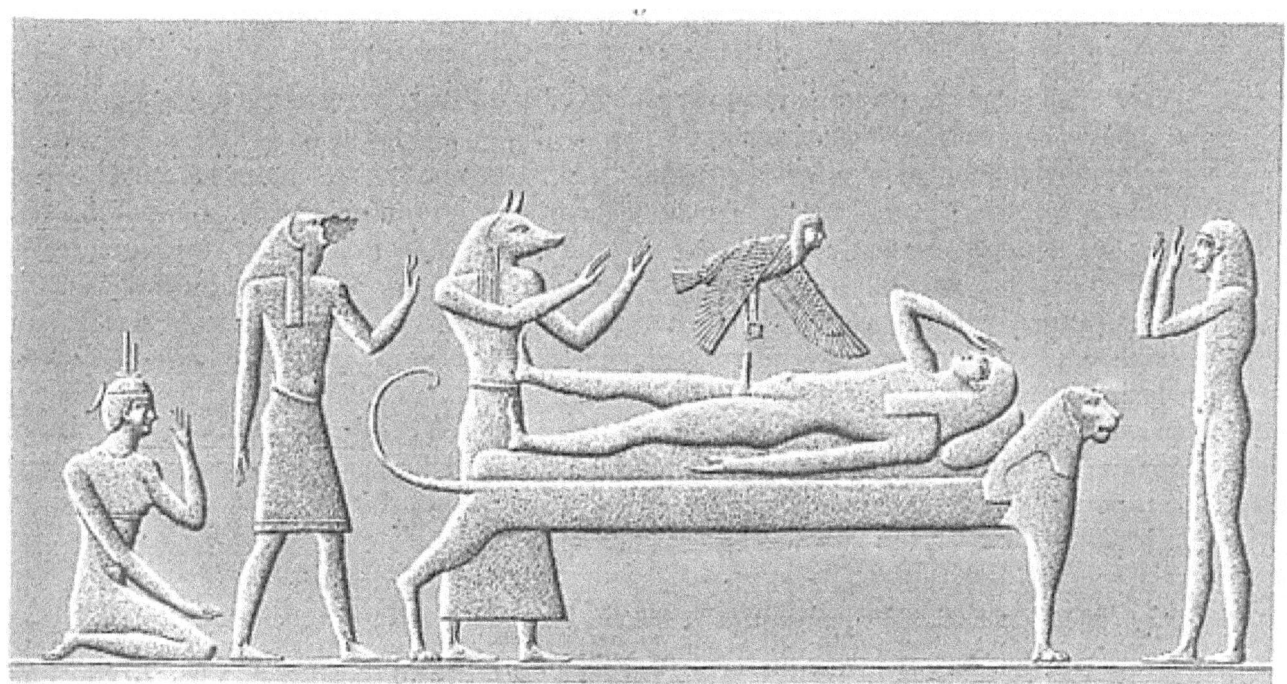

Above: Resurrection scene from the temple of Hetheru (Denderah, Egypt). Asar impregnates Aset (who is in the form of hawk).

Mystical Philosophy of Universal Consciousness

One Last Word

Very often people involved in relationships will be at different levels of evolution. Sometimes one spouse will turn towards the teachings of yoga while the other may feel more comfortable with the religion they grew up with or perhaps with no religion at all. In this case the aspirant should not feel that it is necessary to convince the partner or to find another partner if this one cannot be convinced. Remember, you came together for a Karmic reason that you need to fulfill. If a divorce occurs before this fulfillment the karmic entanglement to the world will remain and another relation will be needed in this life or the next. Therefore, you should honor your commitment to that one person while progressing on your own in private and at the same time supporting your partner's practice of religion. You should honor your family responsibilities even as you explore the glory of Yoga and in so doing you will eventually attract the interest and admiration of your family members even without them knowing what you are doing. You will be able to influence them in a subtle way through your inner spiritual strength, virtue and unselfish love.

>May you develop the vision of oneness, the witnessing self within your heart, may you develop the spirit force within you the Horian soul, to overcome and sublimate the Setian tendencies of the lower self.

Index

Abdu, 32, 50, 145, 206
Absolute, 24, 47, 59, 83, 86, 90
Absolute XE "Absolute" Reality, 59, 83
Adultery, 185
Africa, 4, 8, 21, 43, 63, 67, 128, 133, 134
Air, 85
Akhnaton, 33
Akhus, 36
Alexandria, 67
Amen, 157
Amenta, 157, 219
Amentet, 156, 220
Ammit, 142
Amun, 19, 23, 27, 30, 72, 109, 119, 132, 137, 156, 157, 191, 199
Ancient Egypt, 3, 4, 8, 9, 12, 16, 17, 21, 22, 24, 25, 38, 39, 40, 41, 42, 43, 44, 45, 46, 47, 50, 51, 52, 53, 54, 59, 60, 63, 65, 67, 69, 71, 72, 73, 79, 84, 90, 109, 120, 122, 127, 128, 129, 130, 131, 132, 133, 134, 135, 139, 141, 142, 144, 145, 146, 147, 148, 149, 150, 156, 157, 160, 161, 168, 169, 175, 176, 177, 180, 181, 182, 183, 184, 185, 187, 191, 216, 217, 218, 219, 220, 221, 223, 224, 225
Angels, 80
Ani, 89, 127, 136, 150
Ankh, 41, 124, 125, 127
Anpu, 74
Anu, 19, 27, 28, 73, 134, 220
Anu (Greek Heliopolis), 19, 27, 28, 73, 134, 220
Anubis, 74, 76, 78, 87, 89, 98
Anunian Theology, 23, 27, 28, 135
Apedemak, 63
Apep serpent, 35
Apophis, 35, 86
Ardhanari, 65, 127

Ari, 19
Aryan, 217
Asar, 19, 23, 27, 28, 32, 42, 43, 44, 50, 59, 60, 61, 62, 66, 69, 72, 74, 76, 77, 78, 79, 80, 84, 87, 88, 89, 90, 91, 94, 96, 97, 99, 106, 129, 132, 135, 136, 137, 144, 146, 147, 148, 150, 156, 159, 160, 161, 162, 179, 181, 191, 194, 195, 205, 206, 207, 208, 215, 219, 220, 224, 225
Asarian Resurrection, 23, 53, 219, 220, 221
Aset, 4, 23, 28, 31, 32, 42, 44, 46, 47, 50, 59, 60, 61, 66, 69, 72, 74, 76, 77, 78, 79, 80, 87, 89, 90, 91, 97, 98, 99, 106, 129, 132, 135, 137, 144, 147, 148, 149, 159, 160, 179, 180, 181, 183, 186, 191, 194, 195, 205, 206, 207, 208, 219, 220, 224
Aset (Isis), 4, 23, 28, 31, 32, 42, 44, 46, 47, 50, 59, 60, 61, 66, 69, 72, 74, 76, 77, 78, 79, 80, 87, 89, 90, 91, 97, 98, 99, 106, 129, 132, 135, 137, 144, 147, 148, 149, 159, 160, 179, 180, 183, 186, 191, 194, 195, 205, 206, 207, 208, 219, 220
Ashoka, 63

Asia, 1, 43

Asians, 187
Asoka, 63
Astral, 55, 107, 120, 158, 219
Astral Plane, 55, 107, 120, 158, 219
Aton, 19, 27, 33
Atonism, 33
Atum, 23, 74, 130, 148
Augustus, 8
Awareness, 11

Ba (also see Soul), 51, 60, 106, 146
Babylon, 135
Being, 18, 20, 24, 26, 27, 28, 29, 30, 32, 33, 38, 43, 61, 73, 74, 80, 82, 148, 181, 220
Bhagavad Gita, 38
Bible, 69, 220
Blackness, 9
Book of Coming Forth By Day, 89, 127, 154, 182, 219
Book of Enlightenment, 51, 181
Book of the Dead, see also Rau Nu Prt M Hru, 23, 27, 179, 182, 220
Brahman, 47
Breathing exercises, 86
Buddha, 61
Buddhism, 4, 63, 65, 66
Buddhist, 61, 66, 67, 68, 161
Bull, 162
Buto, 86
C, 85
Caduceus, 78, 144, 145, 146, 147, 148, 149
Caribbean, 4
Catholic, 69, 187, 220
Causal Plane, 107, 120
Celibacy, 104, 154, 165, 166, 177, 178, 179
Chakras, 147
Chakras (see energy centers of the body), 147
Chanting, 47
Chi, 86, 192

China, 1, 39, 41, 76

Christ, 67, 69, 150, 219
Christ Consciousness, 150
Christianity, 12, 44, 63, 68, 69, 125, 150, 180, 216, 220
Church, 187, 220
Civilization, 39, 41
Coffin Texts, 10, 23
Company of gods and goddesses, 73
Conception, 60
Conflict, 169
Consciousness, 8, 36, 39, 43, 44, 58, 147, 219

Contentment (see also Hetep), 21
Coptic, 22, 67, 219
Cosmic consciousness, 38
Cosmogony, 73
Cosmos, 59
Cow, 31
Creation, 16, 21, 23, 24, 27, 28, 29, 30, 31, 32, 33, 44, 55, 59, 61, 62, 67, 68, 72, 73, 80, 83, 84, 85, 91, 109, 119, 128, 130, 131, 137, 145, 167, 175, 188, 191, 219, 220

Crete, 1

Cross, 69
Culture, 21, 35, 218
Cymbals, 224, 225
Death, 90
December, 220
Demotic, 8
Denderah, 91, 110, 113, 115, 116, 117, 159, 207, 208, 219
Desire, 100
Dharmakaya, 61, 68
Diet, 182, 194, 217
Diodorus, 8, 10
Discipline, 4, 46, 49, 104
Divine Consciousness, 36, 195
Djed Pillar, see also Pillar of Asar, 156
Djehuti, 42, 44, 74, 78, 136, 145, 146, 161
DNA, 101, 153
Duat, 156, 157, 219
Dynastic Period, 134, 180
Earth, 80, 83, 85, 157
Edfu, 32, 48, 110, 159, 198, 199, 219
Egoism, 35
Egyptian Book of Coming Forth By Day, 1, 89, 135, 136, 156, 219
Egyptian civilization, 16, 44, 133, 134
Egyptian Mysteries, 12, 44, 217, 221
Egyptian Physics, 220

Mystical Philosophy of Universal Consciousness

Egyptian proverbs, 42, 218
Egyptian religion, 16, 43, 67
Egyptian Yoga, 2, 4, 8, 11, 30, 37, 38, 39, 40, 41, 42, 43, 44, 54, 62, 67, 192, 216, 217, 219, 223, 224, 225
Egyptian Yoga see also Kamitan Yoga, 2, 4, 8, 11, 30, 37, 38, 39, 40, 41, 42, 43, 44, 54, 62, 67, 192, 216, 217, 219
Egyptologists, 8, 35, 43, 134
Electric, 95
Elohim, 85
Enlightenment, 8, 11, 13, 21, 34, 39, 43, 44, 51, 67, 104, 122, 159, 181, 191, 215, 217, 218, 219, 220, 221
Ennead, 74, 79, 80, 98
Ethics, 48
Ethiopia, 8, 9, 63
Ethiopian priests, 8
Eucharist, 219
Evil, 70
Exercise, 192, 194, 219
Eye of Heru, 36
Eye of Horus, 132, 141
Eye of Ra, 79, 136
Fear, 191
Female, 95
Feuerstein, Georg, 53, 54
Forgiveness, 170
Geb, 28, 53, 54, 59, 61, 69, 74, 76, 80, 81, 82, 83, 85, 86, 96, 129, 149, 194, 219
Giza, 133, 134, 141
Gnostic, 12, 67, 69, 70
Gnostic Christianity, 12, 67
Gnostic gospels, 70
God, 16, 20, 21, 24, 36, 38, 42, 43, 44, 45, 47, 49, 51, 59, 64, 65, 66, 67, 68, 78, 83, 84, 85, 86, 87, 96, 99, 102, 118, 119, 120, 127, 128, 130, 132, 136, 137, 139, 141, 142, 145, 148, 149, 150, 158, 161, 162, 164, 169, 170, 174, 177, 188, 215, 218, 219, 220, 225
Goddess, 16, 19, 23, 24, 27, 31, 59, 66, 79, 83, 86, 113, 118, 123, 127, 129, 142, 164, 183, 220, 223, 225, 226
Goddesses, 17, 18, 24, 28, 30, 31, 55, 73, 84, 132, 219
Gods, 8, 17, 18, 24, 28, 30, 55, 73, 78, 79, 80, 84, 119, 132, 148, 156, 219
Good, 175
Gospels, 67, 220
Great Pyramid, 141
Great Truths, 16, 17, 18, 19, 20
Great Year, 134
Greece, 9, 39, 41, 135, 187, 217
Greek philosophy, 216
Greeks, 145, 180, 186, 187
Gregory, 69
Hatha Yoga, 53, 54
Hathor, 69, 70, 74, 79, 80, 89, 98, 99, 122, 160, 219, 220, 221
Hatshepsut, Queen, 197
Health, 4, 216
Heart, 19, 221
Heart (also see Ab, mind, conscience), 19, 221
Heaven, 68, 80, 83, 157, 220
Hebrew, 67, 85
Hekau, 51, 161, 225
Hell, 157
Hermes, 145
Hermes (see also Djehuti, Thoth), 145
Hermetic, 147
Herodotus, 9, 180
Heru, 23, 27, 28, 32, 36, 40, 41, 42, 44, 48, 54, 60, 62, 72, 78, 79, 106, 110, 113, 130, 131, 134, 135, 148, 169, 179, 186, 191, 194, 195, 198, 199, 205, 219, 220, 224, 225
Heru (see Horus), 23, 27, 28, 32, 36, 40, 41, 42, 44, 48, 54, 60, 62, 72, 78, 79, 106, 110, 113, 130, 131, 134, 135, 148, 169, 179, 186, 191, 194, 195, 198, 199, 205, 219, 220, 224, 225
Heru in the Horizon, 134
Heru XE "Heru (see Horus)" XE "Heru" -m-akhet (Sphinx XE "Sphinx"), 134, 135
Hetep, 41, 127, 128
Hetep Slab, 127, 128
Hetheru, 23, 27, 31, 42, 44, 53, 54, 72, 91, 109, 113, 115, 116, 117, 118, 123, 191, 195, 198, 199, 207, 208, 221, 224
HetHeru (Hetheru, Hathor), 224
Hetheru (Hetheru, Hathor), 23, 27, 31, 42, 44, 53, 54, 72, 91, 109, 113, 115, 116, 117, 118, 123, 191, 195, 198, 199, 207, 208, 221
Het-Ka-Ptah, see also Men-nefer, Memphis, 27
Hieroglyphic Writing, language, 65, 218
High God, 148
Hindu, 51, 69, 78, 87, 96, 127, 131
Hindu mythology, 96
Hinduism, 63, 65, 66, 69, 125, 130, 180
Holy of Holies, 160
Hor-m-Akhet, 133
Horus, 23, 32, 60, 69, 70, 74, 76, 78, 79, 80, 87, 89, 91, 95, 97, 98, 99, 129, 132, 135, 136, 159, 161, 186, 224
Horushood, 96
I, 84
Iamblichus, 161
Ida and Pingala, 147
Identification, 39
Ignorance, 174
Illusion, 215

India, 1, 9, 10, 38, 39, 40, 41, 43, 46, 47, 50, 53, 54, 59, 61, 65, 66, 67, 68, 69, 76, 128, 130, 142, 148, 149, 217, 218, 225
Indian Yoga, 4, 38, 216, 217, 225
Indus, 39, 41, 65, 134, 217
Indus Valley, 39, 41, 65, 217
Initiate, 161, 217
Isis, 23, 31, 32, 46, 47, 60, 179, 180, 181, 219, 220, 224
Isis, See also Aset, 31, 32, 46, 47, 60, 179, 180, 181, 219, 220
Islam, 180, 216
Jainism, 65
Jesus, 68, 69, 70, 186, 219, 220
Jesus Christ, 219
Jnana Yoga, 46, 47
Joy, 21, 149
Judaism, 180, 216
Jyotirmayananda, Swami, 51
Ka, 27, 195
Kabbalah, 216
Kali, 60, 61, 66, 69
Kali XE "Kali" position, 61, 66
Kali Position, 60
Kamit, 18, 21, 24, 25, 31, 32, 77, 109, 133, 194
Kamit (Egypt), 18, 21, 24, 25, 31, 32, 77, 109, 133, 194
Kamitan, 4, 18, 22, 23, 24, 26, 34, 39, 49, 54, 56, 59, 61, 62, 63, 131, 133, 147, 148, 217
Karma, 10, 39, 218
Karnak, 109, 118, 199
Keeping the balance, 150
Kemetic, 4, 56, 59, 61, 63, 78, 80, 83, 109, 121, 131, 133, 142, 147, 148, 149, 162, 175, 177, 182, 190, 194, 195, 223, 224, 225
Khonsu, 30
Kingdom, 9, 30, 33, 44, 54, 68, 220
Kingdom of Heaven, 68, 220
Kingdom of the Father, 68
Kmt, 77, 78
KMT (Ancient Egypt). See also Kamit, 9
Know thyself, 34
Know Thyself, 41
Krishna, 69, 220
Kundalini, 4, 10, 39, 61, 65, 66, 67, 68, 86,

211

142, 146, 147, 149, 151
Kundalini XE "Kundalini" Yoga see also Serpent Power, 4, 65, 66, 67, 68, 86, 142, 146
Life Force, 10, 19, 42, 65, 67, 85, 86, 87, 107, 120, 122, 134, 142, 146, 147, 149, 156, 158, 181, 191, 192, 219
Lingam-Yoni, 128
Listening, 19, 27, 46, 47, 49, 215
Lotus, 42, 130, 192
Love, 3, 11, 38, 39, 49, 85, 106, 120, 152, 218
Lower Egypt, 40, 41, 42
Luxor, 109, 199
Maakheru, 17, 18
Maat, 17, 18, 19, 23, 39, 48, 74, 89, 91, 99, 134, 142, 148, 154, 172, 178, 187, 218, 220, 221
MAAT, 79, 98, 100, 101, 140, 142, 218
MAATI, 218
Madonna, 186
Magnetic, 95
Mahabharata, 38
Male, 95, 194
Manetho, 10
Manetho, see also History of Manetho, 10
Mantras, 51, 66
Mary Magdalene, 69, 70
Matter, 102, 220
Maya, 120
Meditating, 46
Meditation, 2, 19, 20, 31, 38, 39, 47, 48, 50, 52, 72, 191, 217, 218, 225

Mediterranean, 1

Mehurt, 31
Memphite Theology, 23, 29, 31
Menat, 122, 123
Metaphysics, 220
Middle East, 216
Min, 69, 80, 87, 88, 89, 129, 194, 219
Modern science, 120
Mookerjee, Ajit, 1
Moon, 9, 148, 162

Music, 109, 154, 224, 225
Muslims, 194
Mut, 30, 31, 72, 109, 191
Mysteries, 11, 31, 44, 84, 159, 217, 221
Mysticism, 4, 43, 49, 121, 127, 148, 217, 219, 220, 221
Mythology, 8, 43, 127
Nature, 22, 96, 102, 153, 168, 172
Neberdjer, 17, 18, 84
Nebertcher, 129
Nebethet, 74, 76, 78, 80, 87, 90, 96, 97, 144, 147, 148, 149, 159, 160, 194
Nebthet, 28
Nefer, 41, 224, 225
Nefertari, Queen, 54
Nefertem, 29, 131
Nehast, 36, 164
Neolithic, 134
Net, goddess, 23, 31
Neter, 16, 17, 18, 19, 21, 22, 23, 24, 25, 27, 33, 34, 36, 38, 42, 43, 44, 80, 83, 137, 160, 177, 178, 219
Neterian, 18, 19, 27, 31, 35, 36, 84, 148, 177, 178, 179
Neterianism, 16, 19, 24, 63, 130, 162, 178
Neters, 43, 45, 59, 74, 80, 83
Neteru, 17, 18, 20, 22, 24, 25, 26, 35, 36, 54, 59, 148, 177, 224, 225
Netherworld, 55, 156
New Kingdom, 30, 33, 54, 119
New Testament, 69
Nile River, 21
Nirvana, 67
Nu, 74
Nubia, 9, 183
Nubians, 21
Nun, 27, 55
Nun (primeval waters-unformed matter), 27, 55
Nun (See also Nu), 27, 55
Nut, 28, 54, 55, 59, 61, 69, 74, 76, 80, 81, 82, 83, 85, 86, 96, 149, 194, 219
Obelisk, 81, 83, 197
Old Kingdom, 183

Old Testament, 67
Om, 224, 225
Origen, 67
Orion Star Constellation, 220
Orthodox, 68, 69, 134, 178, 185
Osiris, 8, 9, 23, 31, 32, 60, 181, 219, 224, 225
Pa Neter, 17, 18, 83
Papyrus of Any, 23
Parvati, 69
Passion, 152
Patanjali, 38, 52
Paut, 19, 54
Pautti, 73
Peace (see also Hetep), 13, 21, 127, 156
Persia, 187
Persians, 186
Pert Em Heru, See also *Book of the Dead*, 42, 179, 219
phallus, 78, 80, 83, 87, 128, 164, 194
Pharaoh, 9, 134, 187
Pharaonic headdress, 135
Philae, 50, 159, 219
Philosophy, 2, 3, 4, 8, 11, 12, 15, 16, 20, 23, 39, 40, 41, 42, 44, 45, 51, 58, 67, 72, 102, 139, 142, 217, 218, 219, 220, 221
Pillar of Asar, 142, 143
Plutarch, 159, 160, 179, 180
Prana (also see Sekhem and Life Force), 85, 86, 192
Priests and Priestesses, 25, 109, 177, 217
Primeval Ocean, 137
Ptah, 19, 23, 27, 29, 72, 118, 132, 137, 149, 156, 191, 220
Ptahotep, 23
Ptolemy, Greek ruler, 135
Puerto Rico, 4
Pyramid, 132
Ra, 19, 23, 27, 28, 30, 35, 51, 55, 73, 74, 76, 79, 80, 86, 129, 130, 132, 134, 137, 146, 148, 157, 215, 219, 224, 225
Radha, 69
Rauch, 85
Reality, 59

Realization, 20
Reflecting, 46
Reflection, 47
Relationships, 138, 165, 166
Religion, 4, 8, 15, 16, 17, 22, 36, 42, 43, 44, 219, 220, 224
Resurrection, 23, 53, 72, 79, 80, 87, 89, 129, 156, 159, 161, 206, 207, 208, 219, 220, 221
Righteous action, 19
Righteousness, 48, 102, 187
Ritual, 19, 23, 39, 49, 72, 109, 113, 118, 128
Rituals, 220
Roman, 12, 23, 68, 69, 185, 187
Roman Catholic, 12, 68
Roman Empire, 69, 185
Rome, 187
Sages, 11, 44, 65, 104, 148, 187, 219, 221
Sahu, 89, 195
Saints, 219
Salvation, 43, 45
Salvation, See also resurrection, 43, 45
Sanskrit, 39, 41, 67
Sebai, 4, 33, 179, 182
See also Ra-Hrakti, 19, 23, 27, 28, 30, 35, 51, 55, 73, 74, 76, 79, 80, 86, 129, 130, 132, 134, 137, 146, 148, 157, 215, 219
See Nat, 23, 31
See Nefertum, 29, 131
Seers, 11
Sekhem, 19, 85, 86, 146, 149, 162, 192
Sekhmet, 129
Self (see Ba, soul, Spirit, Universal, Ba, Neter, Heru)., 2, 19, 35, 39, 40, 41, 42, 43, 44, 45, 46, 47, 48, 54, 59, 60, 65, 72, 84, 85, 90, 91, 96, 97, 99, 103, 104, 107, 120, 130, 131, 132, 133, 137, 138, 139, 141, 143, 148, 149, 153, 154, 156, 167, 170, 172, 174, 179, 191, 194, 217, 218, 219
Self (seeBasoulSpiritUni

versal BaNeterHorus)., 19, 39, 41, 46, 47, 48, 54, 59, 131, 148
Sema, 2, 3, 4, 15, 18, 19, 40, 41, 42, 43, 54, 216
Sema XE "Sema" Paut, see also Egyptian Yoga, 19, 54
Sema Tawi, 15
Semitic, 183
Septuagint, 67
Serpent, 38, 39, 50, 65, 66, 142, 143, 144, 145, 146, 147, 149, 150, 156, 191, 192
Serpent Power, 38, 39, 50, 65, 66, 142, 143, 144, 145, 146, 147, 149, 150, 156, 191, 192
Serpent Power (see also Kundalini and Buto), 38, 39, 50, 65, 66, 142, 143, 144, 145, 146, 147, 149, 150, 156, 191, 192
Serpent Power see also Kundalini Yoga, 38, 39, 50, 65, 66, 142, 143, 144, 145, 146, 147, 149, 150, 156, 191, 192
Set, 17, 18, 28, 35, 40, 41, 42, 44, 70, 74, 76, 78, 79, 80, 87, 89, 91, 95, 96, 97, 98, 136, 156, 159, 160, 161, 169, 181, 215
Seti I, 48, 50, 52, 145, 218
Sex, 64, 89, 129, 141, 151, 190, 194, 215, 219
Sexual energy, 64, 67, 99, 138
Sexuality, 62, 88, 89, 100, 101, 102, 138, 177, 181, 185, 191, 215
Shakti (see also Kundalini), 61, 65, 66, 67, 86, 96, 147
Shen, 127
Shetaut Neter, 3, 4, 8, 15, 16, 17, 21, 23, 27, 34, 38, 43, 162, 219

Shetaut Neter See also Egyptian Religion, 3, 4, 8, 15, 16, 17, 21, 23, 27, 34, 38, 43, 162, 219
Shiva, 61, 62, 65, 66, 69, 78, 86, 87, 96, 128
Shiva XE "Shiva" and Shakti, 61, 66
Shu, 84
Shu (air and space), 28, 55, 74, 76, 80, 83, 84, 85, 149
Sin, 98
Sirius, 220
Skin, 101
Sky, 83
Sma, 19, 40, 42
Smai, 18, 38, 40, 41, 42, 45, 54
Smai Tawi, 38, 40, 41, 45, 54
Society, 138, 155
Soul, 8, 43, 45, 82, 90, 97, 106, 107, 137, 159, 167, 168, 170, 172, 173, 174
Space, 85
Sphinx, 44, 133, 134, 135, 168
Spinal twist, 55
Spirit, 18, 27, 42, 51, 61, 85, 89, 90, 96, 97, 127, 130, 134, 144, 148, 159
Spiritual discipline, 16, 217
Spiritual Preceptor, 4
Study, 19, 43, 151, 191
Sublimation, 190, 194, 215, 219
Sumer, 39, 41, 134
Sun, 99, 148
Sundisk, 51, 55, 62, 161
Supreme Being, 17, 18, 20, 24, 26, 27, 28, 29, 30, 31, 32, 33, 38, 43, 61, 64, 68, 73, 74, 80, 82, 83, 96, 148, 151, 157, 220
Supreme Divinity, 146, 151, 161, 162
Survival, 191
Sushumna, 147
Swami, 51
Swami Jyotirmayananda, 51
Syria, 76, 77, 156
Tantra, 2, 58, 59, 65, 71, 72, 78, 80, 83, 86,

87, 101, 106, 120, 121, 142, 149, 165, 179, 182, 191, 219
Tantra Yoga, 2, 50, 59, 72, 80, 83, 86, 120, 142, 149, 165, 179, 182, 191, 219
Tantric Yoga, 11, 38, 39, 64, 145
Tao, 127
Taoism, 216
Tawi, 18, 38, 40, 41, 45, 54
Tefnut, 28, 74, 80, 84
Tefnut (moisture), 28, 74, 80, 84
Tem, 74, 84, 110
Temple, 4
Temple XE "Temple" of Aset, 4
Temple of Aset, 32, 46, 47, 50, 179, 180, 219
Temu, 89
The All, 129
The God, 28, 31, 83, 130, 131, 137, 149, 219
The Gods, 28, 219
The Hymns of Amun, 132
The Pyramid Texts, 10
The Self, 73, 85, 91, 107, 137, 149
Theban Theology, 23
Thebes, 50, 218
Thoth, 78
Thoughts (see also Mind), 48
Tobacco, 141
Tomb, 50, 52, 54, 218
Tomb of Seti I, 50, 52, 218, 225
Tradition, 19, 27, 28, 29, 30, 31, 32, 33, 144
Tree, 148, 156
Tree of Life, 148, 156
Triad, 159, 205
Trilinga, 62
Trinity, 29, 30, 32, 73, 80, 132, 148, 219, 225
Truth, 20
Tutankhamon, 185
Union with the Divine, 72
Universal Consciousness, 43, 44, 219
Upanishads, 220
Upper Egypt, 40, 41, 42
Ur, 17, 28, 161

Uraeus, 39, 86, 149, 151
Utchat, 136
Vatican, 69
Vedanta, 11, 43, 44, 46, 47, 51, 148
Vedic, 65, 217
Vegetarianism, 179
Veil, 120
Veil of Aset, 120
Waset, 19, 27, 50, 118, 183, 199
Western civilization, 189
Western Culture, 35
Will, 99, 101, 191
Wisdom, 19, 20, 23, 38, 39, 46, 47, 50, 168, 191, 219
Wisdom (also see Djehuti), 19, 20, 23, 39, 46, 47, 50
Wisdom (also see Djehuti, Aset), 19, 20, 23, 38, 39, 46, 47, 50, 168, 191, 219
Wisdom teachings, 46, 47
Words of power, 51
Ying and Yang, 127
Yoga, 2, 4, 8, 11, 12, 30, 37, 38, 39, 40, 41, 42, 43, 44, 46, 47, 50, 53, 54, 59, 62, 64, 65, 66, 67, 83, 86, 102, 143, 145, 146, 148, 155, 168, 169, 191, 209, 216, 217, 218, 219, 220, 221, 223, 224, 225
Yoga of Action, 39
Yoga of Devotion (see Yoga of Divine Love), 11, 38, 39, 168
Yoga of Divine Love (see Yoga of Devotion), 39
Yoga of Meditation, 11, 38, 39, 168
Yoga of Righteous. See also Karma Yoga, 168
Yoga of Selfless Action. See also Yoga of Righteous, 11, 38, 39
Yoga of Wisdom, 46
Yoga of Wisdom (see also Jnana Yoga), 11, 38, 39, 46
Yoga Sutra, 38
Yogic, 38, 53, 67

EGYPTIAN TANTRIC YOGA

Audio Seminar Workshop Series
Presentation of

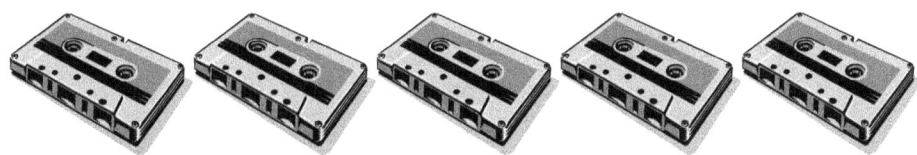

322 Class 21 Illusion of Desires, Tantrism, Sexuality and Enlightenment 4/26/98.
7021 Unity of Asar and Ra, Tantrism God is male and female, Attaining Enlightenment by going beyond love and hate (duality and egoism) V. 7-10
324-325 Class 23 Conclusion Two tape Set 5/10/98: Desperation, Sexuality, Spiritual Victory - Verse 163 to conclusion.
3002 Inspiration for Teenagers (dealing with anger, sex and discovering the purpose of life.)

4045 Class 45 – Principle of Sex Sublimation Part 1
4046 Class 46 – Principle of Sex Sublimation Part 2
4047 Class 47 – Principle of Sex Sublimation Part 3
4047A Class 47A – Principle of Sex Sublimation Part 3 Q and A
4048 Class 48 – Principle of Sex Sublimation Part 4
4049 Class 49 – Principle of Sex Sublimation Part 5 Workshop How to handle conflicts – Righteous Speaking and Listening
4050 Class 50 – Principle of Sex Sublimation Part 6
4051 Class 51 – Principle of Sex Sublimation Part 7
4051A Class 51A – Principle of Sex Sublimation Part 7 Q and A
4052 Class 52 – Principle of Sex Sublimation Part 8
4053 Class 53 – Principle of Sex Sublimation Part 9
4053A Class 53A – Principle of Sex Sublimation Part 9 Q and A
4054 Class 54 – Principle of Sex Sublimation Part 10
4055 Class 55 – Principle of Sex Sublimation Part 11
4056 Class 56 – Principle of Sex Sublimation Part 12

Mystical Philosophy of Universal Consciousness

Other Books From C M Books

P.O.Box 570459
Miami, Florida, 33257
(305) 378-6253 Fax: (305) 378-6253

This book is part of a series on the study and practice of Ancient Egyptian Yoga and Mystical Spirituality based on the writings of Dr. Muata Abhaya Ashby. They are also part of the Egyptian Yoga Course provided by the Sema Institute of Yoga. Below you will find a listing of the other books in this series. For more information send for the Egyptian Yoga Book-Audio-Video Catalog or the Egyptian Yoga Course Catalog.

Now you can study the teachings of Egyptian and Indian Yoga wisdom and Spirituality with the Egyptian Yoga Mystical Spirituality Series. The Egyptian Yoga Series takes you through the Initiation process and lead you to understand the mysteries of the soul and the Divine and to attain the highest goal of life: ENLIGHTENMENT. The *Egyptian Yoga Series*, takes you on an in depth study of Ancient Egyptian mythology and their inner mystical meaning. Each Book is prepared for the serious student of the mystical sciences and provides a study of the teachings along with exercises, assignments and projects to make the teachings understood and effective in real life. The Series is part of the Egyptian Yoga course but may be purchased even if you are not taking the course. The series is ideal for study groups.

Prices subject to change.

1. EGYPTIAN YOGA: THE PHILOSOPHY OF ENLIGHTENMENT An original, fully illustrated work, including hieroglyphs, detailing the meaning of the Egyptian mysteries, tantric yoga, psycho-spiritual and physical exercises. Egyptian Yoga is a guide to the practice of the highest spiritual philosophy which leads to absolute freedom from human misery and to immortality. It is well known by scholars that Egyptian philosophy is the basis of Western and Middle Eastern religious philosophies such as *Christianity, Islam, Judaism,* the *Kabala*, and Greek philosophy, but what about Indian philosophy, Yoga and Taoism? What were the original teachings? How can they be practiced today? What is the source of pain and suffering in the world and what is the solution? Discover the deepest mysteries of the mind and universe within and outside of your self. 8.5" X 11" ISBN: 1-884564-01-1 Soft $19.95

2. EGYPTIAN YOGA: African Religion Volume 2- Theban THeology by Dr. Muata Ashby ISBN 1-884564-39-9 $23.95 U.S. In this long awaited sequel to *Egyptian Yoga: The Philosophy of Enlightenment* you will take a fascinating and enlightening journey back in time and discover the teachings which constituted the epitome of Ancient Egyptian spiritual wisdom. What are the disciplines which lead to the fulfillment of all desires? Delve into the three states of consciousness (waking, dream and deep sleep) and the fourth state which transcends them all, Neberdjer, "The Absolute." These teachings of the city of Waset (Thebes) were the crowning achievement of the Sages of Ancient Egypt. They establish the standard mystical keys for understanding the profound mystical symbolism of the Triad of human consciousness.

3. THE KEMETIC DIET: GUIDE TO HEALTH, DIET AND FASTING Health issues have always been important to human beings since the beginning of time. The earliest records of history show that the art of healing was held in high esteem since the time of Ancient Egypt. In the early 20th century, medical doctors had almost attained the status of sainthood by the promotion of the idea that they alone were "scientists" while other healing modalities and traditional healers who did not follow the "scientific method' were nothing but superstitious, ignorant charlatans who at best would take the money of their clients and at worst

EGYPTIAN TANTRIC YOGA

kill them with the unscientific "snake oils" and "irrational theories". In the late 20th century, the failure of the modern medical establishment's ability to lead the general public to good health, promoted the move by many in society towards "alternative medicine". Alternative medicine disciplines are those healing modalities which do not adhere to the philosophy of allopathic medicine. Allopathic medicine is what medical doctors practice by an large. It is the theory that disease is caused by agencies outside the body such as bacteria, viruses or physical means which affect the body. These can therefore be treated by medicines and therapies The natural healing method began in the absence of extensive technologies with the idea that all the answers for health may be found in nature or rather, the deviation from nature. Therefore, the health of the body can be restored by correcting the aberration and thereby restoring balance. This is the area that will be covered in this volume. Allopathic techniques have their place in the art of healing. However, we should not forget that the body is a grand achievement of the spirit and built into it is the capacity to maintain itself and heal itself. Ashby, Muata ISBN: 1-884564-49-6 $28.95

4. INITIATION INTO EGYPTIAN YOGA Shedy: Spiritual discipline or program, to go deeply into the mysteries, to study the mystery teachings and literature profoundly, to penetrate the mysteries. You will learn about the mysteries of initiation into the teachings and practice of Yoga and how to become an Initiate of the mystical sciences. This insightful manual is the first in a series which introduces you to the goals of daily spiritual and yoga practices: Meditation, Diet, Words of Power and the ancient wisdom teachings. 8.5" X 11" ISBN 1-884564-02-X   Soft Cover $24.95 U.S.

5. *THE AFRICAN ORIGINS OF CIVILIZATION, MYSTICAL RELIGION AND YOGA PHILOSOPHY* HARD COVER EDITION ISBN: 1-884564-50-X $80.00 U.S.   81/2" X 11"   Part 1, Part 2, Part 3 in one volume 683 Pages Hard Cover First Edition Three volumes in one. Over the past several years I have been asked to put together in one volume the most important evidences showing the correlations and common teachings between Kamitan (Ancient Egyptian) culture and religion and that of India. The questions of the history of Ancient Egypt, and the latest archeological evidences showing civilization and culture in Ancient Egypt and its spread to other countries, has intrigued many scholars as well as mystics over the years. Also, the possibility that Ancient Egyptian Priests and Priestesses migrated to Greece, India and other countries to carry on the traditions of the Ancient Egyptian Mysteries, has been speculated over the years as well. In chapter 1 of the book *Egyptian Yoga The Philosophy of Enlightenment,* 1995, I first introduced the deepest comparison between Ancient Egypt and India that had been brought forth up to that time. Now, in the year 2001 this new book, *THE AFRICAN ORIGINS OF CIVILIZATION, MYSTICAL RELIGION AND YOGA PHILOSOPHY,* more fully explores the motifs, symbols and philosophical correlations between Ancient Egyptian and Indian mysticism and clearly shows not only that Ancient Egypt and India were connected culturally but also spiritually. How does this knowledge help the spiritual aspirant? This discovery has great importance for the Yogis and mystics who follow the philosophy of Ancient Egypt and the mysticism of India. It means that India has a longer history and heritage than was previously understood. It shows that the mysteries of Ancient Egypt were essentially a yoga tradition which did not die but rather developed into the modern day systems of Yoga technology of India. It further shows that African culture developed Yoga Mysticism earlier than any other civilization in history. All of this expands our understanding of the unity of culture and the deep legacy of Yoga, which stretches into the distant past, beyond the Indus Valley civilization, the earliest known high culture in India as well as the Vedic tradition of Aryan culture. Therefore, Yoga culture and mysticism is the oldest known tradition of spiritual development and Indian mysticism is an extension of the Ancient Egyptian mysticism. By understanding the legacy which Ancient Egypt gave to India the mysticism of India is better understood and by comprehending the heritage of Indian Yoga, which is rooted in Ancient Egypt the Mysticism of Ancient Egypt is also better understood. This expanded understanding allows us to prove the underlying kinship of humanity, through the common symbols, motifs and philosophies which are not disparate and confusing teachings but in reality expressions of the same study of truth through metaphysics and mystical realization of Self. (HARD COVER)

6. AFRICAN ORIGINS BOOK 1 PART 1 African Origins of African Civilization, Religion, Yoga Mysticism and Ethics Philosophy-Soft Cover $24.95 ISBN: 1-884564-55-0

7. AFRICAN ORIGINS BOOK 2 PART 2 African Origins of Western Civilization, Religion and Philosophy(Soft) -Soft Cover $24.95 ISBN: 1-884564-56-9

Mystical Philosophy of Universal Consciousness

8. EGYPT AND INDIA (AFRICAN ORIGINS BOOK 3 PART 3) African Origins of Eastern Civilization, Religion, Yoga Mysticism and Philosophy-Soft Cover $29.95 (Soft) ISBN: 1-884564-57-7

9. THE MYSTERIES OF ISIS: **The Ancient Egyptian Philosophy of Self-Realization** - There are several paths to discover the Divine and the mysteries of the higher Self. This volume details the mystery teachings of the goddess Aset (Isis) from Ancient Egypt- the path of wisdom. It includes the teachings of her temple and the disciplines that are enjoined for the initiates of the temple of Aset as they were given in ancient times. Also, this book includes the teachings of the main myths of Aset that lead a human being to spiritual enlightenment and immortality. Through the study of ancient myth and the illumination of initiatic understanding the idea of God is expanded from the mythological comprehension to the metaphysical. Then this metaphysical understanding is related to you, the student, so as to begin understanding your true divine nature. ISBN 1-884564-24-0 $22.99

10. EGYPTIAN PROVERBS: TEMT TCHAAS *Temt Tchaas* means: collection of ——Ancient Egyptian Proverbs How to live according to MAAT Philosophy. Beginning Meditation. All proverbs are indexed for easy searches. For the first time in one volume, ——Ancient Egyptian Proverbs, wisdom teachings and meditations, fully illustrated with hieroglyphic text and symbols. EGYPTIAN PROVERBS is a unique collection of knowledge and wisdom which you can put into practice today and transform your life. 5.5"x 8.5" $14.95 U.S   ISBN: 1-884564-00-3

11. GOD OF LOVE: THE PATH OF DIVINE LOVE The Process of Mystical Transformation and The Path of Divine Love   This Volume focuses on the ancient wisdom teachings of "Neter Merri" –the Ancient Egyptian philosophy of Divine Love and how to use them in a scientific process for self-transformation. Love is one of the most powerful human emotions. It is also the source of Divine feeling that unifies God and the individual human being. When love is fragmented and diminished by egoism the Divine connection is lost. The Ancient tradition of Neter Merri leads human beings back to their Divine connection, allowing them to discover their innate glorious self that is actually Divine and immortal. This volume will detail the process of transformation from ordinary consciousness to cosmic consciousness through the integrated practice of the teachings and the path of Devotional Love toward the Divine. 5.5"x 8.5" ISBN 1-884564-11-9 $22.99

12. INTRODUCTION TO MAAT PHILOSOPHY: Spiritual Enlightenment Through the Path of Virtue Known as Karma Yoga in India, the teachings of MAAT for living virtuously and with orderly wisdom are explained and the student is to begin practicing the precepts of Maat in daily life so as to promote the process of purification of the heart in preparation for the judgment of the soul. This judgment will be understood not as an event that will occur at the time of death but as an event that occurs continuously, at every moment in the life of the individual. The student will learn how to become allied with the forces of the Higher Self and to thereby begin cleansing the mind (heart) of impurities so as to attain a higher vision of reality. ISBN 1-884564-20-8 $22.99

13. MEDITATION The Ancient Egyptian Path to Enlightenment   Many people do not know about the rich history of meditation practice in Ancient Egypt. This volume outlines the theory of meditation and presents the Ancient Egyptian Hieroglyphic text which give instruction as to the nature of the mind and its three modes of expression. It also presents the texts which give instruction on the practice of meditation for spiritual Enlightenment and unity with the Divine. This volume allows the reader to begin practicing meditation by explaining, in easy to understand terms, the simplest form of meditation and working up to the most advanced form which was practiced in ancient times and which is still practiced by yogis around the world in modern times. ISBN 1-884564-27-7 $24.99

14. THE GLORIOUS LIGHT MEDITATION TECHNIQUE OF ANCIENT EGYPT ISBN: 1-884564-15-1 $14.95 (PB) New for the year 2000. This volume is based on the earliest known instruction in history given for the practice of formal meditation. Discovered by Dr. Muata Ashby, it is inscribed on the walls of the Tomb of Seti I in Thebes Egypt. This volume details the philosophy and practice of this unique system of meditation originated in Ancient Egypt and the earliest practice of meditation known in the world which occurred in the most advanced African Culture.

EGYPTIAN TANTRIC YOGA

15. THE SERPENT POWER: The Ancient Egyptian Mystical Wisdom of the Inner Life Force. This Volume specifically deals with the latent life Force energy of the universe and in the human body, its control and sublimation. How to develop the Life Force energy of the subtle body. This Volume will introduce the esoteric wisdom of the science of how virtuous living acts in a subtle and mysterious way to cleanse the latent psychic energy conduits and vortices of the spiritual body. ISBN 1-884564-19-4 $22.95

16. EGYPTIAN YOGA *The Postures of The Gods and Goddesses* Discover the physical postures and exercises practiced thousands of years ago in Ancient Egypt which are today known as Yoga exercises. Discover the history of the postures and how they were transferred from Ancient Egypt in Africa to India through Buddhist Tantrism. Then practice the postures as you discover the mythic teaching that originally gave birth to the postures and was practiced by the Ancient Egyptian priests and priestesses. This work is based on the pictures and teachings from the Creation story of Ra, The Asarian Resurrection Myth and the carvings and reliefs from various Temples in Ancient Egypt 8.5" X 11" ISBN 1-884564-10-0 Soft Cover $21.95   Exercise video $20

17. SACRED SEXUALITY: EGYPTIAN TANTRA YOGA: The Art of Sex Sublimation and Universal Consciousness This Volume will expand on the male and female principles within the human body and in the universe and further detail the sublimation of sexual energy into spiritual energy. The student will study the deities Min and Hathor, Asar and Aset, Geb and Nut and discover the mystical implications for a practical spiritual discipline. This Volume will also focus on the Tantric aspects of Ancient Egyptian and Indian mysticism, the purpose of sex and the mystical teachings of sexual sublimation which lead to self-knowledge and Enlightenment. 5.5"x 8.5" ISBN 1-884564-03-8 $24.95

18. AFRICAN RELIGION Volume 4: ASARIAN THEOLOGY: RESURRECTING OSIRIS The path of Mystical Awakening and the Keys to Immortality NEW REVISED AND EXPANDED EDITION! The Ancient Sages created stories based on human and superhuman beings whose struggles, aspirations, needs and desires ultimately lead them to discover their true Self. The myth of Aset, Asar and Heru is no exception in this area. While there is no one source where the entire story may be found, pieces of it are inscribed in various ancient Temples walls, tombs, steles and papyri. For the first time available, the complete myth of Asar, Aset and Heru has been compiled from original Ancient Egyptian, Greek and Coptic Texts. This epic myth has been richly illustrated with reliefs from the Temple of Heru at Edfu, the Temple of Aset at Philae, the Temple of Asar at Abydos, the Temple of Hathor at Denderah and various papyri, inscriptions and reliefs. Discover the myth which inspired the teachings of the *Shetaut Neter* (Egyptian Mystery System - Egyptian Yoga) and the Egyptian Book of Coming Forth By Day. Also, discover the three levels of Ancient Egyptian Religion, how to understand the mysteries of the Duat or Astral World and how to discover the abode of the Supreme in the Amenta, *The Other World*   The ancient religion of Asar, Aset and Heru, if properly understood, contains all of the elements necessary to lead the sincere aspirant to attain immortality through inner self-discovery. This volume presents the entire myth and explores the main mystical themes and rituals associated with the myth for understating human existence, creation and the way to achieve spiritual emancipation - *Resurrection.* The Asarian myth is so powerful that it influenced and is still having an effect on the major world religions. Discover the origins and mystical meaning of the Christian Trinity, the Eucharist ritual and the ancient origin of the birthday of Jesus Christ. Soft Cover ISBN: 1-884564-27-5 $24.95

19. THE EGYPTIAN BOOK OF THE DEAD MYSTICISM OF THE PERT EM HERU $28.95   ISBN# 1-884564-28-3 Size: 8½" X 11" I Know myself, I know myself, I am One With God!–From the Pert Em Heru "The Ru Pert em Heru" or "Ancient Egyptian Book of The Dead," or "Book of Coming Forth By Day" as it is more popularly known, has fascinated the world since the successful translation of Ancient Egyptian hieroglyphic scripture over 150 years ago. The astonishing writings in it reveal that the Ancient Egyptians believed in life after death and in an ultimate destiny to discover the Divine. The elegance and aesthetic beauty of the hieroglyphic text itself has inspired many see it as an art form in and of itself. But is there more to it than that? Did the Ancient Egyptian wisdom contain more than just aphorisms and hopes of eternal life beyond death? In this volume Dr. Muata Ashby, the author of over 25 books on Ancient Egyptian Yoga Philosophy has produced a new translation of the original texts which uncovers a mystical teaching underlying the sayings and rituals instituted by the Ancient Egyptian Sages and Saints. "Once the

Mystical Philosophy of Universal Consciousness

philosophy of Ancient Egypt is understood as a mystical tradition instead of as a religion or primitive mythology, it reveals its secrets which if practiced today will lead anyone to discover the glory of spiritual self-discovery. The Pert em Heru is in every way comparable to the Indian Upanishads or the Tibetan Book of the Dead." Muata Abhaya Ashby

20. ANUNIAN THEOLOGY THE MYSTERIES OF RA The Philosophy of Anu and The Mystical Teachings of The Ancient Egyptian Creation Myth Discover the mystical teachings contained in the Creation Myth and the gods and goddesses who brought creation and human beings into existence. The Creation Myth holds the key to understanding the universe and for attaining spiritual Enlightenment. ISBN: 1-884564-38-0 40 pages $19.95

21. MYSTERIES OF MIND Mystical Psychology & Mental Health for Enlightenment and Immortality based on the Ancient Egyptian Philosophy of Menefer -Mysticism of Ptah, Egyptian Physics and Yoga Metaphysics and the Hidden properties of Matter. This volume uncovers the mystical psychology of the Ancient Egyptian wisdom teachings centering on the philosophy of the Ancient Egyptian city of Menefer (Memphite Theology). How to understand the mind and how to control the senses and lead the mind to health, clarity and mystical self-discovery. This Volume will also go deeper into the philosophy of God as creation and will explore the concepts of modern science and how they correlate with ancient teachings. This Volume will lay the ground work for the understanding of the philosophy of universal consciousness and the initiatic/yogic insight into who or what is God? ISBN 1-884564-07-0 $22.95

22. THE GODDESS AND THE EGYPTIAN MYSTERIES THE PATH OF THE GODDESS THE GODDESS PATH The Secret Forms of the Goddess and the Rituals of Resurrection The Supreme Being may be worshipped as father or as mother. *Ushet Rekhat* or *Mother Worship*, is the spiritual process of worshipping the Divine in the form of the Divine Goddess. It celebrates the most important forms of the Goddess including *Nathor, Maat, Aset, Arat, Amentet and Hathor* and explores their mystical meaning as well as the rising of *Sirius*, the star of Aset (Aset) and the new birth of Hor (Heru). The end of the year is a time of reckoning, reflection and engendering a new or renewed positive movement toward attaining spiritual Enlightenment. The Mother Worship devotional meditation ritual, performed on five days during the month of December and on New Year's Eve, is based on the Ushet Rekhit. During the ceremony, the cosmic forces, symbolized by Sirius - and the constellation of Orion ---, are harnessed through the understanding and devotional attitude of the participant. This propitiation draws the light of wisdom and health to all those who share in the ritual, leading to prosperity and wisdom. $14.95 ISBN 1-884564-18-6

23. *THE MYSTICAL JOURNEY FROM JESUS TO CHRIST* $24.95   ISBN# 1-884564-05-4 size: 8½" X 11" Discover the ancient Egyptian origins of Christianity before the Catholic Church and learn the mystical teachings given by Jesus to assist all humanity in becoming Christlike. Discover the secret meaning of the Gospels that were discovered in Egypt. Also discover how and why so many Christian churches came into being. Discover that the Bible still holds the keys to mystical realization even though its original writings were changed by the church. Discover how to practice the original teachings of Christianity which leads to the Kingdom of Heaven.

24. THE STORY OF ASAR, ASET AND HERU: An Ancient Egyptian Legend (For Children)   Now for the first time, the most ancient myth of Ancient Egypt comes alive for children. Inspired by the books *The Asarian Resurrection: The Ancient Egyptian Bible* and *The Mystical Teachings of The Asarian Resurrection, The Story of Asar, Aset and Heru* is an easy to understand and thrilling tale which inspired the children of Ancient Egypt to aspire to greatness and righteousness. If you and your child have enjoyed stories like *The Lion King* and *Star Wars* you will love *The Story of Asar, Aset and Heru*. Also, if you know the story of Jesus and Krishna you will discover than Ancient Egypt had a similar myth and that this myth carries important spiritual teachings for living a fruitful and fulfilling life. This book may be used along with *The Parents Guide To The Asarian Resurrection Myth: How to Teach Yourself and Your Child the Principles of Universal Mystical Religion*. The guide provides some background to the Asarian Resurrection myth and it also gives insight into the mystical teachings contained in it which you may introduce to your child. It is designed for parents who wish to grow spiritually with their children and it serves as an introduction for those who would like to study the Asarian Resurrection Myth in depth and to practice its teachings. 41 pages   8.5" X 11"   ISBN: 1-884564-31-3 $12.95

EGYPTIAN TANTRIC YOGA

25. THE PARENTS GUIDE TO THE AUSARIAN RESURRECTION MYTH: How to Teach Yourself and Your Child the Principles of Universal Mystical Religion. This insightful manual brings for the timeless wisdom of the ancient through the Ancient Egyptian myth of Asar, Aset and Heru and the mystical teachings contained in it for parents who want to guide their children to understand and practice the teachings of mystical spirituality. This manual may be used with the children's storybook *The Story of Asar, Aset and Heru* by Dr. Muata Abhaya Ashby. ISBN: 1-884564-30-5 $16.95

26. HEALING THE CRIMINAL HEART BOOK 1 Introduction to Maat Philosophy, Yoga and Spiritual Redemption Through the Path of Virtue Who is a criminal? Is there such a thing as a criminal heart? What is the source of evil and sinfulness and is there any way to rise above it? Is there redemption for those who have committed sins, even the worst crimes? Ancient Egyptian mystical psychology holds important answers to these questions. Over ten thousand years ago mystical psychologists, the Sages of Ancient Egypt, studied and charted the human mind and spirit and laid out a path which will lead to spiritual redemption, prosperity and Enlightenment. This introductory volume brings forth the teachings of the Asarian Resurrection, the most important myth of Ancient Egypt, with relation to the faults of human existence: anger, hatred, greed, lust, animosity, discontent, ignorance, egoism jealousy, bitterness, and a myriad of psycho-spiritual ailments which keep a human being in a state of negativity and adversity. 5.5"x 8.5" ISBN: 1-884564-17-8 $15.95

27. THEATER & DRAMA OF THE ANCIENT EGYPTIAN MYSTERIES: Featuring the Ancient Egyptian stage play-"The Enlightenment of Hathor' Based on an Ancient Egyptian Drama, The original Theater - Mysticism of the Temple of Hetheru $14.95 By Dr. Muata Ashby

28. GUIDE TO PRINT ON DEMAND: SELF-PUBLISH FOR PROFIT, SPIRITUAL FULFILLMENT AND SERVICE TO HUMANITY Everyone asks us how we produced so many books in such a short time. Here are the secrets to writing and producing books that uplift humanity and how to get them printed for a fraction of the regular cost. Anyone can become an author even if they have limited funds. All that is necessary is the willingness to learn how the printing and book business work and the desire to follow the special instructions given here for preparing your manuscript format. Then you take your work directly to the non-traditional companies who can produce your books for less than the traditional book printer can. ISBN: 1-884564-40-2 $16.95 U. S.

29. Egyptian Mysteries: Vol. 1, Shetaut Neter ISBN: 1-884564-41-0 $19.99 What are the Mysteries? For thousands of years the spiritual tradition of Ancient Egypt, S*hetaut Neter,* "The Egyptian Mysteries," "The Secret Teachings," have fascinated, tantalized and amazed the world. At one time exalted and recognized as the highest culture of the world, by Africans, Europeans, Asiatics, Hindus, Buddhists and other cultures of the ancient world, in time it was shunned by the emerging orthodox world religions. Its temples desecrated, its philosophy maligned, its tradition spurned, its philosophy dormant in the mystical *Medu Neter*, the mysterious hieroglyphic texts which hold the secret symbolic meaning that has scarcely been discerned up to now. What are the secrets of *Nehast* {spiritual awakening and emancipation, resurrection}. More than just a literal translation, this volume is for awakening to the secret code *Shetitu* of the teaching which was not deciphered by Egyptologists, nor could be understood by ordinary spiritualists. This book is a reinstatement of the original science made available for our times, to the reincarnated followers of Ancient Egyptian culture and the prospect of spiritual freedom to break the bonds of *Khemn,* "ignorance," and slavery to evil forces: *Såaa* .

30. EGYPTIAN MYSTERIES VOL 2: Dictionary of Gods and Goddesses ISBN: 1-884564-23-2 $21.95 This book is about the mystery of neteru, the gods and goddesses of Ancient Egypt (Kamit, Kemet). Neteru means "Gods and Goddesses." But the Neterian teaching of Neteru represents more than the usual limited modern day concept of "divinities" or "spirits." The Neteru of Kamit are also metaphors, cosmic principles and vehicles for the enlightening teachings of Shetaut Neter (Ancient Egyptian-African Religion). Actually they are the elements for one of the most advanced systems of spirituality ever conceived in human history. Understanding the concept of neteru provides a firm basis for spiritual evolution and the pathway for viable

Mystical Philosophy of Universal Consciousness

culture, peace on earth and a healthy human society. Why is it important to have gods and goddesses in our lives? In order for spiritual evolution to be possible, once a human being has accepted that there is existence after death and there is a transcendental being who exists beyond time and space knowledge, human beings need a connection to that which transcends the ordinary experience of human life in time and space and a means to understand the transcendental reality beyond the mundane reality.

31. EGYPTIAN MYSTERIES VOL. 3 The Priests and Priestesses of Ancient Egypt ISBN: 1-884564-53-4 $22.95 This volume details the path of Neterian priesthood, the joys, challenges and rewards of advanced Neterian life, the teachings that allowed the priests and priestesses to manage the most long lived civilization in human history and how that path can be adopted today; for those who want to tread the path of the Clergy of Shetaut Neter.

32. THE KING OF EGYPT: The Struggle of Good and Evil for Control of the World and The Human Soul ISBN 1-8840564-44-5 $18.95 This volume contains a novelized version of the Asarian Resurrection myth that is based on the actual scriptures presented in the Book Asarian Religion (old name –Resurrecting Osiris). This volume is prepared in the form of a screenplay and can be easily adapted to be used as a stage play. Spiritual seeking is a mythic journey that has many emotional highs and lows, ecstasies and depressions, victories and frustrations. This is the War of Life that is played out in the myth as the struggle of Heru and Set and those are mythic characters that represent the human Higher and Lower self. How to understand the war and emerge victorious in the journey o life? The ultimate victory and fulfillment can be experienced, which is not changeable or lost in time. The purpose of myth is to convey the wisdom of life through the story of divinities who show the way to overcome the challenges and foibles of life. In this volume the feelings and emotions of the characters of the myth have been highlighted to show the deeply rich texture of the Ancient Egyptian myth. This myth contains deep spiritual teachings and insights into the nature of self, of God and the mysteries of life and the means to discover the true meaning of life and thereby achieve the true purpose of life. To become victorious in the battle of life means to become the King (or Queen) of Egypt.Have you seen movies like The Lion King, Hamlet, The Odyssey, or The Little Buddha? These have been some of the most popular movies in modern times. The Sema Institute of Yoga is dedicated to researching and presenting the wisdom and culture of ancient Africa. The Script is designed to be produced as a motion picture but may be adapted for the theater as well. $19.95 copyright 1998 By Dr. Muata Ashby

33. AFRICAN DIONYSUS: FROM EGYPT TO GREECE: The Kamitan Origins of Greek Culture and Religion ISBN: 1-884564-47-X $24.95 U.S. FROM EGYPT TO GREECE This insightful manual is a reference to Ancient Egyptian mythology and philosophy and its correlation to what later became known as Greek and Rome mythology and philosophy. It outlines the basic tenets of the mythologies and shoes the ancient origins of Greek culture in Ancient Egypt. This volume also documents the origins of the Greek alphabet in Egypt as well as Greek religion, myth and philosophy of the gods and goddesses from Egypt from the myth of Atlantis and archaic period with the Minoans to the Classical period. This volume also acts as a resource for Colleges students who would like to set up fraternities and sororities based on the original Ancient Egyptian principles of Sheti and Maat philosophy. ISBN: 1-884564-47-X $22.95 U.S.

34. THE FORTY TWO PRECEPTS OF MAAT, THE PHILOSOPHY OF RIGHTEOUS ACTION AND THE ANCIENT EGYPTIAN WISDOM TEXTS <u>ADVANCED STUDIES</u> This manual is designed for use with the 1998 Maat Philosophy Class conducted by Dr. Muata Ashby. This is a detailed study of Maat Philosophy. It contains a compilation of the 42 laws or precepts of Maat and the corresponding principles which they represent along with the teachings of the ancient Egyptian Sages relating to each. Maat philosophy was the basis of Ancient Egyptian society and government as well as the heart of Ancient Egyptian myth and spirituality. Maat is at once a goddess, a cosmic force and a living social doctrine, which promotes social harmony and thereby paves the way for spiritual evolution in all levels of society. ISBN: 1-884564-48-8 $16.95 U.S.

EGYPTIAN TANTRIC YOGA

Music Based on the Prt M Hru and other Kemetic Texts

Available on Compact Disc $14.99 and Audio Cassette $9.99

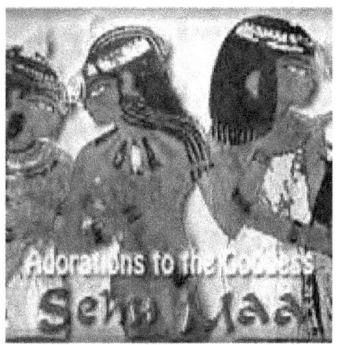

Adorations to the Goddess

Music for Worship of the Goddess

NEW Egyptian Yoga Music CD
by Sehu Maa
Ancient Egyptian Music CD
Instrumental Music played on reproductions of Ancient Egyptian Instruments– Ideal for meditation and
reflection on the Divine and for the practice of spiritual programs and Yoga exercise sessions.

©1999 By Muata Ashby
CD $14.99 –

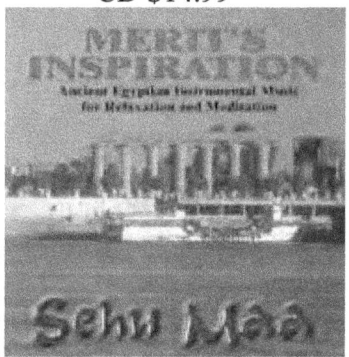

MERIT'S INSPIRATION
NEW Egyptian Yoga Music CD
by Sehu Maa
Ancient Egyptian Music CD
Instrumental Music played on
reproductions of Ancient Egyptian Instruments– Ideal for meditation and
reflection on the Divine and for the practice of spiritual programs and Yoga exercise sessions.
©1999 By

Mystical Philosophy of Universal Consciousness

Muata Ashby
CD $14.99 –
UPC# 761527100429

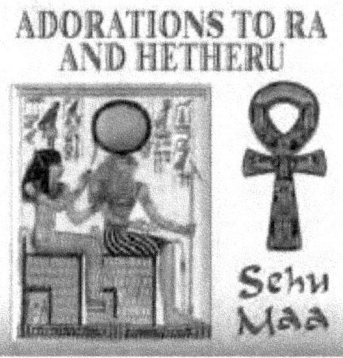

ANORATIONS TO RA AND HETHERU
**NEW Egyptian Yoga Music CD
By Sehu Maa (Muata Ashby)
Based on the Words of Power of Ra and HetHeru**
played on reproductions of Ancient Egyptian Instruments **Ancient Egyptian Instruments used: Voice, Clapping, Nefer Lute, Tar Drum, Sistrums, Cymbals** – The Chants, Devotions, Rhythms and Festive Songs Of the Neteru – Ideal for meditation, and devotional singing and dancing.

©1999 By Muata Ashby
CD $14.99 –
UPC# 761527100221

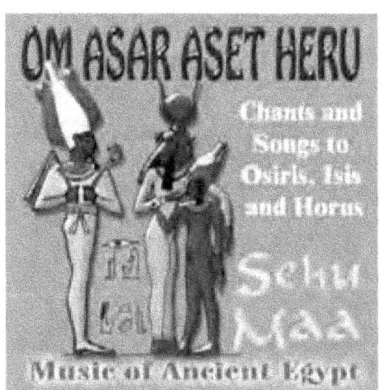

SONGS TO ASAR ASET AND HERU
**NEW
Egyptian Yoga Music CD
By Sehu Maa**
played on reproductions of Ancient Egyptian Instruments– The Chants, Devotions, Rhythms and Festive Songs Of the Neteru - Ideal for meditation, and devotional singing and dancing.
Based on the Words of Power of Asar (Asar), Aset (Aset) and Heru (Heru) Om Asar Aset Heru is the third in a series of musical explorations of the Kemetic (Ancient Egyptian) tradition of music. Its ideas are based on the Ancient Egyptian Religion of Asar, Aset and Heru and it is designed for listening, meditation and worship. ©1999 By Muata Ashby
CD $14.99 –
UPC# 761527100122

EGYPTIAN TANTRIC YOGA

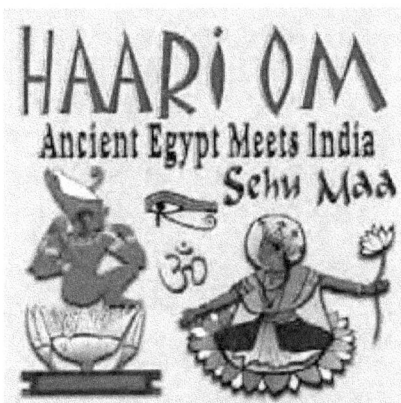

HAARI OM: ANCIENT EGYPT MEETS INDIA IN MUSIC
NEW Music CD
By Sehu Maa

The Chants, Devotions, Rhythms and Festive Songs Of the Ancient Egypt and India, harmonized and played on reproductions of ancient instruments along with modern instruments and beats. Ideal for meditation, and devotional singing and dancing.

Haari Om is the fourth in a series of musical explorations of the Kemetic (Ancient Egyptian) and Indian traditions of music, chanting and devotional spiritual practice. Its ideas are based on the Ancient Egyptian Yoga spirituality and Indian Yoga spirituality.

©1999 By Muata Ashby
CD $14.99 –
UPC# 761527100528

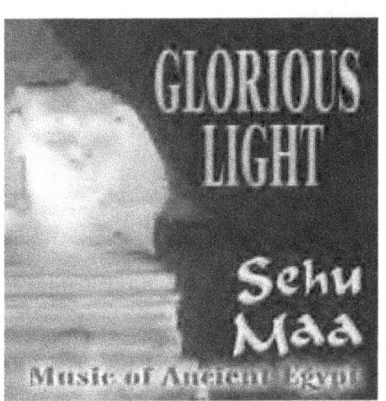

RA AKHU: THE GLORIOUS LIGHT
NEW
Egyptian Yoga Music CD
By Sehu Maa

The fifth collection of original music compositions based on the Teachings and Words of The Trinity, the God Asar and the Goddess Nebethet, the Divinity Aten, the God Heru, and the Special Meditation Hekau or Words of Power of Ra from the Ancient Egyptian Tomb of Seti I and more...

played on reproductions of Ancient Egyptian Instruments and modern instruments - Ancient Egyptian Instruments used: Voice, Clapping, Nefer Lute, Tar Drum, Sistrums, Cymbals

– The Chants, Devotions, Rhythms and Festive Songs Of the Neteru – Ideal for meditation, and devotional singing and dancing.

©1999 By Muata Ashby
CD $14.99 –
UPC# 761527100825

Mystical Philosophy of Universal Consciousness

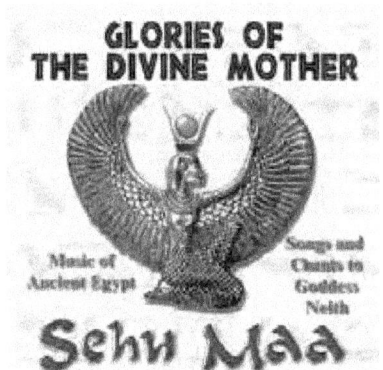

GLORIES OF THE DIVINE MOTHER
Based on the hieroglyphic text of the worship of Goddess Net.
The Glories of The Great Mother
©2000 Muata Ashby
CD $14.99 UPC# 761527101129`

EGYPTIAN TANTRIC YOGA
Order Form

Telephone orders: Call Toll Free: 1(305) 378-6253. Have your AMEX, Optima, Visa or MasterCard ready.

Fax orders: 1-(305) 378-6253   E-MAIL ADDRESS: Semayoga@aol.com

Postal Orders: Sema Institute of Yoga, P.O. Box 570459, Miami, Fl. 33257. USA.

Please send the following books and / or tapes.

ITEM

_____ Cost $_____
_____ Cost $_____
_____ Cost $_____
_____ Cost $_____
_____ Cost $_____

Total $_____

Name:_____
Physical Address:_____
City:_____ State:_____ Zip:_____

Sales tax: Please add 6.5% for books shipped to Florida addresses
_____ Shipping: $6.50 for first book and .50¢ for each additional
_____ Shipping: Outside US $5.00 for first book and $3.00 for each additional

_____Payment:_____
_____Check -Include Driver License #:
      _____

_____Credit card: _____ Visa, _____ MasterCard, _____ Optima, _____ AMEX.

Card number:_____
Name on card:_____ Exp. date:_____/_____

Copyright 1995-2005 Dr. R. Muata Abhaya Ashby
Sema Institute of Yoga
P.O.Box 570459, Miami, Florida, 33257
(305) 378-6253 Fax: (305) 378-6253

www.ingramcontent.com/pod-product-compliance
Lightning Source LLC
Chambersburg PA
CBHW080248030426
42334CB00023BA/2738